Community
Support Systems
and Mental Health

David E. Biegel, A.C.S.W., is Assistant Professor, University of Pittsburgh School of Social Work, and a doctoral candidate at the University of Maryland School of Social Work and Community Planning. Recently he served as Director of the Neighborhood and Family Services Project, University of Southern California, Washington Public Affairs Center. He has held a variety of organizing, planning, and administrative positions in mental health and human services agencies.

The author of a number of reports and articles related to mental health and neighborhoods, he is the co-author (with Arthur Naparstek and Herzl Spiro) of a forthcoming book on neighborhood-based mental health.

Arthur J. Naparstek, Ph.D., is Professor of Public Administration and Director of the University of Southern California, Washington Public Affairs Center. He has served as a member of the National Commission on Neighborhoods and as a Task Panel member of the President's Commission on Mental Health. A consultant to numerous federal and local organizations, he has been the Principal Investigator of grants relating to mental health, aging, capacity building, and human service delivery. He has written a number of monographs and other publications focusing on neighborhoods and empowerment.

Community Support Systems and Mental Health

Practice, Policy, and Research

David E. Biegel, A.C.S.W.
Arthur J. Naparstek, Ph.D.
Editors

with contributors

Foreword by Gerald Caplan, M.D.

SPRINGER PUBLISHING COMPANY
New York

Springer Publishing Company, Inc.
200 Park Avenue South
New York, New York   10003

82 83 84 85 86 / 10 9 8 7 6 5 4 3 2 1

Library of Congress Cataloging in Publication Data

Main entry under title:

Community support systems and mental health.

   Chiefly papers from 2 USC-sponsored Conferences
on Neighborhood Support Systems and Mental Health,
held in Baltimore, Md. and Milwaukee, Wis., winter
1980.
   Bibliography: p.
   Includes index.
   1. Community mental health services—Congresses.
I. Biegel, David E.   II. Naparstek, Arthur.
III. University of Southern California.   IV. Con-
ference on Neighborhood Support Systems and Mental
Health (1980 : Baltimore, Md.) V. Conference on
Neighborhood Support Systems and Mental Health
(1980 : Milwaukee, Wis.) [DNLM: 1. Community
mental health services—United States. WM 30
C7345]
RA790.C681226   362.2'0425   81-23296
ISBN 0-8261-3420-3   AACR2
ISBN 0-8261-3421-1 (pbk.)

Printed in the United States of America

Contents

v

Foreword

During the past fifteen years research evidence has been accumulating which proves that exposure to acute and chronic stress usually increases vulnerability to bodily illness and psychopathology only if the individual does not at the same time receive appropriate social support. The essential element of this support is also becoming clear. It has two main components: the individual is helped to reduce his stress-induced emotional reactions so that they do not unduly interfere with his coping efforts; and he is given cognitive guidance and help with tasks to enable him more effectively to grapple with his current problems.

Most people do not face stress on their own; their adaptive efforts are strengthened by the supportive intervention of members of their nuclear and extended family, friends, neighbors, workmates, a variety of informal caregivers (the so-called natural helpers), self-help and mutual-help groups, and religious and social institutions, as well as professionals and community caregiving agencies. Those individuals who live in neighborhoods where people are bound together by common history and cultural identity are especially well supported. But until recently caregiving professionals labored under the erroneous belief, amounting almost to a myth, that not only was the protective extended family a thing of the past in our large cities, but that people in general were nowadays relatively cut off from effective supporters apart from health and welfare professionals.

On the contrary, as this book demonstrates, most ordinary people in the United States have available to them a wide range of adequate nonprofessional supporters on whom they can call in a predicament; and some of these supporters can usually be relied upon to ameliorate the stresses of life through buffering emotion and providing cognitive guidance, as well as concrete help with tasks, thus preventing increased vulnerability to bodily and mental disorder. Moreover, a sense of well-being that is a central element of positive mental health is induced in most individuals, particularly those who live in cohesive neighborhoods, by their roles within the ubiquitous rubric of community life that provide them with a meaningful sense of belonging and worth.

It is mainly the socially deviant and alienated, the stigmatized, the transients and the newcomers to a community, and those who have become isolated because of inactive old age, bereavement, or divorce who run a special risk of illness because of exposure to stress. It is these individuals who should be the main target of professionals interested in prevention, whose primary mission it should be to identify them and to link them with the available nonprofessional supporters in their neighborhood.

Unfortunately, many caregiving professionals have little knowledge of the existence or the identity of such supportive individuals and groups in their community, nor do they have a proper respect for their potency in reducing the harmful effects of stress. This book should help to remedy this. It also reveals how routine professional intervention may sometimes weaken instead of strengthen the helpful operation of natural support networks and mutual-help organizations. The book makes a most valuable contribution by emphasizing how important it is for professionals to understand the supportive social matrix in which they and their clients live, which was invisible until recently. It provides rich details of relevant research; and it suggests how practitioners and program planners may utilize the results of this research in preventing illness and promoting health through building up mutually respectful partnerships with community supporters.

I believe that an increased understanding of support systems is probably the most important current development in the field of prevention. It is certainly one of the most exciting, as this book so well demonstrates.

Gerald Caplan, M.D.
Professor of Child Psychiatry;
Chairman, Dept. of Child Psychiatry;
Hadassah University Hospital,
Jerusalem, Israel

Acknowledgments

This book developed out of the Neighborhood and Family Services Project, a four-year research and demonstration effort funded by grant #R01MH2653 from the Mental Health Services Development Branch, National Institute of Mental Health, to the University of Southern California, Washington Public Affairs Center. We would like to give special thanks to our Project Officer, Dr. Howard R. Davis, Chief, Mental Health Services Development Branch, whose interest, commitment, and support made our work possible. A particular debt of gratitude is also owed to Msgr. Geno Baroni, under whose leadership the project was sponsored in the first grant year at the National Center for Urban Ethnic Affairs.

We are also indebted to the work of the Community Support Systems Task Panel of the President's Commission on Mental Health (1978b), chaired by June Jackson Christmas and directed by Marie Killilea. The report of the Task Panel was a pioneer effort in defining the field of Community Support Systems and pulling together for the first time in one place research findings and program examples from a wide variety of areas.

Most of the papers in this book were prepared for two USC-sponsored Conferences on Neighborhood Support Systems and Mental Health held in Baltimore, Maryland, and Milwaukee, Wisconsin, during the winter of 1980. So many individuals and organizations helped make those Conferences successful that individual recognition and appreciation is not possible here. We would like, however, to acknowledge the work of the South East Community Organization, Inc., Baltimore, Maryland, and the South Community Organization, Inc., Milwaukee, Wisconsin, who served both as local community sponsors of the Conferences and also as the local sponsors of the Neighborhood and Family Services Project during the entire four-year grant period.

This book would not have been possible without the support and encouragement of our respective schools. We therefore thank the University of Pittsburgh, School of Social Work and the University of Southern California, School of Public Administration for allowing us time to complete this volume.

Contributors

Martha Baum, Ph.D., is Professor of Social Work at the University of Pittsburgh. She teaches courses in Social Science Theory, Gerontology, Justice Policy Research, and Family Policy. Her research centers on aging with special emphasis on retirement and kinship networks and on victimology.

Rainer C. Baum, Ph.D., Professor of Sociology at the University of Pittsburgh, has contributed to the fields of action theory, macro-sociology, and the sociology of aging. He is currently teaching courses in the areas of death and aging.

Nancy J. Chapman, Ph.D., is Associate Professor in the School of Urban Affairs at Portland State University, and Co-Principal Investigator of the "Natural Helping Networks and Service Delivery" grant, funded by the Office of Human Development Services, DHHS. She is an environmental and social psychologist and has written in the areas of social networks, privacy, and assessing the environmental needs of specific populations such as the elderly and families living in public housing.

James P. Comer, M.D., is Maurice Falk Professor of Child Psychiatry at the Yale Child Study Center and Associate Dean of the Yale Medical School. He received his A.B. from Indiana University in 1956, his M.D. from Howard University College of Medicine in 1960, and his M.P.H. from the School of Public Health at the University of Michigan in 1964. Since 1968, he has directed a school intervention project in New Haven, Connecticut, which is a collaborative effort between the Yale Child Study Center and the New Haven School System. Dr. Comer writes a weekly syndicated newspaper column and a monthly column for *Parent's Magazine* on issues of child development, education, and social policy. He has written three books: *Beyond Black and White*, (Quadrangle/New York Times Books, 1972); *Black Child Care* (co-authored with Dr. Alvin Poussaint) (Simon and Schuster, 1975); and *School Power* (Free Press,

1980). Dr. Comer is one of five recipients of the 1980 Rockefeller Foundation Public Service Award.

Anthony R. D'Augelli, Ph.D., is Associate Professor of Human Development in the Division of Individual and Family Studies at Pennsylvania State University. He received his Ph.D. in community-clinical psychology from the University of Connecticut in 1972. He is co-author of *Helping Others* (Brooks/Cole, 1981) and *Helping Skills: A Basic Training Program* (Human Sciences, 1980). His interests are in training nonprofessional and paraprofessional helpers, improving rural mental health, developing community-oriented prevention programs, and innovation in mental health service design.

Charles Froland, D.P.H., is Assistant Professor at the School of Social Work and the Regional Research Institute for Human Services, Portland State University, Portland, Oregon. He is the project director of a national study for DHHS's Office of Human Development Services of agencies working to develop natural helping systems, self-help efforts, or informal networks of social support. His interests include mental health, program evaluation, and income-maintenance programs.

Donald E. Gelfand, Ph.D., is Associate Professor at the School of Social Work and Community Planning of the University of Maryland at Baltimore and Research Coordinator of the National Policy Center on Women and Aging. A sociologist, he has been extensively involved in many applied areas of sociology including mental health, community sociology, and aging. Formerly co-director of the Community Sociology Training Program at Boston University, his current research focuses on changes in the family related to aging and the role of ethnicity in the aging process. During 1979–1980 he was on leave at the National Council on the Aging in Washington, D.C.

Judy R. Gelfand, M.S., O.T.R., is presently Director of the Holiday Park Multipurpose Senior Center in Montgomery County, Maryland. Previously, she organized and directed one of the early adult day-care centers in Maryland. She is acting vice president of the Maryland Association of Senior Centers and serves on the steering committee of the National Institute of Adult Day Care, a program of the National Council on the Aging.

Benjamin H. Gottlieb, Ph.D., is Associate Professor in the Department of Psychology at the University of Guelph, Guelph, Ontario, Canada.

He holds a joint Ph.D. in Social Work and Psychology from the University of Michigan. His research interests center on the role of social support in moderating stress, the study of informal helping behaviors, and the relation between natural and professional forms of helping.

David Guttmann, D.S.W., Associate Professor, is the Director of the Center for the Study of Pre-retirement and Aging of the Catholic University of America. Formerly serving as Assistant Dean for Academic Affairs of the National Catholic School of Social Service, Dr. Guttmann has been the Principal Investigator of four large-scale studies in aging, funded by the Administration on Aging. He is the author of numerous publications on aging, as well as on education in social work, and has taught and conducted workshops on aging in major national conferences in the past ten years.

Muriel E. Hamilton-Lee, Ed.D., is currently a postdoctoral fellow at the Yale Child Study Center. She received her Ed.D. from Atlanta University in 1979 and her M.S. from Bank Street College of Education in 1973. Her primary research activities have been in both early childhood education and social policy as related to educational administration and governance. At present, Dr. Hamilton-Lee is investigating collaborative working relationships between universities and urban school systems.

Abraham M. Jeger, Ph.D., received his degree in Psychology from SUNY at Stony Brook in 1977. He is Assistant Professor and Co-Director, Long Island Self-Help Clearinghouse in the Human Resources Development Center of the New York Institute of Technology, Old Westbury, New York. He is co-editor (with R. S. Slotnick) of *Community Mental Health: A Behavioral-Ecological Perspective* (Plenum, 1981) and *Social Ecology in Community Psychology* (with R. S. Slotnick and E. J. Trickett), Special Issue of the APA Division of Community Psychology Newsletter (Summer, 1980). His recent papers have been in the areas of community mental health and social ecology.

Mohammad M. Khan, Ph.D., is Research Associate, Boys Town Center, Catholic University of America. Formerly, he served as Research Director of the Neighborhood and Family Services Project, University of Southern California, Washington Public Affairs Center. His areas of specialization are urban studies, demography, and research methods. He has held research positions with the University of Hawaii and the University of North Carolina. Dr. Khan has published in several national and international journals.

Harold Lewis, D.S.W., is Professor and Dean, Hunter College School of Social Work, New York. He received his Doctorate from the University of Pennsylvania in 1959 and has held a number of agency and academic positions over the past twenty years. Dr. Lewis is the author of numerous monographs, research reports, and articles in professional journals. He is currently serving on the editorial boards of five journals.

Tom Choken Owan, A.C.S.W., is the Chief, Services for Minorities Program, Mental Health Services Development Branch, NIMH. He received his B.S. and M.S.W. degrees from Ohio State University, Columbus, Ohio. For the past thirteen years he has worked extensively in the development of methodologies to overcome the present inequities in the delivery of health and welfare services targeted to minority groups.

Diane L. Pancoast is a social worker and a Research Associate at the Regional Research Institute for Human Services, Portland State University. She has written and taught extensively on natural helping networks. She was Principal Investigator of the "Natural Helping Networks and Service Delivery Project," funded by the Office of Human Development Services, Department of Health and Human Services.

Kenneth I. Pargament, Ph.D., received his doctorate in clinical-community psychology at the University of Maryland. He completed a post-doctoral program in mental health epidemiology and program evaluation at the School of Public Health and Hygiene at Johns Hopkins University. Currently Assistant Professor of Psychology at Bowling Green State University, he is actively involved in the areas of community psychology, the psychology of religion, and the development of competence-enhancing programs.

Stanley R. Platman, M.D., is currently the Assistant Secretary for Mental Health, Mental Retardation, Addictions, and Developmental Disabilities, State Department of Health and Mental Hygiene, Baltimore, Maryland. Formerly, he was the Regional Director for the Department of Mental Hygiene, Buffalo, New York, and then Acting Deputy Commissioner, Division of Mental Health, New York State Department of Mental Hygiene. Dr. Platman, who received his M.D. in 1959 from Queens University in Belfast, is a member of the Royal College of Psychiatry and is a Fellow of the American Psychiatric Association. He has served as the Coordinator of the Task Panel on Deinstitutionalization, Rehabilitation, and Long-Term Care for the President's Commission on Mental Health and has authored a wide range of publications.

Thomas Plaut, Ph.D., received his doctorate from the Department of Social Relations and his M.P.H. from Harvard School of Public Health. He served on the staff of the Harvard School of Public Health Community Mental Health Program (1955–1962) and was Director of the Massachusetts Division of Alcoholism prior to moving to Stanford University (Institute for the Study of Human Problems) in the early 1960s. He joined the National Institute of Mental Health in 1967 and has served there since then in a number of positions. He is currently Director of the Office of Prevention at NIMH. He is co-author of *Personality in a Communal Society: The Mental Health of the Hutterites* (University of Kansas Press, 1956) and author of over forty articles in professional and scientific journals.

Matthew Schure, Ph.D., received his degree in Psychology from Columbia University in 1976. He is Director of the Human Resources Development Center of the New York Institute of Technology and Visiting Clinical Associate Professor of Community Medicine, New York College of Osteopathic Medicine, of the New York Institute of Technology, Old Westbury, New York. He serves as the Chairperson of the Classroom and Skills Training Subcommittee, Nassau County Office of Employment and Training (CETA). He has published in the areas of violence and infertility, including a book (with Judith Schure), *Hannah's Trial: Our Triumph Over Infertility* (Nova University, New York Institute of Technology Press, 1981).

Phyllis R. Silverman, Ph.D., is on the faculty of the Social Work and Health Program of the Institute of Health Professions of Massachusetts General Hospital. She also holds an appointment in the Department of Psychiatry at Harvard Medical School. She served as consultant to the National Institute of Mental Health and has consulted with agencies across the country on issues of bereavement, mutual help, and prevention. In addition to her Social Work degree from Smith College School of Social Work, she holds an M.S. in hygiene from Harvard School of Public Health and a Ph.D. from the Florence Heller School for Advanced Studies in Social Welfare at Brandeis University. Her most recent publication is *Mutual Help Groups: Organization and Development* (Sage Publishing Co., 1980).

Robert S. Slotnick, Ph.D., is Assistant Professor and Co-Director, Long Island Self-Help Clearinghouse in the Human Resources Development Center of the New York Institute of Technology, Old Westbury, New York. He received his Ph.D. in Psychology from Stanford University in

1967. He is co-editor (with A. M. Jeger) of *Community Mental Health: A Behavioral-Ecological Perspective* (Plenum, 1981), and *Social Ecology in Community Psychology* (with A. M. Jeger and E. J. Trickett), Special Issue of the APA Division of Community Psychology Newsletter (Summer, 1980). His previous papers have appeared in numerous scholarly journals in the field of psychology. He has held positions with the City University of New York as well as various community mental health agencies.

David Spiegel, M.D., is Assistant Professor of Psychiatry and Behavioral Sciences and Director of the Adult Psychiatric Outpatient Clinic at Stanford University School of Medicine. He received his M.D. from Harvard in 1971, did his Psychiatric Residency at Massachusetts Mental Health Center and Cambridge Hospital, and completed a Fellowship at the Laboratory of Community Psychiatry, Harvard Medical School.

Theodore R. Vallance, Ph.D., has been Professor of Human Development at Pennsylvania State University, College of Human Development, since 1967 and Associate Dean of Research and Graduate Study until 1979. Dr. Vallance holds joint appointments in the Departments of Community Development and Man–Environment Relations and is on the faculty of the graduate program in Community Systems Planning and Development. Prior to going to Penn State, he was Chief of the Office of Planning at the National Institute of Mental Health. His most recent publication is a policy sourcebook entitled *Mental Health Services in Transition* (Human Sciences, 1981), co-edited with Ru M. Sabre. His doctorate is in social and political psychology from Syracuse.

Donald I. Warren, Ph.D., is a sociologist who has been involved in urban community research and has authored many articles as well as three recent books on neighborhood social structure and citizen action. He is currently Director of the Community Effectiveness Institute and Associate Professor of Sociology and Anthropology at Oakland University. As a member of the President's Commission on Mental Health he was active on the "community support" task panel. Professor Warren is currently engaged in studies of community acceptance and along with Rachelle Warren is conducting training programs on neighborhood-based outreach and citizen participation programs. He is also involved in a nine-nation comparative study of the strength of locality attachment in urban society.

Introduction

David E. Biegel and
Arthur J. Naparstek

The mental health system in the United States has taken conflicting and confusing approaches to the role of "community" in service delivery over the past 150 years. At times the community has been the problem, at other times it has been the solution. Though there has been a gradual shift toward community-based care and toward viewing the community's role in mental health in a positive sense, the mental health system has neither fully understood the concept of community nor been aware of the important roles that the community does and should play in mental health service delivery.

In the early nineteenth century, mental health care was focused on the "insane." The insane were removed from the chaotic conditions of Jacksonian society which were felt to be causing their insanity and placed into the controlled, ordered, and secure environment of the asylum located far from the community. Family, friends, and other community members were allowed few if any visiting privileges lest they bring reminders of the disordered community that was seen as the cause of the problem. These characteristics, combined with other attributes, constituted the treatment philosophy known as "moral treatment." By the Civil War this philosophy was in disrepute and shortly thereafter disregarded. The asylums, which were often located at great distances from population centers, over 150 built between 1860 and 1900, remain in place to this day, however. During the period from 1860 to 1900, the asylums were transformed from places of first resort—for treatment—to places of last resort—for custody.

By the turn of the twentieth century, there were the beginnings of a movement that viewed the community not as the source of the problem but as an important component of the solution. The seeds of the community mental health movement were being planted. Dr. Adolph Meyer of

This introduction is based in part upon Biegel, D., *Help seeking and receiving in urban ethnic neighborhoods*, unpublished doctoral dissertation, University of Maryland School of Social Work and Community Planning, 1982.

Johns Hopkins Hospital did pioneering work in this area at the beginning of the century, believing that effective treatment of mental health problems required a focus on environmental and community factors. In a 1907 lecture given at the New York Academy of Medicine, Dr. Meyer stated concerning the care of the insane, "It opens the way to what is sorely needed: a closer relation between the hospitals and the communities which have too long stood aloof, in mutual ignorance and lack of sympathy. It is bound to call on the forces that work for the best hygienic conditions in the community."

Dr. Meyer's call for greater involvement with the community went largely unheeded. For the next fifty years, mental health care was provided to the "mentally ill" in large understaffed and underfunded state hospitals that provided more custody than treatment and maintained few if any linkages with the community.

The year 1963 marked a milestone in the mental health system with the passage of the Community Health Centers Act. The Act was to be "a bold, new approach" with a focus on prevention, community involvement, and a shift in treatment locus from the state hospital to the community, President Kennedy told Congress in a major speech introducing the proposed new legislation.

Thus mental health care has made a complete turnabout in a century and a half, from a negative view of community to a positive one, and from institutional to community-based care as the treatment modality of choice. Yet several decades later, despite significant accomplishments in some areas, the promise has not been fulfilled. The network of federally funded Community Mental Health Centers (CMHCs), envisioned as 2,000 in number by 1980, has failed to fully materialize. Today only one-third of the Centers are in place. The bold, new approach of the 1960s has become the target of significant attacks on a broad range of issues by both consumers and professionals. Among the concerns are the following: the lack of coordination between state hospitals and local communities; the lack of understanding of "community" by professionals; lack of accountability to the public; and the failure to account for ethnic and class differences among population groups in the design and delivery of services.

Central to all of these problems has been the lack of clear conceptualization of community and its support systems. In fact, the term *community* in community mental health has been a misnomer from the beginning. The service or "catchment" area for community mental health centers has been between 75,000 and 200,000 persons. People do not live in catchment areas, they live in neighborhoods. Yet many community mental health center catchment areas have split neighborhoods in half.

Further evidence of the inability to fully comprehend the nature of community can be seen in the deinstitutionalization movement of the

1960s and 1970s. Thousands of chronic mental patients were released to
the community by mental health planners without real consultation with
the affected neighborhoods on the assumption that strong communities
would accept the chronically ill. When few welcomed large numbers of
these troubled people, patients were steered to transitional neighborhoods that would not put up a fuss, but the strong community support
factor essential for effective aftercare was absent. Attempts to remedy
these past errors have focused upon the coordination of professional
services with still too little attention to the role of informal systems of
community support.

Community involvement in mental health has been sought first
through Community Advisory Boards and then through CMHC Governing Boards with legislatively mandated majority consumer representation. But there has been little understanding of the role of "Community
Support Systems"—friends, family, neighbors, "natural helpers," clergy,
self-help groups, civic and voluntary organizations, neighborhood organizations, co-workers, and so on, in mental health. In fact, services are
often "parachuted" into communities, bypassing personal, organizational,
and cultural networks in the community that have the capacity to support
individuals in times of need. CMHCs have fragmented, threatened, or
undermined existing community support systems by ignoring them.

An example of how CMHCs have ignored support systems is the
Consultation and Education (C & E) program. The original 1963 mental
health legislation mandated five essential services that all CMHCs had to
provide in order to receive federal funding. Of the five, C & E was the
only nontreatment service. C & E offers an excellent opportunity for mental health professionals to work with informal support systems through
consultation with natural helpers, self-help groups, neighborhood organizations, and the like. Yet NIMH reports indicate that almost 100 percent
of consultation time by mental health center staff is to other professionals.
There is little or no involvement with community support systems.

The lack of appreciation of community support systems by the mental health system is further indicated by the fact that the President's
Commission on Mental Health's emphasis on "Community Support Systems" in their 1978 report was the "first time that a prestigious nationwide study group has afforded such prominence to the role of such
non-mental health system supports in mental health" (HEW Implementation Committee Report, 1979). It is perhaps too easy to indict the
mental health system for not knowing in the 1960s what we now know in
the 1980s. This is not our purpose, rather we want to show how some of
the problems of the mental health system can be traced to lack of
knowledge about the "community." Further conceptualization of community is one of the goals of this book.

Often the more things change, the more they remain the same. Community support systems are not a new phenomenon. The first mutual aid group, the Scots Charitable Society, was formed in 1657. Strengthening neighborhood support systems was a major goal of the Settlement House Movement led by social workers in the early twentieth century. What is new in the 1980s, however, is renewed interest and involvement with such support systems, coupled with an expanding knowledge base in this area. This has occurred for a number of reasons.

First, there is growing awareness that mental health needs cannot be met by professionals alone. In any given year, at least 15 percent of the population shows symptoms of such severity as to be considered mentally ill (President's Commission on Mental Health, 1978a). If mild or moderate anxieties and emotional upsets are included, the rates go much higher. If all the available professional mental health resources were maximally deployed, no more than 3 percent of the population could receive professional care at any given time. It is clear that alternative strategies, such as utilization of community support systems, must be developed to counter our overreliance on clinical treatment by professionals if those in need are to be adequately served.

Second, there is an increasing societal interest in individuals' assuming more responsibility for the maintenance of their own health. The U.S. Surgeon General's annual report in 1979 on the status of the health of the population placed heavy emphasis on prevention of illness and promotion of positive health. "Doing it yourself," an outgrowth of the human-potential movement of the 1970s, is in vogue.

Third, America, the land of "good and plenty," has had to realize, painful as it may be, that its resources, fiscal and human, are not unlimited. We have begun to acknowledge that dollars alone cannot meet human needs and that government agencies and programs are "limited" in their ability to solve pressing social problems. This has led to a sense of frustration but also a willingness to explore alternative approaches to meeting human needs.

We are beyond the point of arguing in the '80s whether or not mental health professionals should work with the community. This has now been accepted as proper and appropriate. Therefore the issue is not whether, but how, mental health professionals should interact with the community. Conceptualization and operationalization of such interaction is an important goal. Unanswered questions include: What are community support systems and what are the proper roles they can play in the mental health system? What are the similarities and differences between the roles of community support systems and the roles of professionals in mental health? What should the relationship/interaction be between community support systems and mental health professionals? What obstacles may inhibit/prevent such relationships? And are there any dangers that linkages between community support systems and mental health professionals could be detrimental to community support systems and/or mental health professionals?

We attempt to address many of these issues in this book. Our aim is to share with the student, mental health or human service professional, and lay members of the community some exciting recent developments in knowledge and practice about community support systems and their relationship to mental health. There is a critical need for a new policy and program framework for community mental health that is based on the strengths, resources, and diversities existing in local communities. We believe that a community-support-systems approach to mental health that recognizes the unique contribution of both the lay community and professionals in mental health and that formalizes such contributions through partnerships can be the basis for this new framework.

The book presents a comprehensive overview of community support systems by a multidisciplinary group of researchers and practitioners that crosscuts various types of support systems and population groups. It is impossible to cover this subject matter fully in any one volume, and we do not claim to do so here. The book is divided into four parts. Part I discusses theory and research about community support systems; Part II presents examples of programmatic interventions that provide an overview of existing practice with support systems; Part III discusses professional roles with support systems from both conceptual and practice perspectives; Part IV discusses policy implications of community support systems and presents recommendations for enhanced public policy in this area.

Too often researchers, practitioners, and policy makers speak to different audiences, resulting in a lack of integration of theory, practice, and public policy. The book takes an integrative approach because we believe that theory, practice, and policy issues are interrelated and should not be considered in isolation from each other.

At this point, it will be helpful to shift gears and attempt to define the term *community support systems* since it is used in an ambiguous and often conflicting manner in the professional literature and in practice. Our discussion will be at some length to ensure that our approach to support systems is clear to the reader.

Examples of community support systems are:

- The woman in her sixties on the block that neighbors turn to for help and support when their welfare checks are late.

- The bartender that customers talk to about their marital problems.
- The widowed-persons group the church sponsors to provide mutual support and socialization.
- The neighbor who takes in the fourteen-year-old girl who has been thrown out of her house by her family.
- The clergyman that parishioners talk to about family problems.
- The community organization that helps residents develop a needed community-based hotline.
- The ethnic organization that helps the middle-aged parent with the strains caused by value conflicts with their children.
- The co-worker who helps with the problems of caring for aged parents.

In a pluralistic society, people seek help, solve problems, and meet needs in different ways. Family, friends, neighbors, co-workers, clergy, neighborhood organizations, and mutual-aid groups can all provide meaningful assistance in times of need and are encompassed in the term *community support systems*. Community support systems can serve preventive, treatment, and rehabilitative functions. On a preventive level, they can contribute to an individual's sense of well-being and of competent functioning. They can assist in reducing the negative consequences of stressful life events. On a treatment level, they can play an adjunctive role to professional care through positive reinforcement and assisting individuals to follow treatment plans. They can also be directly involved in treatment. For example, social network therapy utilizes extended networks of family, friends, and other significant individuals in providing treatment to an individual client. On a rehabilitative, or "tertiary prevention," level community support systems even help to reintegrate the formerly ill back into the community. This can be especially important for the "deinstitutionalized" chronically mentally ill who need assistance in recovering from the isolation of institutional life.

Community support systems operate on both one-to-one and group levels. On the one-to-one level, community support systems are "natural" caregiving efforts that are ongoing and develop and function without support or assistance from mental health professionals. Supportive relationships may exist between a friend and neighbor, a nephew and uncle, a pastor and parishioner, teacher and parent, neighborhood leader and group member, co-workers, to name but a few.

Group forms of community support systems such as support groups for the divorced, widowed, alcoholic, or former mental patient are "organized" as opposed to "natural." Sometimes these groups are organized with the support of professionals; many times they develop without professional intervention. These groups help the individuals in need realize that they are not alone, that others share their problems and needs. Participation in these groups varies by need and interest of the group member. Some individuals stay in the group for a short period of time until they can cope on their own with their situation, while others remain for ongoing friendship and social activities. In fact, the type of participation also varies by group. In some groups, members are expected to remain for long periods of time, for example, Alcoholics Anonymous. Alcoholics, the A.A. philosophy assumes, can never be cured and thus need an ongoing support group. Other groups like Parents Without Partners, a support group for single parents, fully expect a rapid turnover in membership as many members either remarry or are able to function independently as a result of the help of the group and of the informal relationships and friendships they made through the group. Though individuals receive assistance through formal group activities and programs, much of the support in these groups is informal as particular individuals develop friendships, relationships, and support systems. Many of the individuals who join these groups and receive help would never go to professionals for assistance.

Other groups exist that may not be organized for self-help purposes, but participation in these groups becomes an important element of an individual's support system providing much help and sustenance. Ethnic clubs, PTAs, neighborhood organizations, social and fraternal groups can all provide important levels of support. There is evidence that individuals who are members of organizations experience fewer symptoms of mental illness than individuals who are not group members.

Community support systems are found in all places. They exist in low-, middle-, and high-income communities and in rural, suburban, and urban areas. Support systems cut across age, sex, class, ethnic, and racial lines. Thus community support systems serve all of us in some degree and in different ways. More specifically, however, community support systems serve many population groups that are unable or unwilling to seek professional help, or for whom professional services are currently lacking. Community support systems offer help in a culturally acceptable manner without stigma or loss of pride. The individual seeking help does not need to identify himself as having a problem, being weak, sick, a client, or a patient as he would when seeking professional help. There is often much less "stigma" in relying on community support systems for assistance as compared with seeking help from mental health professionals. We now turn to some theoretical and conceptual formulations of community support systems.

Part I
Theory and Research

The first part of this volume provides an overview of conceptual and research issues related to community support systems. The interdisciplinary perspective of the psychiatrists, psychologists, social workers, and sociologists who have authored chapters in this section adds richness and diversity to the subject matter. There is much we do not know about support systems, and our attempt is to explore a number of key issues here related to defining and conceptualizing what support systems are, how they operate, and what their effect is upon the mental health status of particular population groups.

As a starting point, we begin with the chapter by Warren, who provides a conceptual analysis of the role of social networks in urban areas. Warren's work is based upon a recently completed NIMH-funded study of help seeking and receiving in fifty-nine neighborhoods in the Metropolitan Detroit area. He finds evidence of strong links among family, friends, neighbors, relatives, and other associates. Warren notes that having problems is not necessarily associated with having poorer mental health than not having problems, since networks can help individuals cope positively with the problems of daily living and in so doing revitalize and reaffirm their attachment to the community. Warren's analysis makes clear that mere number of helpers is not correlated with positive well-being; rather both size and types of assistance provided by the helpers are key factors. He also contributes the important notion that helping networks can be analyzed on community as well as individual levels and that such analysis can help to identify gaps in provision of informal and formal services.

Biegel, Naparstek, and Khan's chapter continues the attempt at conceptualizing support systems by examining the relationship between social support, mental health, and life stress in urban white ethnic communities. They define social support as consisting of three components: direct (family, friends, co-workers), indirect (group participation and interaction), and social adjustment (work satisfaction and neighborhood attachment). Their findings show that for all population groups the higher the level of social support the more positive the mental health status, and for elderly and ethnic populations in particular, neighborhood attachment is the most important component of social support. The finding that the components of social support vary in importance for particular population groups suggests that preventive strategies to enhance support systems should be population specific.

1

Gottlieb focuses on social support in the workplace, presenting research findings documenting that social support systems in the workplace can moderate life stress and promote positive mental health. He presents a four-stage framework that examines the effect of social support by work associates in the help-seeking and -receiving process and demonstrates (as do Jeger, Slotnik, and Schure, and Froland in later chapters) the interdependence between formal and informal systems of support. Gottlieb concludes by calling for professionals to reach out and assist workers who are isolated from systems of support to develop ties with each other and by admonishing professionals to be careful that their interventive efforts do not weaken or undermine existing systems of informal support.

The next two chapters, by Baum and Baum and by Guttmann, discuss support systems among the elderly, a group that is "at risk" for developing mental health problems. The Baum and Baum chapter presents a sociological perspective on the search for "community" in society which assists the aging person to find meaning and acceptance in their life and thus to experience positive well-being. They examine the relationship between social network embeddedness—operationalized in terms of ethnicity, religion, and social class—and mental health status, as measured by the Erikson concept of integrity in old age. Utilizing a mixed ethnic sample of approximately a hundred individuals aged about seventy and over, this exploratory study finds confirming evidence for the hypothesis that embeddedness in social networks is correlated with an enhanced sense of well-being.

Guttmann's chapter, which focuses on the aged in white ethnic communities, is based upon a recently completed three-year project funded by the Administration on Aging which examined the use of formal and informal support systems among eight white ethnic population groups. He finds that in times of need the family and ethnic neighborhood are extremely important resources with little use of formal services. Guttmann notes, however, that about one-fifth of the respondents in his study seem to be lacking any social support and are thus at a great risk of developing mental health problems. He suggests, as do a number of authors in the book, the need for professional services to build upon the positive strengths of informal support systems with special emphasis upon developing strategies to reach the isolated, at-risk, white ethnic elderly.

Community support systems can play especially significant roles in the prevention area. Plaut synthesizes recent developments in prevention and discusses the relationship between prevention and community support systems. He sees support systems as enhancing and maximizing psychosocial growth and development and also as providing a buffering effect to stress during times of crisis. Plaut warns that barriers such as limited fiscal resources, the overwhelming clinical orientation and training of mental health professionals, and the crisis-oriented nature of our society may inhibit the future development of prevention and community-support-system initiatives. He says that support systems can serve a dual emphasis, helping people adjust and cope with life crises and conditions and also helping people organize to change inhumane systems.

The final chapter, by Spiegel, presents a very comprehensive and systematic review of professional literature related to self-help and mutual help. Noting the deep historical underpinnings for self-help, Spiegel discusses the important roles that such groups perform in assisting individuals to cope with life stresses. He notes that there is general consensus by professionals that self-help is an important and complementary approach to professional mental health and health services. Although there is a vast descriptive literature in the self-help area, Spiegel notes that there are too few scientific studies evaluating the effectiveness of self-help groups. The few studies that do exist, however, show that self-help groups can indeed be effective. He supports the call by Killilea and other self-help experts for further scientific research in this important area.

Using Helping Networks: A Key Social Bond of Urbanites

Donald I. Warren

The quest for, loss of, and need to seek community are among the most pervasive themes of modern life. Yet social scientists and many "doomsday" prophets foretell the virtual demise of such ties. It appears that the twenty-first century will arrive with urban society devoid of cohesive families, work groups, or neighborhoods—and with only a complex of highly specialized and bureaucratic systems providing the help and social support individuals need to cope with daily problems.

How valid is this image of a "nation of strangers" (to quote Vance Packard) in which sense of community and mutual help will disappear? At every hand evidence mounts that hot lines and impersonal human service systems are the key if not the only means urbanites have to deal with the stresses or "future shock" of our society.

In this chapter we shall discuss and utilize research recently completed in one large metropolitan area to provide new clues about the rich and diversified and yet almost invisible links that bind near strangers, close friends, occasional acquaintances, and social service professionals. We call these ties "problem-anchored helping networks" (PAHNs).

From that vague, indeterminant point at which a problem begins to the receipt of effective help is often a long road. The symptomatic

This chapter is based upon a study entitled "Helping Networks in the Urban Community," which was sponsored by the Center for the Study of Metropolitan Problems of the National Institute of Mental Health, USPHS-3R01-MH24982. A newly published book based on the study is entitled *Helping Networks: How People Cope with Problems in the Metropolitan Community*, The University of Notre Dame Press. I wish to express my gratitude to the study sponsors for their support in developing a follow-up monographic analysis.

manifestation of psychological or social problems often represents the culmination of a long period of accumulated symptoms, events, or behaviors. In other words, problems do not just happen, they develop through a process over time. Similarly, help-seeking and -receiving need to be examined not in terms of specific behavioral occurrences or events but instead as a helping process.

The network study of helping processes in an urban metropolitan area upon which this paper is based was guided by three essential questions:

1. What are the helping resources individuals utilize for a range of frequently experienced problems—and how are these distributed between "informal" and "formal" helping systems?

2. How are the patterns of help-seeking of the individual related to the individuals' social context—class, race, age, local neighborhood, and community social organization?

3. What are the effects of using particular kinds of helping resources (or not using them) on the individuals' well-being?

The study was conducted from 1973 to 1976, with field surveys taking place during 1974–75. To carry out the substantive task of the study, survey interviews with over 4,000 persons were conducted. An initial baseline sample included approximately 2,500 persons. Twelve months later, follow-up interviews were made with 1,500 additional persons. Each interview took approximately eighty minutes and was administered in person by trained interviewers. The study sample covered fifty-nine neighborhoods in eleven cities. Once the data were collected and analyzed, we were led to modify very substantially the ideas with which we started. The image of isolated and distressed people lacking in contact with neighbors, friends, kin, and other key helpers did not emerge. Instead, insights from the "Helping Network" study along with the wealth of research conducted over the past decade or so are now being applied to understand how "natural helping systems" offer a basis of optimism about new forms of community within the traditional settings of neighborhood, town, and larger city that is our urban society.

Problem-Anchored Helping Networks

The research conducted in the Detroit metropolitan area has provided—beyond its original intent—a basis for defining a distinct "network" in which the linkage between types of helpers such as friends, neighbors, relatives, co-workers, and professional agency helpers is defined by the reported "talking about a recent concern or problem." Specifically, we have distinguished as Problem-Anchored Helping Networks (PAHNs):

Social contacts that an individual makes with any number of other persons (not necessarily intimates or status equals) in a number of helping arenas (kin, kith, neighborhood, work, voluntary association, etc.) with the result that a particular "problem" or "concern" or "crisis" is discussed and advice or help provided.

Problem-anchored helping networks are composed of a single thread between one individual and another because of a specific problem. This tie can be extended as the first helper mentions information provided to him or her by yet another individual. The original help seeker need never directly be in touch with this third link in the chain. Thus, helping network analysis is not simply looking at the *direct* contact that an individual makes with a helper. An individual is part of a system of networks that can provide resources or pathways to help. So the various behavior settings of neighborhood, workplace, and organizations that a person is attached to can actually themselves—as arenas—be linked. In fact, a different neighbor, co-worker, or organization member can be tapped for each unique problem. This indirect linkage between social contexts forms a new basis of community solidarity. We see the individual as help-seeker being tied to a variety of behavior arenas. Within each setting the PAHN user may potentially be linked to a variety of networks simultaneously.

Being part of a helping network can direct an individual's attention to the needs of others in a community. Yet the helping that is indigenous to a community is not self-conscious or necessarily instrumental—it grows out of sociability; it becomes an expression of a potential, unspoken reciprocity.

Helping networks are characterized by people moving across different social arenas—out of their neighborhood, out of their work setting, out of the PTA group or whatever organization they belong to that might be the basis of close social bonds. They are now linked to a range of others outside these intimate circles.

That we all may become referral agents in problem helping is one indicator of community health. From one perspective a problem-anchored helping network is based on entering into the larger community through a series of steps or pathways (combinations or resources) that are based, not on intimacy, but simply the sharing of the same problem with another individual. The links are indirect—a form of "organic" wholeness which is often experienced only as a helping transaction between two individuals but is, in fact, an intricate web of ties that forms a viable social structure of helping.

A basic implication of the PAHN process is that when professional services bypass existing helping structures within the community, the effect may be to systematically lower the adaptive capacity of that community. The result is to weaken such indigenous resources so that in times of crisis natural systems may not be available and only professional services may be operative. Let us now turn to the specific research out of which the key ideas and hypotheses we shall develop in this chapter have emerged.

The List of "Recent Concerns": Active Coping with One's Life Context

As part of the Detroit study design, a set of helping behaviors were associated with a series of nine "concerns," developed out of initial in-depth interviews. People were asked, "Tell me if this has happened to you recently: In the last month or so, not recently, or never." The following experiences were then listed:

1. Wanted to change the way you and your wife/husband divide the family activities.
2. Wanted to get a completely different job.
3. Concerned about suspicious people in the neighborhood.
4. Felt it's no use trying to do things because so many things go wrong.
5. Thought about going back to school.
6. Thought about how it would be to retire.
7. Felt so "blue" it ruined your whole day.
8. Got so tense at work you blew your stack.
9. Thought about moving from the neighborhood because of the crime problem.

In utilizing these recent concerns as a major test of the help-seeking behavior of individuals we, in effect, employed a conceptually different type of problem than the more conventional life crisis. In the former instance, individuals are coping with problems that involve change in their life-style, including desired and not yet realized future alterations of life-style. Thus, thinking about retirement, wanting to go back to school, thinking about moving from a neighborhood because of crime, and wanting a different job are potential life changes. Some of these are a means to eliminate a negative condition in the present life of the individual; others are looking toward change without knowing whether this is a positive or a negative adjustment.

Recent concerns are experiences that individuals report that may or may not presume the use of helping resources. Often, an individual's helping networks may be taxed beyond their current limits. But the search for help can serve to increase the variety and strength of networks available and thereby strengthen the individual's sense of well-being and social integration.

Key Qualities of Helping
Networks: Range and Depth

We begin with a consideration of the size or scope of helping networks in terms of the variety of helpers sought out by the individual. Each respondent who indicated that any of the above-specified concerns had happened to them recently was then asked to describe with whom they had talked about it. Three-quarters of the sample indicated at least one recent concern. The following list of helpers was given to respondents who were asked to identify which, if any, they contacted for each recent concern.

Your spouse
A relative   } Primary Helpers
A friend

A neighbor
A co-worker   } Proximal Helpers

A doctor
A clergyman
A counselor   } Professional/Formal Agency Helpers
A teacher
The police

The definitions were specified in the case of relative to be someone related by blood not living in the same household. For counselor, this included a family counselor, psychiatrist, psychologist, and social worker.

Range of Helping Networks

Of those respondents experiencing a recent concern, almost two-thirds (62 percent) contacted a spouse (of married respondents only, over four-fifths [82 percent] contacted a spouse), approximately two-fifths contacted a friend or relative (41 percent and 37 percent, respectively), and over one-quarter (28 percent) contacted a co-worker. Neighbors were contacted by more than one-quarter (27 percent) of the sample. The five categories of informal/formal agency helpers were each contacted by less than 10 percent of those persons expressing recent concerns.

We also focused upon how many helpers were brought into play on any given problem. Of those with at least one recent concern, about one in seven (14 percent) used no help at all and about one in four (24 percent) used only a single type of helper. More than half (62 percent) used two or more different kinds of helpers. Overall, people who sought help for recent concerns used an average of 2.7 unique kinds of helpers per problem experienced.

Depth of Helping Networks

A second major quality of helping concerns the content—what kind of help is obtained. Based on a very simplistic coding of therapeutic modalities, we included six different helper behaviors in the interview for each instance of using a helper: just listened to me, asked me questions, showed me a new way to look at things, took some action about the matter, told me who else to see, took me to someone who could take action. The specific question was: "Which of these things happened when you talked with that person?" Persons surveyed were given the set of six different types of helping behaviors and could indicate that *any or all* were part of a given transaction. Results show that the typical problem coping sequence involved more than a single form of help received from a given helper.

The most typical helping behavior—the one that occurs in the largest number of helping situations—is that of listening: nearly four out of five contain such help. A majority of helping includes the more active kind of social support defined by asking questions. Redirecting of the help seekers' thinking—that is, "showing a new way to look at the problem"—is found in one of three helping transactions. Taking direct action as part of the helping process occurs in somewhat more than one out of four situations. Finally, the two types of referral helping—giving information about another helper or taking the person directly to that individual—is found in approximately one out of five of all transactions.

The typical pattern of using PAHNs can be stated as follows:

For both the scope and the depth of helping networks, the modal pattern is a multiple one: More than one type of helper is utilized and more than one type of helping behavior is provided.

The Consequences of
Help-Seeking on Well-being

Our discussion of the form of help-seeking has led almost logically to the issue of the effect of such patterns on the individual with problems. While our study was mainly aimed at tracing the pathways of helping—the form and variety of resources people use to cope with a range of common concerns—we employed several measures of self-reported mental and physical health that can be correlated with the use of helpers.

Basically, the question posed is: What is the effect of help-seeking on the helpee? The number of different helpers utilized as well as the variety of helping behaviors they provide tends to limit the negative impact of problem load on individual well-being. Help that is only listening and is not linked simultaneously to more active behaviors, such as asking questions, referring, intervening by taking the individual to someone for help or providing a new way to look at the problem, is not much better than the individual coping alone.

Such refinement of the depth measure—by showing the role of helping which may include, but must go beyond, passive social support (just listening)—provides important insights about the role of helping in problem-coping. An absence of problems is not necessarily correlated with well-being. In fact, those individuals having both problems and an effective helping network are not any less well than those having no problems. Our findings suggest a proper range of optimal patterning of helping resources to maximize the level of well-being when an individual experiences problems: Using more than three different types of helpers does not appear to reduce the stress of problem coping any more than having no helpers or only using one form; risk to well-being is reduced most effectively with two or three types of helpers. At the same time, where a combination of listening and some other more active form of help is utilized, such as referral or showing a new way to look at a problem, risk to individual well-being is reduced more than if only one type of help is provided—especially if that help is only listening or asking questions.

Diagnosing PAHN Patterns

The Detroit study not only pinpoints the modal type of help-seeking but also underscores the variability in what type of helper is available and used and whether he or she offers the kind of help that will be effective. For example, we find that many low-income and minority women are heavily reliant on neighbor helping. Often this means a kind of locked-in pattern where alternative PAHNs are not available or accessible. Moreover, often such help as neighbors provide is of a commiserative variety—everyone listens to everyone else's problems, but no one has the linkages to other resources or more active forms of helping.

In Table 1.1 we have depicted a set of six different situations in which an individual may fit in terms of how "strong" or "weak" his or her PAHN is. Our criterion is simply the index of stress—the self-

TABLE 1.1. Forms of Helping Networks and Their Effectiveness

DEFICIT	Used 1 or 2 different kinds of helpers; listening and asking questions the only types of help provided--good social support but too narrow a range of systems used; risk to well-being may increase rapidly with higher "problem load."
VULNERABLE	Used 1 or 2 different kinds of helpers; at least 3 different kinds of helping-- a "small world" that is fragile if any network members are lost.
TOO SPECIALIZED	Used 3 to 4 different kinds of helpers; listening and asking questions are the only types of help provided--good social support but the repertoire is too narrow in what helpers do--may prolong needs and lead to dependency.
BALANCED	Used 3 to 4 different kinds of helpers; 3 or more different types of help pro- vided--good scope and depth to PAHN.
CRISIS ORIENTED	Used 5 or more kinds of helpers; listen- ing and asking questions are the only types of help provided--almost a random search which may mean heavy reliance over an extended period without adequate problem resolution.
COMPLEX	Used 5 or more kinds of helpers; 3 or more different helping behaviors pro- vided--extensive system requires a great deal of personal energy to main- tain; high-cost system.

reported well-being questions that were associated with particular numbers of and kinds of helping. We start with the "Deficit" pattern. Here, the individual may have a spouse and a neighbor as helpers and they provide social support but nothing beyond this. As the problem load goes up or a life crisis situation emerges, their PAHN system may be limited in its capacity to prevent or treat the emergent distress of the individual. No matter how sympathetic a spouse may be to the need to find an effective employment role, or supportive of the desire of wife or husband to return to school, finding out how to apply and the early steps of coping with the new role may be beyond their experience, knowledge base, or understanding.

In the case of the "vulnerable" PAHN situation, there is a rich repertoire of personal experience and helping skills to rely on, but kin and spouse may be too overloaded themselves or may be hard to replace if the individual faces a new situation without them being present or available.

At the opposite end, a "complex" PAHN pattern means that the individual engages in a kind of ransacking of all available helpers and seeks out so many different points of view and helping options that no effective progress in solving the problem may be made. This situation often reflects the trauma of a given situation and the almost random search for help under crisis-like conditions. When that mental outlook becomes a habit, we may speak of the "crisis-oriented" PAHN pattern.

Table 1.1 also contains a form of PAHN that is too specialized, in which the help-seeker may look for or receive only very similar kinds of advice or information—which provides a comforting sense of reinforcement but may not be effective problem coping. This overreliance on a tight-knit network—perhaps a clique of friends—may result in relatively uninspired or noninnovative problem coping. Granovetter (1973) describes this in his analysis of job-seeking: The best new opportunities do not come from close friends but from some former acquaintance or occasional chance meeting with a person who can bring a new slant or new information to an old problem.

The "balanced" problem-anchored helping network is one in which a sufficiently wide variety of helpers is accessible and used—primary, proximal, or professional—and in which, like the pieces of a mosaic, each offers a unique insight and distinct type of help tailored to the situation at hand. This rich tapestry of effective helping is the one associated with the least stress. Both social support—expressive reinforcement of the self and active helping—and instrumental activities are suggested or actually initiated by one's PAHN.

Assessing Community Helping

Just as we have illustrated varieties of PAHN at the individual level, it is also possible to describe the prototypical patterns for an entire group of people, such as those living in a given neighborhood or community.

From the Detroit study a set of eight municipalities may be compared in terms of their profile and helping capacity. Here, the average or modal patterns dealing with how each of ten different kinds of helpers are used is the basic descriptive tool. When use of one helper was statistically correlated with use of another, that is, when two helpers are simultaneously used for one recent concern, this is designated as a *linkage*. When a negative correlation exists between two different kinds of helpers, we have called this a *barrier*. Figure 1.1 schematically depicts the patterns obtained for each community sampled. Thus we see that in Troy, use of friend helping is also significantly associated with using co-workers, formal helpers, neighbors, and kin. But in that same community if the spouse is used as a helper for a given problem, that tends to preclude the use of a range of other helpers. The configurations contained in Figure 1.1 provide network maps that serve to diagnose pathways of help-seeking and their unique forms.

Figure 1.1 shows the resulting patterns for the three communities sampled. On an overall basis, Royal Oak, Michigan—a mixed blue- and white-collar older community—emerges as the most healthy in terms of helping resources. It has a linkage among four different kinds of helpers including primary and proximal types and no barriers. By contrast, Mt. Clemens, Michigan—a relatively low-income, blue-collar community—comes out as least healthy in terms of network patterns. It has no links and many barriers between helpers. Troy—a fast growing white-collar suburb—shows a dichotomous pattern of spouse helping versus help from many other sources. It contrasts with another white-collar suburb—Livonia—where spouse help is highly correlated with help from neighbors, kin, friends, and formal helpers.

The patterns shown in Figure 1.1 can serve as diagnostic profiles that bring into focus points of needed strengthening of particular helping arenas—such as neighborhood or workplace—and also where a particular system may be overloaded. In addition, such network analysis identifies underutilization patterns for professional service agencies.

FIGURE 1.1. Network Linkages and Barriers for Sample Communities

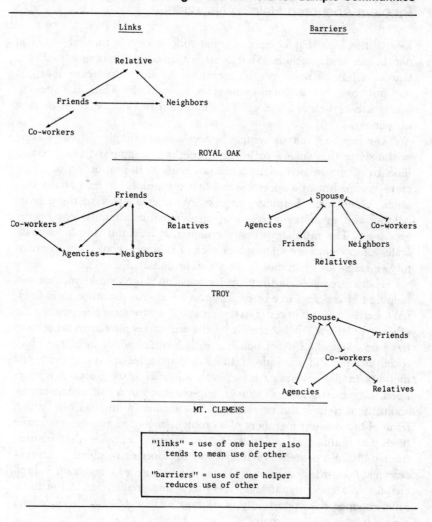

Links   Barriers

ROYAL OAK

TROY

MT. CLEMENS

"links" = use of one helper also
    tends to mean use of other

"barriers" = use of one helper
    reduces use of other

The Bridging Roles of
Problem-Anchored Helping Networks

Key to the idea that helping is a network process is the link between one helper and another. What is so critical about helping networks is that a variety of resources is assembled by the help-seeker much as one puts together a model of an atom or molecule. Thus, the simultaneous use of helpers is a critical dimension in the system of helping networks.

The bridging role of helping networks is not simply a structural one in the sense that such a pattern of sometimes temporary, non-intimate links to others in several social arenas leads to the formation of a concrete group, but in a special sense that the process of community emerges within such helping networks. Without a problem there is no helping and even the very social meaning of community may not be expressed. The intimate primary groups that bind individuals to small-scale components are themselves part of a larger whole—the community. PAHNs knit together these different potential elements.

There are at least three major ways in which problem-anchored helping networks act in a bridging or brokerage role between an individual's loose- and tight-knit ties by creating or strengthening one or the other type. First, this is shown by the fact of keeping alive (as a loose tie) some aspect of a relationship with former members of close-knit social groups. For example, instead of geographic movement or social mobility totally severing contact with a former work group, neighborhood, or organization, occasional help-seeking can maintain knowledge about the activities and whereabouts of a former intimate. Even though none of the present members of a problem-anchored network may have been part of that earlier close-knit group, there is a greater-than-random probability of a present neighbor knowing a former neighbor, a present workmate knowing a prior one, or the people now active in a local chapter of a civic organization knowing a former member. All of these links enhance the opportunity of present social contact with those who are no longer one's intimates.

Second, problem-anchored helping networks serve as potential spawning grounds for the creation of new close-knit ties by virtue of the shared problems and crises that occasionally emerge. These infrequent events intensify the social ties that are otherwise relatively dormant and bring together members of the network so that they come to know each other. For instance, a severe winter (not just a bad snow storm) may require neighbors to help each other in larger numbers or over a longer problem sequence than is the case for such helping as watching a home when a neighbor is on vacation or keeping an eye on children playing in the street.

A threat of school bussing, urban renewal clearance, or traffic hazards may bring neighbors together in ways that were previously lacking in collective dimensions and enduring social action. These potential problem incidents can be found in the work setting and the voluntary-association context as well. Such events are idiosyncratic and are not the normal basis of helping. Moreover, they generally do not spill over into linkages with other groups or individuals. But individuals rooted in a single setting may begin to call upon helpers outside of that milieu and to therefore mobilize a network of helping ties that may bring together individuals in a face-to-face and intimate sense as a "social web" who were previously linked solely by their having been referrals from one person in a proximity-based social setting.

The third way in which problem-anchored helping networks bridge or strengthen other social ties is by creating a base of reciprocity in terms of past favors or help. While there are no requirements for such reciprocity, these are relationships in which the norm of reciprocity is implied even if it is not immediately satisfied. It is this future contingency of a social tie that provides continuity to loose-knit relationships and may require the cashing-in of favors precisely in one of the problem or crisis situations where close-knit ties are likely to be built.

PAHNs are so variable in structure that they can be creative forms of new community identity. Considered in terms of a continuum, PAHNs may be generative of self-help organizations at one extreme (which replace or supplant reliance on formal agencies or organizations) or at the opposite pole PAHNs may be stepping stones to the use of formal services.

For any given behavior arena, one can visualize a pool of potential helpers whose capacity to form a network is based on the single individual who seeks aid in that setting. To the degree that the same person also goes to other arenas for problem coping, these otherwise disparate spheres are tied together. This process is one of the very indirect versus direct social integration. Neither the seeker of help nor the giver of aid need be in a close social relationship for linkage to occur.

Specifically we argue that community and individual health or well-being (or effectiveness in problem coping) is a function of the range of informal social ties utilized by members and the diversity of pattern characterizing a population.

Programmatic Uses of PAHN Analysis

There is a wide range of roles and functions related to using helping networks:

1. Overcoming the isolation and loneliness of individuals, particularly in urban settings.
2. Coping with personal and family problems associated with contemporary life, such as those associated with life crises (loss of job), life concerns (getting a better education), and life conditions (social isolation).
3. Improving the knowledge residents have about community services and resources—making contact with and using such services and resources.
4. Providing a method for diagnosing the local community and identifying its weaknesses—effects or causes of problems (such as uneven distribution of resources or lack of needed services in the community).

We cannot explore in this single chapter the full panoply of policy issues raised by network analysis. We at the same time, however, feel that the design of social intervention projects aimed at improving human services and problem-solving resources of individuals must address the following:

1. Can "natural networks" be built by professionals?
2. What is the range of strategies for linking networks of informal/communal helping with professional service programs?
3. How effective are social/helping networks?
4. Does the helping-network approach offer a substitute for, a complement to, or a supplement to professional helping?
5. Can or should natural networks be built by public agencies?

As researchers and practitioners learn more about the positive functions of informal social support systems in helping people cope with stress and a variety of life concerns, the importance of assuring that public and private agencies offering services are not destroying or discouraging the natural support systems becomes very important. Some of the functions that have been performed by formal services may devolve back onto the informal systems due to rising costs. Hospital stays, for example, are growing shorter, placing a greater burden on the informal systems to provide convalescent care. Thirty years ago, women commonly spent ten days in the hospital after having a baby. Now they are routinely discharged after two or three days. The community is also being asked to care for chronically disabled persons who were previously institutionalized.

Let us consider the utilization of PAHN analysis in the specific context of a problem-solving sequence (derived from health and mental health foci):

In prevention: Identifying and mapping the density, distribution, and vitality of PAHNs can aid in program planning and evaluation, directing attention to where professional services should be expanded or may be appropriately reduced to avoid duplication. Thus, an informal PAHN solution may be equally or more successful than use of a formal service system.

In treatment: Since most professionals see the indivdual after he or she has been in touch with many PAHNs first, it is often only as a last resort or because the person trusts the advice of that informal "referral agent" that the individual—otherwise fearful and misinformed about formal helpers—ends up using such formal professional services.

So-called self-referral really involves, in 90 percent of cases, a person who has talked with at least one natural helper first—a spouse, neighbor, co-worker, or friend—before going to an agency for help. The pathway to the professional is either blocked or facilitated by the role of the informal PAHN helpers.

In the vast majority of instances, the therapy or treatment process itself relies for ultimate success on the role of informal helpers—family, friends, co-workers. The professional is always in an invisible partnership with a host of colleagues in the natural environment of the patient. The absence or subversion of the natural helpers is a major obstacle to treatment and often to diagnosis itself.

Aftercare: Here the case for PAHNs is especially strong. Many kinds of illnesses and social-service help require the cooperation of natural helpers in the environment of the patient or client. Monitoring of symptoms, therapeutic interventions, and medical regimens such as dieting or other behavior controls cannot be mainly dependent on professional visitations and contact. All of the patterns of patient behavior and treatment that are out of the hands of the professional depend on natural helping systems.

In many programs of outpatient placement, returning the person to the community is dependent for its success on the strength and role of informal helping networks. Agencies that use and understand these dynamics can make maximum use of their staffs and insure the highest level of success in deinstitutionalization and general outpatient care. Often informal helping networks are used because of the intuitive insight of administrators. But the need is to have all health and social welfare agencies using informal helping networks by locating and seeking to build relationships with key members of such networks.

A Closing Note

We need to underscore a key finding in the helping network study that becomes a basic proposition about understanding the role of PAHNs in contemporary society. Essentially, we suggest that meeting the challenge of life dissatisfactions is a sign of mental health, not pathology. To have problems is not necessarily associated with being worse off than having none. If the problem load gets too large too quickly, an individual is going to express distress and a decline in well-being. But, as a number of researchers have shown, the buffering of support networks is one way the individual can cope with problems and not be a candidate for mental illness.

Coping with a range of concerns can be healthy in the short run as well as for the longer haul. Helping networks appear to reinforce a person's motivation to recognize an unsatisfactory condition in his or her life and not sweep it under the rug. Furthermore, people who have effective helping networks can find ways to deal with and to take significant steps toward the resolution of a problem.

There is also a hidden benefit in using helping networks. Without reaching out to build such ties, an individual may develop a sense of isolation and alienation from life. Seniors and youth are both especially prone to such a syndrome. By becoming entwined in helping networks, the individuals may come to revitalize and reaffirm their sense of belonging—their attachment to community. This is one way to avoid the anomie so often described as a disease of urban life.

2

Social Support and Mental Health in Urban Ethnic Neighborhoods

David E. Biegel,
Arthur J. Naparstek, and
Mohammad M. Khan

In recent years there has been a growing interest in the relationship between social support and mental health. Research studies reviewed by Cobb (1976), Dean and Lin (1977), Kaplan, Cassel, and Gore (1977), and the President's Commission on Mental Health (1978b) indicate that social support is an important correlate of mental health status. These studies show that social support plays a major role in moderating the harmful effects of life stress such that at times of high stress, those having high social support are likely to experience fewer symptoms of psychological distress. However, our knowledge about the dynamics of the relationship between social support and mental health is still very limited. We do not know, for example, how this relationship varies by levels of stress when age, ethnicity, and socioeconomic status are controlled. We also do not know enough about the relative importance of different components of social support. The aim of the present study is to address these gaps in our knowledge with specific attention to urban ethnic communities.

A number of operational definitions of social support can be traced in the literature (e.g., Caplan, 1974; Weiss, 1974; Cobb, 1976; Kaplan et

An earlier version of this paper was presented at the Eighty-Eighth Annual Meeting, American Psychological Association, Montreal, Canada, 1980. This research was supported by a grant #R01-MH26531-03, from the Mental Health Services Development Branch, National Institute of Mental Health.

al., 1977; Andrews, Tennant, Hewson, Vaillant, 1978). One of the most recent and useful definitions is offered by Lin, Simeone et al. (1979). According to them, "Social support is defined as support accessible to an individual through social ties to other individuals, groups, and the larger community" (p. 109). This definition and those of others (e.g., Andrews et al., 1978) suggest that social support may consist of three distinct components. First, an individual may derive support from other individuals such as family, friends, and co-workers. This component, as proposed by Andrews et al. (1978), may be referred to as "direct support." Second, one may obtain support from groups through interaction and participation processes. This component may be termed "indirect support." Finally, individuals may derive support from the community at large through their attachments to place of residence and to work. These attachments are a proxy of adjustment to one's environment, an essential dimension of social support (Nuckolls, Cassel, & Kaplan, 1972; Lin and colleagues, 1979). Following the terminology of Lin and colleagues this component may be called "social adjustment."

Thus by its very definition, social support consists of three components. Individuals may experience varying levels of support from each of these components depending on their socioeconomic, cultural, and demographic backgrounds. It is logical, therefore, to expect that the relationship between social support and mental health may vary by the importance individuals attach, consciously or subconsciously, to each component. Furthermore, this relationship may also vary by levels of stress an individual may face, as social support has been found to provide a significant "buffering effect" at times of high life stress (Nuckolls et al., 1972; Cassel, 1974; Kaplan et al., 1977). While there has been research examining each of these variables-components of social support, life stress, and socioeconomic, cultural, and demographic background, individual studies have tended to focus only on one or two variables (see reviews by Dean & Lin, 1977; Kaplan et al., 1977; Hamburg & Killilea, 1979).

Nuckolls and associates (1972) studied the joint effect of social support and life stress on the outcome of pregnancies. The data were obtained from 170 pregnant women between the ages of eighteen and twenty-nine of similar social class. Nuckolls and co-workers found that taken alone, neither social support nor life stress had any significant effect on pregnancy complications. However, when considered jointly, they found that 91 percent of the women with high life stress and low social support had experienced one or more complications. The importance of joint effect of social support and life stress on mental health is also emphasized by Cassel (1974) and Kaplan and colleagues (1977). While their studies are an important step forward, they did not take into account the effects of socioeconomic, cultural, or demographic background.

Henderson and colleagues (1978) and Andrews and co-workers (1978) are two of the few groups who studied the relative importance of components of social support. Henderson and his colleagues, using a general population sample in Australia and building upon Weiss' work (1974) on provisions of social relations, found that the "available attachment" (an equivalent of direct support in the present study) explained the greatest amount of variance in mental health status. However, the authors did not control for levels of life stress. Also, the sample size in Henderson's study is small for a multivariate analysis ($N = 41$).

Andrews and his colleagues (1978), who used a relatively large suburban population sample in Australia ($N = 863$) and controlled for levels of life stress, also found that direct support is the most important correlate of psychological well-being. However, both the Henderson and the Andrews studies did not control for individuals' socioeconomic, cultural, or demographic backgrounds.

Our review of the literature indicates that there has been little examination of the relationship between social support and mental health in the context of urban neighborhoods. Lin and colleagues (1979), however, did study this relationship in an urban (Washington, D.C.) Chinese community. They found that the effect of social support upon mental health status was greater in magnitude than the effect of life stress. Although Lin and colleagues showed that social support may have a direct effect on mental health in urban ethnic communities, they did not examine the relative importance of components of social support.

The study drawn upon in this chapter is part of a larger research and demonstration project focusing on issues of delivery of mental health services in urban ethnic communities (Biegel & Naparstek, 1979). Urban ethnic communities contain large numbers of elderly and lower-class individuals. Support systems of these population subgroups differ significantly from those of the general population (Biegel & Sherman, 1979). Neighborhood, for example, is a locus of activities for elderly (Mann, 1965), ethnics (Gans, 1961), and the lower class (Mann, 1965; Lee, 1968) and hence constitutes an important aspect of their support system. Neighborhood attachment, especially in urban ethnic communities, provides a sense of belonging, reduces alienation, and enhances ability to solve problems and to maintain the motivation to overcome modern-day frustrations (Warren, 1977; Stuart, 1979). Thus it is our feeling that it is helpful to examine the relationship between social support and mental health by taking into account neighborhood attachments and individuals' sociocultural and demographic background. Similarly, the question raised by some researchers (Hamburg & Killilea, 1979; Lin and colleagues, 1979) regarding interaction of social support and mental health should also be examined in sociocultural and demographic contexts.

Using data from two urban ethnic communities, the present study examines (1) the relationship between various indicators of social support and mental health controlling for levels of life stress and individuals' background; (2) the relative importance of different components of social support for different population groups; and (3) the interaction of social support and life stress. While our study attempts to address some of the literature gaps we have noted, no one study can adequately examine all of these issues. Rather, we see our work as just one step in adding to knowledge in this area.

Methodology

The data used in the present study are derived from a random sample survey of residents of two urban ethnic communities ($N = 400$), the south side of Milwaukee, Wisconsin, and southeast Baltimore, Maryland. These communities consist of white, working-class ethnic neighborhoods, with most of the ethnic population descending from Southern and Eastern Europe. The sample consists of 27 percent first- and second-generation ethnics and about 26 percent elderly. The average number of school years completed by the respondents is 9.2 and the median family income is approximately $12,000 per year.

It may be noted here that our sample has a relatively high proportion of elderly and lower-class individuals which, though not atypical of urban ethnic communities, may limit generalizability of the findings to other communities. The data were collected in 1977 by professionally trained interviewers as a part of the Neighborhood and Family Services Project, a four-year research and demonstration effort funded by NIMH, which focused upon improving neighborhood and family life by identifying and rectifying help-seeking and -receiving obstacles.

The survey instrument consisted of approximately a hundred open- and closed-ended questions focusing upon various aspects of neighborhood and family life. The sections of the instrument most relevant to the present analysis focused on the following: mental health status (self-administered psychological symptom checklist scale); social support (relations with family, friends, and co-workers; neighborhood interaction and organizational participation; activities in the neighborhood and neighborhood attachments; life crises events; and the respondents' background, such as age, ethnicity, and socioeconomic status.

Measurement of Variables

Mental health status, the dependent variable, was measured by a symptom checklist scale known as the SCL-90. This scale consists of ninety Likert-type items measuring frequency of various psychological symptoms. The scale contains nine dimensions; namely, Somatization, Obsession–Compulsion, Interpersonal Sensitivity, Depression, Anxiety, Hostility, Phobia, Paranoia, and Psychoticism. These dimensions are combined into global indices such as the Positive Symptoms Index, the Global Severity Index, and the Positive Distress Index, with the dimensions and indices scored according to specific procedures outlined in the SCL-90 manual (see Derogatis, 1976). In the present analysis, we used the Global Severity Index (GSI) as an indicator of an individual's psychological state because its construct validity is greater than that of the other two indices. Boieloucky and Horvath (1974), for example, correlated GSI with symptom scores of the Middlesex Hospital Questionnaire (MHQ) and found a correlation coefficient of .92. The correlation for other dimensions or indices of the SCL-90 were either less than .74 or were not comparable with other scales. Furthermore, Derogatis, Yevzeroff, and Wittelsberger (1975) state that the GSI represents the best single indicator of current depth of a disorder, and, therefore, its use is preferred when a single summary measure is called for.

Life stress was measured by Holmes and Rahe's (1967) Social Readjustment Rating Scale (SRRS). The SRRS is designed to measure the magnitude of life stress created by a certain life event. The score for each event is based on the perceived amount of adjustment required to cope with the event. The original scale consisted of forty-four items, but following Warren's (1976) framework, we have used only fourteen items in the present analysis. The stress scores were categorized into high and low by taking the median of the sample scores as the cutting point.

An adequate scale for social support is yet to be developed. Dean and Lin (1977, p. 408) noted, "A thorough search in the social and psychological inventories of scales has failed to uncover any measures of social support with either known and/or acceptable properties. . . ."

Our own review of the literature confirms that there is still no standard scale to measure social support (i.e., different authors have measured social support differently—Nuckolls et al., 1972; Lin & Simeone, 1979; etc.). In the absence of a standard scale, we have attempted to measure social support using conceptual frameworks proposed by Andrews and co-workers (1978) and Lin and Simeone (1979).

Based on Breslow's (1972) quantitative approach to the World Health Organization's definition of physical, mental, and social health and the work of Renne (1974), Andrews and colleagues (1978) conceptualized social support in terms of direct support from the individual's relationship with other individuals and indirect support derived from interaction in the neighborhood and participation in community organizations. In the present analysis we have extended the framework of Andrews' group to include the social-adjustment component, not only because it is an important source of social support (Lin & Simeone, 1979), but also because our study is focused upon an urban ethnic population which exhibits stronger attachment to place (Gans, 1961; Mann, 1965; Lee, 1968) as compared with the general population. Following Lin and colleagues we have measured the adjustment component by attachment to neighborhood and by work satisfaction.

Social support in the present study is thus measured by three components: (1) direct support—relationships with family, friends, and co-workers; (2) indirect support—interaction with neighbors and organizational participation; and (3) social adjustment—measured by neighborhood attachment and work satisfaction. Each of these components is operationalized through several indicators (Table 2.1). Direct support, for example, is operationalized by an individual's marital status (married vs. others) and living alone (yes vs. no), friends in the neighborhood (> 50 percent vs. < 50 percent) and co-workers (working vs. nonworking). Indirect support is measured by two separate variables. The first variable, neighborhood interaction, is operationalized through a six-item *summated* scale providing a score of an individual's interaction with neighbors, for example, chatting, exchanging favors, informal visiting; the second variable, organizational participation, is operationalized as the number of organizations an individual belongs to. The social adjustment component is operationalized through work satisfaction (yes vs. no) and neighborhood attachments. The attachments consist of five items: consider neighborhood real home (yes vs. no), loyal to neighborhood (yes vs. no), satisfied with neighborhood (yes vs. no), length of residence (number of years), and own home (yes vs. no). It may be mentioned here that neighborhood attachment in previous literature has often been measured by attitudinal questions (see, for example, Kasarda & Janowitz, 1974); however, in the context of social adjustment, it was deemed necessary to include additional items on residential stability and home ownership as well.

Socioeconomic, cultural, and demographic background was measured in terms of ethnicity, education, income, and age. Residents of first- and second-generation Eastern and Southern European background were classified as ethnics. Education and income were combined to measure socioeconomic status (SES) such that an individual having a college education or income above $12,000 per year (median for our sample) was classified as the higher SES group; whereas the remaining sample was classified as the lower SES group. Age was dichotomized into less than sixty years and sixty years and older.

It should be noted that most of the study variables are continuous (e.g., age, SES). However, using them as continuous variables in the present analysis would not allow us to examine how the relationship between social support and mental health is different among elderly as compared with younger populations.

The relationship between various indicators of social support and mental health, within each category of population subgroups, was examined using zero-order correlations. Obviously, there are a few categorical indicators of social support (e.g., married vs. nonmarried, satisfied with job vs. not). Generally, categorical variables are not used in a correlational analysis. However, by coding the category representing favorable support as one and the remaining category as zero, these variables can conceptually be treated as continuous for the purposes of the present analysis. Furthermore, to undertake a categorical data analysis (e.g., Chisquare) would have necessitated categorizing the symptom scale and risking a greater loss of information. Thus it was decided to use effect codes one and zero for the dichotomous indicators of social support.

In order to examine the relative importance of the components of social support, a score for each component was computed by a linear combination of its indicators. For example, "indirect support" component was measured by neighborhood interaction and organizational participation. It should be noted here that although "social adjustment" is labeled as one component, it has two distinct subcomponents, work satisfaction and neighborhood attachment. It was decided to use the two subcomponents separately in the subsequent analysis. The relative importance of each of the components of social support was then examined using multiple-regression models (Table 2.2). The statistical significance of the interaction of life stress and social support was examined using Goodman's log-linear analysis (Table 2.3).

Results

Correlation between Mental
Health Status and Social Support

Table 2.1 presents zero-order correlation coefficients between various indicators of social support and mental health status. Only statistically significant correlations ($p < .05$) have been presented. These correla-

TABLE 2.1. Correlation between Mental Health Status and Social Support by Stress, Ethnicity, Age, and SES

Indicators of Social Support	Overall	Ethnicity						Age				SES			
		Overall		Ethnics		Nonethnic		Elderly		Others		Low		High	
		LS	HS	LS	HS	LS	HS	LS	HS	LS	HS	LS	HS	LS	HS
		(363)	(183)	(180)	(51)	(53)	(130)	(48)	(129)	(50)	(130)	(60)	(66)	(123)	(114)
Direct Support															
1. Married	-.112	—	-.130	—	—	—	—	—	-.154	—	—	—	—	-.159	—
2. Living alone	—	—	—	—	—	—	—	—	—	—	—	—	—	—	—
3. Friends	—	—	—	—	-.269	-.128	—	—	—	—	—	—	—	—	-.168
4. Co-workers	-.106	—	-.118	—	—	—	-.173	—	-.188	—	-.178	—	—	—	—
Indirect Support															
1. Neighborhood interaction	—	—	—	—	-.236	—	—	—	—	—	—	—	—	—	—
2. Organization participation	—	—	-.129	—	—	—	—	—	-.147	—	-.142	—	—	—	—

Social Adjustment

1. Work satisfaction	-.132	-.191	---	-.304	-.196	-.168	---	-.235	---	-.145
2. Neighborhood attachment										
(a) Neighborhood real home	-.095		-.251		-.343					---
(b) Loyal to neighborhood		-.238		-.346		-.454	-.274			---
(c) Satisfaction w/neighborhood	-.211	-.267	-.152	-.332	-.267	-.243	-.491	-.247	-.486	-.325	-.197
(d) Length of residence		-.144		-.266		-.168		-.227			
(e) Own home	-.157		-.118	-.282	-.393		-.235	-.204			

Key: LS = Low Stress   ( ) = Sample
      HS = High Stress

tions are presented for the overall sample as well as controlling for levels of life stress, ethnicity, SES, and age.

Focusing on the overall sample, the results in Table 2.1 show that there is a small but statistically significant correlation between mental health status and various indicators of social support. The negative sign of the coefficients indicates that the higher the score on the indicators of social support, the lower the score on the symptom scale. The results show that indicators of the social-adjustment component are most related with mental health status. For example, only two out of four indicators of direct-support component, being married and having co-workers, have a statistically significant correlation, and neither of the two indicators of the indirect-support component are significant, whereas four out of six indicators of social adjustment have statistically significant correlations with mental health status. Also, the magnitude of most of the coefficients of the social adjustment indicators are greater than the coefficients of other component indicators. This is understandable in the context of our sample because, as our literature review has shown, neighborhood constitutes an important aspect of social support.

When controlling for life stress, the importance of satisfaction with neighborhood does not change. The importance of other indicators, however, varies with levels of stress. For example, relationship with co-workers and work satisfaction are important correlates of mental health at low levels of stress, whereas marital status, friends in the neighborhood, organizational participation, length of residence, and home ownership are important at times of high life stress only.

Focusing on population subgroups, it can be seen from Table 2.1 that neighborhood attachment is statistically significant for ethnics, especially at high life stress. Among other indicators of social support for ethnics, neighborhood interaction is significant at low stress, whereas friends in the neighborhood and work satisfaction are significant at high stress. For the nonethnics at times of low stress, work satisfaction and satisfaction with neighborhood are significant; whereas at times of high stress, being married, relationships with co-workers, organizational participation, and work satisfaction are significant.

Examining the correlations between social support and mental health status by levels of stress and age, the results in Table 2.1 show that for the elderly, neighborhood attachment, loyalty to the neighborhood, and satisfaction with the neighborhood are significant at both low and high stress. For adults eighteen to fifty-nine years of age at times of low stress, work satisfaction and satisfaction with neighborhood are important; whereas at times of high stress, being married, organizational participation, and residential stability are important correlates of mental health status. Relationships with co-workers for this subgroup are important regardless of levels of stress.

Focusing on the correlation between indicators of social support and mental health controlling for life stress and socioeconomic status, the results show that for the lower SES group, mental health status is mainly related to residential stability, regardless of levels of stress. For the higher SES group, at times of low stress, being married and work satisfaction are significantly correlated with mental health status, whereas at times of high life stress, friends in the neighborhood are significantly correlated with mental health status. Neighborhood satisfaction is a significant correlate of mental health status at both levels of life stress for the higher SES group.

Thus Table 2.1 shows that indicators of neighborhood attachment, though of small magnitude, are statistically significant correlates of mental health status for ethnics and elderly in urban neighborhoods. While the neighborhood literature has shown that neighborhoods are important resources for elderly and ethnics, there has been little empirical evidence to date demonstrating the relationship between neighborhood attachment and mental health.

It also can be noted from Table 2.1 that the living-alone indicator of social support has no significant relationship with mental health status. Generally, one would expect that people living alone might be lonely and be at greater risk for developing mental health problems (Maguire, 1979). But, as Lin and colleagues (1979) have pointed out, with changing life-styles and increasing ability of individuals to adapt to new situations, it is possible that living alone is not a significant correlate of mental health status.

Relative Importance of the
Components of Social Support

The next step in the analysis was to examine the relative importance of the components of social support. This was done using multiple-regression models. Table 2.2 presents the standardized regression coefficients (beta-values), which can be compared within each column. Each column represents a subpopulation group. Table 2.2 also presents the total variance explained (R-squared) by all components of social support within each subgroup. These values can be compared across subgroups (bottom row) to determine the goodness of fit of each regression equation.

Table 2.2 shows that among the lower SES groups, ethnics, and elderly, neighborhood attachment has the most important effect on

TABLE 2.2 The Effects (β-Values of Components of Social Support upon Mental Health Status by Stress, Ethnicity, Age, and SES)

	Ethnicity				Age				SES				Overall
	Ethnics		Nonethnic		Elderly		Others		Low		High		
Components of Social Support	LS	HS	LS	HS	LS	HS	LS	HS	LS	HS	LS	HS	
Direct	.153	.187	.014	.187	.172	.058	.089	.244	.008	.102	.135	.195	.115
Indirect	.080	.143	.037	.068	.055	.05	.003	.086	.053	.069	.09	.08	.014
Social adjustment													
Work satisfaction	.035	.201	.189	.092	.10	.03	.223	.005	.138	.022	.186	.028	.088
Neighborhood attachment	.310	.471	.089	.005	.354	.327	.011	.039	.219	.266	.03	.094	.139
% of total variance explained	25.4	29.2	4.7	7.0	17.2	11.2	6.4	8.3	8.7	7.8	7.0	7.3	5.4

Key: LS = Low Stress
      HS = High Stress

mental health status regardless of levels of life stress. Among the higher SES group, nonethnics, and younger populations, the relative importance of components of social support varies by levels of life stress. At lower stress, the work satisfaction component of social support has the most important effect on mental health status, whereas at high stress the direct support component has the most important effect.

Focusing on the goodness of the general regression equation, Table 2.2 shows that this equation explains greatest variance for ethnics at high life stress (R^2=29.2 percent). In general it explains more variance for ethnics and elderly than for other population subgroups. It is interesting to note that for the elderly, the model explains more variance at low stress than at high stress, which we would not expect from previous research findings. To ascertain that the relative effects of the components of social support were not spurious, we introduced further controls. The relative importance of components of social support among ethnics was examined controlling for age and SES, among elderly controlling for ethnicity and SES, and among lower SES groups controlling for age and ethnicity. However, due to small sample size, levels of stress could not be used as a control variable. The results of this analysis indicate that neighborhood attachment components still have the most important impact on mental health status among ethnics and elderly even when we controlled for other variables. However, the neighborhood attachment among the lower SES group was no longer important when we controlled for age and ethnicity. This suggests that the effect of neighborhood attachment on mental health status by SES may be spurious.

The observed patterns of relative importance of components of social support among elderly, ethnics, and the lower SES group are different from those for younger population, nonethnics, and the higher SES group. For example, for the former subgroups, neighborhood attachments have relatively greater impact upon mental health status regardless of levels of life stress, whereas for the latter subpopulations (younger adults, nonethnics, and higher SES individuals) work satisfaction and family relations have greater impact on mental health status depending on the level of life stress (see Table 2.2). Thus ethnics, elderly, and lower SES individuals can be considered a homogeneous subpopulation. Similarly, nonethnics, younger adults, and higher SES individuals can be considered a uniform subpopulation. Based on this observation from Table 2.2, we have divided the sample into two broad categories, ethnics–elderly–lower SES and nonethnics–younger adults–higher SES, for the purpose of examining interaction between social support and life stress.

Interaction of Social Support and Life Stress

Some researchers have argued that social support acts as a buffer against harmful effects of life stress (Cassel, 1974; Kaplan et al., 1977). Statistically, this suggests that the interaction of social support and life stress in affecting mental health is important (see, for example, Hamburg & Killilea, 1979). Other researchers have argued that social support has a direct effect upon mental health status regardless of level of life stress (Lin and colleagues, 1979). The present study examines the interaction effect of social support and life stress using an improved methodology (Goodman's log-linear analysis). Table 2.3 shows that this interaction effect is significant only for the nonethnic–younger adults–lower SES subpopulations ($p < .05$).

Table 2.3 also presents main effects of social support and life stress on mental health. Focusing on ethnics–elderly–lower SES individuals, it can be seen that both social support and life stress have significant effects on mental health status. The effects of social support on psycho-

TABLE 2.3. Effects and Interactions (Goodman's γ's) of Social Support and Life Stress among Ethnics, Elderly and Lower Class, and Nonethnics, Younger Adults, and Higher Class

Effect/ Interaction		Model 1 Ethnics, Elderly, and Lower Class		Model 2 Nonethnics, Younger Adults, and Higher Class	
		γ-Effect	% Change in γ	γ-Effect	% Change in γ
Mean (U)		1.29*	---	1.72*	---
Stress (T)	Low	0.82*	49	0.88	28
	High	1.22*		1.13	
Social support	Low	1.53*	-57	1.19	-29
	High	0.65*		0.84	
Interaction (T x S)		0.95		0.71*	

*Sig. at p <.05

logical symptoms is negative, whereas the effect of life stress is positive. This can be seen from the percent change in value of γ, which is the equivalent of the β-value in ordinary regression analysis. The magnitude of variations in γ-effects suggests that for the low SES group, ethnics, and elderly, social support may have a direct effect on mental health.

Focusing on nonethnics–younger adults–higher SES individuals, the results in Table 2.3 show that the magnitude of the effects on social support and life stress are almost equal (28 percent and −29 percent). However, the interaction of social support and life stress for this subpopulation is statistically significant.

Thus we can see from the above results that social support has a direct effect on mental health among elderly, ethnics, and lower SES subpopulations, whereas it acts as a buffer among younger adults–nonethnics–higher SES individuals. This finding is understandable in that the former subpopulation may be much more dependent on social support, especially neighborhood support, as compared with the latter.

Implications

The results of the present study have shown that social support is indeed a positive mental health resource. We have seen that various indicators of social support have small but statistically significant correlations with positive mental health status. This finding is not unique, as a number of previous studies have reported a negative correlation between social support and psychological distress (Cobb, 1976; Dean & Lin, 1977; Hamburg & Killilea, 1979). The present study, however, unlike most previous research, has examined how the relationship between various indicators of social support and mental health status varies by levels of stress and individuals' socioeconomic, cultural, and demographic background.

Kaplan and colleagues (1977), building upon the theoretical foundations of Cassel (1974), argue that social support is important only at times of high life stress. We find that when individual indicators of social support are examined in relation to mental health status, social support is important even at low levels of stress. Thus social support may have an impact upon mental health status regardless of levels of stress. This is especially true concerning the neighborhood-attachment indicators of social support.

Henderson and co-workers (1978) and Andrews and co-workers (1978) suggest that direct support from individuals is the most important component of social support affecting individuals' mental health status. We are in only partial agreement with this view; direct support was the most important social-support component only among the higher SES, nonethnic, and nonelderly populations.

Our finding of the importance of neighborhood attachment in white urban ethnic communities is supported by Lin and Simeone's (1979) research in the Chinese community. This suggests that the neighborhood's importance to urban populations transcends racial and cultural differences. The importance of neighborhood attachment in these communities may be a reflection in part of the large proportion of elderly population in these areas. The neighborhood literature has shown that neighborhood is extremely important in the lives of the elderly, more so than for other age groups (Mann, 1970; Arling, 1976; Biegel & Sherman, 1979).

As stated earlier, there is no agreed-upon scale to measure social support. Thus differences between our findings and previous research may partially be a reflection of differences in measurement of this variable. Differences may also be due in part to variations in sample characteristics and in the measurement of mental health status.

The finding that different social support elements are of varying levels of importance for particular population groups suggests that multiple strategies and approaches are needed in health-promotion programs aimed at strengthening social support systems. Interventions to strengthen support systems should be carefully developed and rigorously evaluated.

3

Social Support in the Workplace

Benjamin H. Gottlieb

In New York City, at the headquarters of the Equitable Life Assurance Society, women employees have been meeting biweekly in small groups and monthly, in larger caucuses, in order to share job experiences and knowledge, provide support to one another, and further their personal and collective career aspirations. Most of the original members of the association they called "Networks" have since been promoted internally or have left Equitable for other positions that have advanced their careers (Welch, 1980). In Oakland, California, union shop stewards have been organizing "Occupational Stress Groups" in which workers begin by discussing the part their job environments play in undermining their feelings of control and efficacy in life, and proceed toward the planning of collective action aimed to improve working conditions and their sense of empowerment (Lerner, 1980). In Cleveland, the Ohio Public Interest Campaign has launched a program involving the creation of support groups on behalf of workers who have been hit by plant closings, groups that initially congeal for the purposes of lobbying for plant-closing legislation and exploring worker takeover of closed plants, and which, in the process, also accomplish health-protective functions for the workers and their families in the face of unemployment (Ohio Public Interest Campaign, 1978).

In each of these instances, workers are talking to workers and are beginning to identify a common image of themselves and their work situations in what they see reflected in the environment they share. Not only does the process of comparing experiences and feelings reduce

their sense of isolation and helplessness, while also raising their consciousness of structural features of the workplace which engender those
feelings, but also these peer groups provide access to a variety of new
resources. As interpersonal networks, their outward branches can be
used to link people to new contacts in new occupational and informa-
tional environments. They provide introductions and referrals to needed
health and welfare services and information about where members'
goods and services can be bartered for those needed; most important,
they represent the building blocks for collective action to change stressful aspects of the environment and to wrest resources from institutions
in the community which few group members would confront alone.

Each of these situations also highlights a different professional stance
toward informal support systems that can develop in the workplace.
Equitable's Networks arose *despite* the existence of a personnel department, which assumed it was the only legitimate channel for resolving the
personal and career issues of employees. Recognizing the inherent threat
posed by Networks, members approached the head of Personnel and
interpreted their association's functions as purely educational; theirs was
simply another avenue toward improving worker morale. Notices of the
meetings of Networks were thenceforth distributed to the staff of the
personnel department, leaving lines of communication open between the
two groups but eschewing direct collaboration. In contrast, both in Oakland and in Cleveland, professionals played a major role in stimulating the
development of support systems among workers. They mounted their
support groups by first identifying key influentials in the workplace, such
as shop stewards and leaders of employee organizations, and capitalized
on the latters' existing influence among employees to train them in the
initiation and conduct of the groups. In Oakland, Occupational Stress
Groups were chosen as the means of counteracting worker demoralization
and self-blame through the expression of mutual support and the planning
of organizational change, and this vehicle was deemed to be more congruent with the workers' culture and needs than the traditional stigmatizing
forms of help such as family therapy. In Cleveland, professionals took a
two-pronged approach. They not only assisted indigenous leaders to establish Displaced Workers Groups as supportive social structures but also
designed a training program for mental health professionals and other
"community caregivers" to educate them about how they might improve
their effectiveness in serving the needs of terminated workers and their
families. Considered together, the strategies used in these three employment contexts reflect a continuum of professional involvement ranging
from a "separate camps" position to professional activism in the creation
of worker-led support systems.

The events taking place in New York, Oakland, and Cleveland are instances of how lay persons form networks of mutual aid both to forestall and to deal with mental health problems arising in and from the workplace. However, these peer networks and support groups are only the most visible and organized outcroppings of a phenomenon that is as ubiquitous in the workplace as it is in the open community and that is just beginning to receive attention from organizational psychologists and mental health professionals. They are beginning to recognize the fact that most people are embedded in a primary group composed of family members and close associates drawn from such settings as their workplaces, neighborhoods, and voluntary associations and that it is within the confines of this network that people seek counsel for their personal problems and validation of their social roles and that they routinely obtain feedback about the adequacy of their performance and the appropriateness of their feelings.

In this chapter I wish first to set out a general framework for viewing the ways in which people's contacts on the job—and in particular those contacts with whom they repeatedly interact on the job—can moderate the occupational stress they experience, can influence their workmates' help-seeking behaviors, and can affect people's feelings about the time and effort invested in work. I will then draw out the implications of events occurring in the workers' social system for the tasks undertaken by professionals in personnel departments and in employee assistance programs, professionals who have the "official" mandate to serve the health needs of employees. Specifically, I will discuss aspects of the interdependence that exists between the formal and informal systems of worker support, and I will conclude with some ideas about how the professional sector can become involved, as in Cleveland and in Oakland, in further animating the development of meaningful support systems in the workplace and collaborating with those already in existence.

Before detailing the elements of this framework that capture the influence of work relationships on the course and outcome of employee stress management, I want to clarify the relationship of the framework to the extant corpus of research on occupational stress and, in particular, to research on the effects of social support in moderating the impact of work-environment stressors. I will trace the role that work associates play in providing feedback, guidance, and direct help of both an instrumental and an emotional sort to one of their number who is undergoing stress. In doing so, I will not restrict my discussion only to stressful experiences and strains that arise from conditions in the workplace—the topic addressed in the literature on occupational stress—

but in addition, I will consider how work associates become involved in resolving problems stemming from all spheres of an associate's life. Second, while research on occupational stress concentrates only on how a supportive social context on the job protects workers from the adverse health consequences of job stressors, the framework I will outline considers, in addition, the influence of co-workers on the entire process or course of problem management, including stages prior to and after the provision of support for coping. Hence, I will consider how work associates influence the individual's definition of the problem he or she is experiencing, his or her help-seeking behavior, and his or her reintegration on the job following a period of acute distress which may have temporarily removed the individual. In short, the literature on occupational stress can be subsumed within a broader perspective on the process of coping, one that gives recognition to the influence of workmates on the several stages experienced by the person who is attempting to come to terms with, manage, and resolve life stressors. Consequently, I will review work on the role of job relationships in moderating the effects of job stressors in Stage 3 of my framework, the help-giving stage (see below).

Workmates' Influence on the Course of Problem Management

People who become involved in the process of seeking help and receiving support in dealing with emotional problems in their lives undergo a course of successive movements that I have conceptualized as a series of four consecutive stages: problem recognition and crystallization, help-seeking process, help-giving, and reintegration and normalization. At each stage they are subjected to the influence of lay persons who set the direction for subsequent events. I have developed this framework only for analytic purposes and it should not be construed as designating a fixed sequence or process governing the experience of all help-seekers. Depending on the nature and severity of the problem they face, their past experience in dealing with emotional distress, and the responsiveness of their social networks, people will move through these stages at different rates. For example, feelings of demoralization and helplessness may accumulate only very gradually, over a period of three months, for example, in the life of an autoworker who has been laid off his job, while a middle-manager who fails to receive the promotion he expected and witnesses his peers moving ahead is likely to recognize his anger, hurt feelings, and self-blame within a relatively short interval following the event and will therefore move from Stage 1 to Stage 2 much sooner. Similarly, the temporal distinctions between stages may be blurred in certain cases. For example, people with a history of routinely mobilizing certain network members whenever they face periods of unusual hardships are likely to move directly from Stage 1 to Stage 3, while those who are more inclined toward seeking specialized help from professionals or from their own network of social ties will conduct an extended reconnaissance at Stage 2. In short, the stages are intended only to inform our understanding of the sequence of issues and choice points people may face when dealing with emotional problems and to highlight the kind of influence their lay associates may exert on this sequence. I have tried to define the issues people face at each stage and to introduce the main functions their work associates play by spotlighting the kinds of questions that arise at each stage.

Stage 1: Problem
Recognition and Crystallization

Initially, the individual who is undergoing stress may become aware of discomforting thoughts or feelings, may suffer a loss of work productivity or interest, may have increasingly troublesome relations with others, or may experience a variety of somatic or behavioral symptoms of disequilibrium. At this earliest stage, individuals begin to note their vulnerability and face such questions as: "Is something wrong with me?" "Is it serious?" and "What is the problem?" More often than not, these questions are first prompted by members of the individual's work group who are sensitive even to small deviations from course because of the interdependent nature of their work. Supervisors and peers at work may compare notes with one another about the signs and symptoms of disequilibrium they have observed and may decide to wait it out or share their observations with the distressed party. Hence, this first stage of problem awareness and crystallization either may be reached through the personal sensitivity of the troubled party or may await the message sent by his or her work associates, a message signifying that something is awry and requires attention. It is at this earliest stage that work associates collectively constitute an *informal diagnostic network*. While at a later career stage some of their number may also be mobilized as members of the individual's informal support system, their earliest functions are to answer questions about the nature and severity of the problem the distressed party is experiencing. In particular, the informal diagnostic network helps to define the problem, assesses how lethal it is, offers accounts of the potential causes of the problem, and reacts to whatever self-diagnosis the distressed party offers and to those that may have been offered by professional consultants. An example might help to clarify the influence of the lay diagnostic network.

John Doe, the office manager of an insurance firm, has been working with a group of six field salespersons and two office secretaries. After a year of productive work and amicable relations with the group, he begins to miss planning and review meetings, appears depressed and irritable when he does attend them, and complains about chronic tiredness and headaches. The group responds first by talking among themselves about what they have observed, and subsequently by agreeing that one of their number—most likely, the person who is seen as most trusted by Mr. Doe—should broach the sensitive topic with him. The confidant, acting as a messenger for the informal diagnostic network, shares the group's observations with Mr. Doe, discusses their beliefs about the severity of the problem, offers alternative explanations of the problem's etiology, and through dialogue, the two parties eventually hammer out a shared understanding of the nature of the problem. Naturally, there are variations on this scenario depicting how the informal diagnostic network is mobilized. For example, there are instances when the network is not so compassionate in response to troublesome people. Some networks may simply spit people out, and others may saddle them with a stigmatizing or deviant label. In any case, a diagnostic message of some sort is delivered to the distressed party, and it usually contains an estimate of the extent to which he or she is "at risk" of further deterioration and the losses it entails.

One other clarification is necessary here. Mr. Doe may be approached by other messengers from other regions of the social network who also perform informal diagnostic functions. His wife, for example, may represent the consensus of the family about his condition, and a neighbor or a member of a social club to which he belongs may engage him in a dialogue that hints at certain decrements in performance observed in that setting. The point is that the lay diagnostic network may be composed of several relatively independent subsystems, each composed of associates with whom the individual regularly interacts. To the extent that these subsystems send people similar diagnostic messages, greater cognitive clarity about the situation is achieved. However, conflicting diagnostic messages, especially those that disagree about whether there is cause for concern, may leave people more confused or, worse yet, may leave them immobile. Immobility is the worst outcome of this first stage because it forestalls movement to the second stage—the help-seeking stage when the lay referral network is engaged.

Stage 2: Help-Seeking

The second, help-seeking stage is marked by the questions: "Where should I go for help?" "What kind of help do I need?" An important corollary question that also arises for the help-seeker is, "What are the costs of going to alternative help sources?" These questions are predicated upon a decision, made in concert with the lay diagnostic network, that some sort of outside help is called for, given the nature and proportions of the problem at hand. So the help-seeker is faced with the question, "Who can I turn to?" and if professional help sources are considered, he or she is faced with a maze of agencies, free clinics, private practitioners, and human service information bureaus, not to mention the in-house employee-assistance staff. Few help-seekers take a socially independent approach to making their decisions about service utilization. Most people, instead, talk to their friends and to other community contacts they have, using these people's past experience and accumulated knowledge to help them sift through the agencies and sort out the best match for themselves. Even in a small town where the choices are limited to Country Doctor Brown or Social Worker Jones at the Family Service Agency, people talk to one another and especially to social intimates who know *them* well enough to indicate whose "fireside chat" they would find more helpful, and whose office would afford them the most privacy from public scrutiny. In short, help-seekers use the *lay referral network* as a means of screening potential sources of help, so that screening occurs on both sides of the desk.

While the lay referral system thus exerts great influence on the help-seeker's utilization decisions, it also strongly affects the formal health and human services programs that exist in the workplace. It affects rates of program utilization, it conditions the help-seeker's expectations about the kind and duration of help offered by different programs or by different practitioners, and, most important, the lay referral system can either link people to help sources quickly, or it can involve them in a prolonged referral process with numerous false starts. This latter issue is critical because the speed and accuracy of the lay referral system can determine whether help is received early or late in the problem's evolution and whether the help is suited or mismatched to the presenting problem. Early and appropriate intervention at Stage 3— the help-giving stage—is, of course, most desirable.

Stage 3: Help-Giving

It is important not to lose sight of the fact that the lay referral network not only channels the help-seeker to appropriate professional services but also considers a pool of nonprofessionals as potentially suitable helpers. The latter issue bridges to the topic of informal support systems, since the lay referral network may put the help-seeker in touch not only with people who have the expert knowledge to deal with the problem but also with those possessing experiential knowledge. Another workmate may also have recently experienced a divorce and come through it well, or there may be people in the work force of the organization who are members of a self-help group that addresses the same chronic disease or addiction or the same life transition as the help-seeker's. Hence, at the third stage—the stage that brings us face to face with the key concept of a *social support system*—the helpee is likely to turn to both professional and informal resources for answers to questions concerning the process and outcome of the help that is needed. At this stage, questions of the following order arise: "How can I get back into control of my feelings?" "Do I feel better about myself and my situation?" "How actively am I sharing in this healing experience?"

I offer the following in defense of my argument that at Stage 3 people usually become "clients" of both the informal and the professional service-delivery systems. There is much evidence to suggest that, typically, all but the most isolated people attempt to resolve their problems by first engaging the members of their own informal support system (Gottlieb, 1976). The lay support network is therefore the first line of defense; its provisions are tapped first because they are most accessible and acceptable. If, however, the informal support system is unable to address the problem alone, either because it is so serious that it proves intractable at the hands of untrained persons, or because complementary resources are needed and can be supplied only by professionals, then the helpee will become involved with both the formal and informal systems. While the pattern of involvement will be either sequential or simultaneous, the implication is that each system is affected by and affects the other. An example may help to clarify these reciprocal influences.

Imagine that personnel supervisor Jones has discussed her alcohol problem with her lay diagnostic network and through a sequence of informal referrals has rendered herself to the company's Employee Assistance Program where she has been advised to begin a regimen of Antabuse treatment, supplemented by professional counseling. Imagine, also, that she has begun to attend meetings of the local A.A. chapter, which from my perspective represents the most organized type of lay helping arrangement. Furthermore, her workmates, with whom she regularly drinks at lunch and after work, collectively represent a third source of informal support with ideas of their own about how she can get her drinking under control. This is an instance of the parallel use of three independent sources of help, each exercising its own ideology about the kind of help that really counts. And their relative independence can create a whopping Excedrin headache for Ms. Jones. While her drinking partners are all determined to slow her down but are equally convinced that some drinking is a harmless way for the group to release job tensions, her counselor, the Antabuse, and her A.A. manual with its twelve steps to sobriety all require total abstinence. She now faces the choice of alienating the people who have been the mainstay of her support at work or dropping out of A.A. and the Employee Assistance Program.

While this vignette points out that members of informal support systems are not more gifted with "natural wisdom" about how to help people than professionals are endowed with infallible skills, it also underscores the need for professionals to be cognizant of the fact that their clients may be involved with other sources of help and guidance that may undermine or reinforce the therapeutic regimen they recommend. Later in this chapter I will discuss in more detail how professionals can take greater account of the social ecology in which clients participate. But here I must emphasize the need for professionals to assess the extra-therapeutic social influences on their clients by asking straightforward questions like: "Who else are you talking with about this problem?" "What do *they* think you ought to do about it?" "Are you having trouble reconciling different people's advice to you?" The goal of this inquiry is not to neutralize the work of these informal support systems but, where possible, to try to accommodate their points of view through dialogue with these systems and eventually to contract with all parties for the good of their "client." This process of dialogue with the informal support systems can be very tricky for the professional and hazardous for the client. There may be some initial resistance on the part of some members of the lay system because of fears they may have that the professional will try to colonize them; similarly, the professionals may have trepidations about stepping into a helping culture whose norms and beliefs are markedly different from those held by people in the "business" of helping.

There is, indeed, considerable evidence pointing to the fact that many informal helping relationships are spawned in the workplace, evidence entirely consistent with past research on the importance of informal decision making and communication in organizations (Likert, 1961, 1967). Burke and his colleagues have investigated this topic most extensively. In a series of studies, they asked managers about their use of work associates as sources of informal help in dealing with work tensions and other stressful life events (Burke & Weir, 1975; Burke, Weir, & Duncan, 1976). Their earliest report revealed that 94 percent of their sample of 250 engineers and accountants cited someone at work (e.g., a supervisor, co-worker, subordinate, or secretary) among their first two choices of helpers for work-related tensions, and when asked to explain why they chose particular work associates, the respondents most frequently described personal qualities of these helpers or a process of dialogue which these helpers established which were experienced by the helpees as emotionally sustaining. Later, when the researchers began to explore how varying organizational climates affected aspects of managers' involvement in informal helping relationships at work, they discovered that those organizations that tended toward a "participative-consultative" style of management were those in which (1) norms favored the expression of informal support in work relationships; (2) there was a greater sharing of personal as well as work problems; and (3) problems were disclosed among individuals who occupied different rungs in the organizational heirarchy (Burke & Weir, 1978). This last finding represents the strongest contrast to the normative pattern observed by the authors in other organizations, which proscribes the disclosure of problems to subordinates. Considered alongside other data indicating that managers also tend to view work associates of lower organizational status as most effective helpers, this finding suggests that organizational development programs aimed at establishing more favorable social climates constitute one approach to the enlargement of support systems based in the workplace.

While the workplace thus constitutes a setting in which important helping relationships are formed, the primary groups in which employees are embedded also can provide a *generalized climate of support* capable of moderating the psychological strain induced by stressors in the workplace. Documentation of this phenomenon comes from research on occupational stress, and, as I noted earlier, that research bears upon this third, help-giving stage of the framework. In several studies of occupational stress, employees who perceived the character of their relations with co-workers and with supervisors as "supportive" tended to suffer less from psychological strain, were in better health, and experienced less psychophysiological stress than their counterparts who had poor or unsupportive relations with work associates. For example, Caplan (1972) found that professionals working at NASA had elevated levels of serum cholesterol and experienced other physio-chemical symptoms of strain when they were exposed to subjectively defined job stressors such as role ambiguity and high quantitative and qualitative workload, only while experiencing poor relations with work-mates. Similarly, Wells (1977) found that among a large sample of blue-collar rubber-plant workers, supportive ties to supervisors in par-ticular were found to moderate the adverse health consequences of subjective job stressors. Moreover, supervisor support was especially effective in ameliorating the workers' feeling of deprivation or lack of rewards and served to protect them against developing ulcers arising from perceived job stress. Using a "P E Fit" (Person-Environment Fit) conceptual framework to assess the relations between job stress and health at the Kennedy Space Center, French (1974) found that the quality of relations with work supervisors conditioned the effects of workload size on smoking. Currently, they are examining the processes in supportive relationships that prevent strain, analyses directed to exploring whether ". . . social support reduces the objective environ-mental stresses, . . . whether it only affects the perceived stresses, or perhaps, . . . enables the person to cope more effectively with stresses which are there" (French, 1974, p. 9).

While the studies reviewed here have appeared since the publica-tion of Kiritz and Moos' (1974) literature review on the physiological effects of various work environments, their findings are entirely consis-tent with earlier reports. Specifically, they provide more precise mea-sures of workers' perceptions of the social environment and the ten-dency of this environment to radiate a climate of interpersonal support and cohesion or lack of support and fragmentation. As such, they rein-force Kiritz and Moos' (1974) conclusion that: "The social stimuli asso-ciated with the relationship dimension of *support, cohesion,* and *affilia-tion* generally have positive effects—enhancing normal development and reducing recovery time from illness, for example" (p. 109).

Whether measured in objective or subjective terms, job loss quali-fies equally well as a significant occupational stressor, especially among blue-collar workers, who are so vulnerable to plant shutdowns and lay-offs. Results of a major longitudinal study of the role of social support in moderating the physical and psychological health consequences of job loss reveal that perceived support from spouses, friends (including work-mates), and relatives is associated with relatively lower and more stable cholesterol levels, fewer reported illness symptoms and days not feeling well, and less self-blame. Furthermore, even among the sample of workers who found a new job, thus ending a period of acute financial hardship, those who perceived themselves as inadequately supported continued to feel economically deprived (Gore, 1978). Although the data from this study have not been analyzed to determine the unique role of former workmates in moderating the strains associated with job loss, they are sufficiently conclusive to justify the initiation of programs like Cleveland's Displaced Workers Groups, involving the mobilization of peer supports.

To sum up, at Stage 3 workmates can exert a moderating influence on job stressors in two ways: they can be mobilized as informal sources of help, providing emotional support, cognitive guidance, and instrumental forms of aid to work associates, and they can offer a more general climate of support at work which attenuates the psychological and physiological strains of occupational stressors. While it is clear that much more research must be conducted in order to specify the circumstances under which social support at work buffers against particular job strains (see, for example, Pinneau, 1975), the evidence currently available is sufficiently strong to warrant the introduction of action-research programs involving the creation of social support networks in the workplace. Moreover, events occurring in the informal system at this third stage have important implications for the work of professional helpers. Notably, the lay helping network may contradict or reinforce professional counsel; it can be enlisted to augment professional practices or it can be disregarded or, worse yet, blamed for its intrusion into matters affecting public health.

Stage 4: Reintegration and Normalization

Turning now to the fourth and final stage, the reintegration stage, our analysis centers on the role of the *lay aftercare network*. The questions uppermost now relate to matters of reintegration and normalization on the job: "Can I follow through with this new plan of living without backsliding?" "Will I get back to normal relations with workmates, resume productivity, and restore good feelings about myself?"

It is significant that this reintegration stage has proved to be the nemesis of so many professional treatment programs, and once again this reflects the fact that the professional system works largely in isolation from the social contexts in which its clients are embedded. That is, clients relapse into their disorders or patients lose control over their afflictions in such great numbers because they are unable to maintain the medical and behavioral regimens that have been prescribed for them during the treatment stage. The name that has been given to this problem—patient noncompliance—betrays the tendency among professionals to "blame the victims" of their own incomplete system of patient management. An example from the medical field might help to clarify my point.

Imagine that after a course of diagnostic tests Air Controller Brown is informed by his physician that his blood pressure is chronically high and that all other indications point to a case of hypertension. He is given a series of five appointments with hospital technicians, who instruct him in the use of the blood pressure cuff, show him what exercises are appropriate for his condition, and review the schedule of medication and the new diet with him. They ask him to return in six months for a checkup. It turns out that after two months he sustains a mild myocardial infarction, which is compounded by the stern reaction of his physician when he learns that he has not "complied" with his prescribed treatment regimen. Mr. Brown explains feebly that his supervisor at work was unable, as yet, to reduce his responsibilities; that his wife, though sympathetic, felt unable to prepare two meals, one in accordance with his diet and another for the remainder of the family; that his exercise time interfered with the children's piano and swim lessons; and that he had to abandon his habit of taking blood pressure readings at work because it made everybody squirm and made him feel like a cripple. The doctor's response? "Now, now, I know you've done your best, but we'll just have to try harder. You realize this could be a matter of life or death."

In fact, this "matter of life or death" hinges, in part, upon the role of the family and other members of the patient's primary group who are in a position to either reinforce or undercut the elements of a totally new life-style, which has been calibrated by medical technology. As long as the physician and other medical staff remain oblivious to these extra-therapeutic influences, or to the degree to which their importance is being minimized in the period following an acute disturbance, to that extent have the health professionals failed to mobilize all the forces that undergird recovery. In order to actively promote the health of clients or patients, the professional community must find ways of contracting with the lay aftercare system. That system should become as much a part of the recommended regimen as are the drugs, the diet, and the exercise.

It follows that in the medical health field the lay aftercare system is equally important in speeding the individual's total recovery. Workmates can help to grade the work stress to which the recuperating party is exposed, they can monitor any untoward side effects of the treatment plan, they can help to identify the ambiguous areas of the regimen and encourage the individual to seek clarification from the professional, and, perhaps most important in the mental health field, they can offer the recuperating party an accepting community and neutralize whatever stigma is attached to the individual's condition or to the course of treatment. But in too many cases, people do not know how to respond to the prospect of working with someone who has a chronic disease, such as multiple sclerosis, or who is returning from a period of sick leave, and their immobility is, in part, a function of the implicit message they receive from the professional community—a message that entreats them not to question the "wisdom" of an advanced technology, much less to bargain for alterations in an aftercare plan to make it one with which all parties can live.

Implications for Professional Practice

The framework I have outlined and the examples I have cited reflect an ideal picture of how the lay network can assist people to assess their difficulties, to seek and receive help for them, and to readjust. A more accurate picture of reality is that some people do have access to a responsive network of supportive peers at work, and some people do not. Those who do will probably draw less upon professional resources, whether housed in the employee-assistance program of their organization or in the larger community, than those who do not. In the case of the former people, we need to take certain actions, which I will discuss below, to ensure that we do not undermine or supplant the work of these natural support systems. But the latter people—those who do not participate in a network of supportive ties at work—are the ones on whom we should concentrate. We should be active in reaching out to these people, not only to inform them of the backstopping role professional services are intended to play, but primarily to weave them into the fabric of social support in the workplace.

If we accept the premise that those who are socially isolated are at risk of ill health because they lack the sort of routine feedback and reassurance that human dialogue provides, then we need to think about the conditions under which people become socially isolated in the workplace. In some cases, their isolation is self-imposed; some people have internalized certain frontier norms that favor highly autonomous work-related behaviors. In some instances, their isolation stems from skill deficits; there are those who simply lack the social skills needed to create and maintain supportive social ties. While the former are likely to resist efforts to draw them into group situations, the latter can be invited to join employee organizations and participate in informal social settings that offer nonthreatening first contexts for affiliating. In most cases, however, people are isolated on the job as a result of situational factors.

It is no fault of their own that their jobs were designed along the competitive lines of a zero-sum game, or in such a way as to preclude human contact, much less to provide opportunities for socializing. Still others are isolated because the informal status hierarchy of their workplace dictates that they are marginal people who can make no claim for attention or support from the insiders. Finally, in every organization, there are people who occupy a minority status, by virtue either of their sex or their race or their unorthodox beliefs or behavior. We must find ways of reaching out to the isolated, developing ties with them, and, more important, helping them to develop ties to one another. These have been the goals of the programs in New York, Oakland, and Cleveland, and growing numbers of others like them sponsored by management, unions, or employees themselves that are in the vanguard of a whole new approach to fostering mental health in the workplace.

Another major theme which runs through the framework I have outlined and which deserves further development is that the lay system of diagnosis, referral, treatment, and aftercare also conditions the success of the formal treatment system. It follows that professional helpers should concentrate more on the interface between their own service-delivery system and the lay or informal networks of influence at each of the four stages. The main purpose of efforts to coordinate the two systems should be to get help for people as early as possible and, where feasible, to make this help available in their natural work environment. What follow are some examples of these coordinating functions and some examples of activities that should be avoided because they risk damaging or defeating the purpose of the lay system.

First, the don'ts. My description of the lay diagnostic network emphasizes its role in helping people to get a reading on the nature and severity of the problems they are experiencing. But any campaign aimed at increasing the sensitivity of employees—especially supervisors and department heads—to their people's reactions to stress, and to any indications of deteriorating job performance, must be watchful not to educate them as if they were "junior psychiatrists." In particular, it is important not to alert people to all the early warning signs of mental illness and not to teach them an elaborate system of differential diagnosis, because in the process their threshold for tolerating deviance may be lowered. We do not want to make people into pathology detectives, but we do want them to make themselves more available to people who they think are slipping or to people who approach them, often in very indirect ways, to discuss a problem or the disorienting feelings they are experiencing. And when referrals do come from supervisors and department heads, the diagnostic conclusions we make about these cases should, in part, be informed by the observations of their lay job associates. They may have very helpful information about the history of the client's problem, about how it has affected the client's work performance, and about what they are prepared to do to restore their workmate to normal functioning. Through this process of mutual consultation, a shared understanding of the client's problem can evolve, and any conflicting diagnostic messages can be eliminated.

Second, I think that professionals may also find themselves tempted to extend some training in helping skills to the natural support systems that arise in the workplace. This sort of activity can also be pernicious, because it carries the suggestion that lay forms of support are not effective, and we have no justification for this view. In fact, there is a growing body of evidence that nonprofessionals and volunteers are as effective as and sometimes more effective than professionals at the job of providing "armchair therapy" to people (Durlak, 1979). Moreover, professionals may have as much to learn from lay helpers as vice versa, so that the two parties could come together on an equal footing to learn about the helping tactics they share and those that are unique to each. Elsewhere, I report on a study of informal helping behaviors (Gottlieb, 1978) in which I found that lay persons used a number of Rogerian techniques—they helped by merely reflecting empathy, trust, and real concern for the helpee's problem—but in addition, they offered unique forms of support predicated upon their natural participation in the helpee's life space. For example, they helped by providing material aid and direct services; they intervened in the environment to reduce the source of stress; they acted as models of effective problem-solving and gave direct testimony of how they had coped with a similar situation; and they helped by letting people know that the resources to which they had access and their own personal attention were unconditionally available in the future. Hence, any approach to training in helping skills should cast both parties in the roles of teachers and learners.

In closing I want to accentuate the positive. First, we can and should improve the accuracy of the lay referral system as it affects our "official" employee assistance programs and other professional services in the community. Pamphlets and brochures do not go far enough in letting people know whether their own or an associate's problem can be addressed in confidence by a given service; they do not say enough about who will greet them when they arrive or about what they can expect regarding the form and length of help they will receive. But the way to improve the success of referrals is not to enlarge on our printed words. The whole point of this chapter is that people, not programs and pamphlets, influence the course of help-seeking. So we need to get out and interpret our programs to people—let them ask us questions, give them examples, solicit their opinions about what we can do to clarify misconceptions regarding our role. And rather than taking on the whole workplace at once, we can start by doing some informal reconnaissance directed toward finding a select group of people who serve as more influential points of mediation between help-seekers and the world of professional helpers; people who are the opinion leaders in the lay referral network. We can identify these opinion leaders by asking people whom they would seek out at their workplace for advice about where to go for help with certain problems. Then we need to cooperate closely with the nominees, recognizing that they are the "advance people" of our program.

Second, we need to concentrate on methods of collaborating with the lay aftercare system. We need to prepare people for the returning client; we need to negotiate with them about how to follow through and renew their kinship with the client; and we need to solicit their support for any job changes that may be needed to accommodate the client. If there is anything that most strongly affects the credibility of human service professionals in industry and conditions people's readiness to participate in service programs, it is what they see professionals doing to ensure that employees are returned to healthy functioning and that they reoccupy their places in the informal support systems of their workplace.

In order for professionals to effect a greater rapprochement with the social networks in which employees participate, they must make a deliberate decision to commit a portion of their resources to outreach activities of the sort I have described. They need to improve the "ecological validity" of their diagnostic and helping efforts. It is also clear that professionals must be advocates for tougher, more political forms of environmental action. They must try to change organizational policies that tend to isolate people or that reinforce their marginal statuses at work, and they will have to argue their case with management in terms of the health dollars that can be saved through modification of their institution's social climate in ways that foster the expression of social support. Further, professionals must try to counteract changes in institutional policies and alterations of the organizational map which destroy or weaken existing and responsive support systems among employees. Our goals should be to attenuate those management pronouncements that may sever people's attachments to one another and to amplify those messages that enlarge the fund of mutual aid in the workplace.

4

Psycho-moral Health in the Later Years: Some Social Network Correlates

*Martha Baum and
Rainer C. Baum*

Well-being in old age has been perceived as stemming from an ability to view the life one has lived as meaningful and fulfilling. Contentment with one's life as a whole contributes to "psycho-moral health,"* while dissatisfaction with that life as full of missed opportunities creates a depressed mental state. The term *psycho-moral health*, as contrasted with *life satisfaction* or *morale*, is appropriate here because of the implication of evaluating the past life in order to feel satisfied with the present. While there is some disagreement among investigators as to whether this evaluative process should be labeled *life review*, which seems to entail a more conscious and structured process, or simply

---

*The term *psycho-moral health*, which is used in this chapter, is extrapolated from the work of Erikson (1963) in which he attempts to combine the insights of psychoanalysis with those of cultural anthropology, sociology, and history. From this interdisciplinary perspective, the well-being of the individual is dependent on both psychological and social environmental considerations. To attain psycho-moral health, the person must be able to place him- or herself in a context of interaction with others and to feel that those interactions have been generally positive. One feels good about the self, in large part, because of the meaningful nature of one's relations with associates and social institutions. The social environment feeds back to the person the message that he or she has been a valued, contributing person and therefore should have a sense of moral worth. Emphasizing psycho-moral, rather than simply psychological, health is intended to make very explicit the idea that self-assessment is highly dependent on the individual's perceptions of the evaluations of other persons and institutions that have been important relationships during the life span.

intensive reminiscing, there is general agreement that preoccupation with the past becomes a focal part of the experience of growing old in our culture (Butler, 1970; Sheehy, 1974; Lowenthal, Thurner, & Chiriboga, 1975).

That the process of reconsidering the past life, in turn, directly affects the mental health of older persons has also been found in a number of studies. Looking backward through one's memories can create considerable stress for the older person, as Butler (1963) has shown. Butler, on the basis of extensive clinical experience, has postulated a universal occurrence in old people of a mental process of reviewing one's life as a response to the biological and psychological fact of impending death. Life will soon be coming to an end and little can be done to revise it at this life stage: Has it all been worthwhile? The answer to that question depends on whether the material reviewed can be integrated in such a manner as to lead to a positive acceptance of the past life or is rather perceived as containing a residue of unresolved conflicts and dissatisfaction. The resultant mental state of the older person is highly dependent on the outcome of that evaluation. Beyond the very extensive work of Butler, other investigators have also found significant correlations between reminiscing activity and the mental states of older persons (Costa & Kastenbaum, 1973; Myerhoff & Tufte, 1975; Boylin, Gordon, & Nehrke, 1976). The fact that some of these correlations have been positive, that is, indicating enhanced well-being, and others negative attests to Butler's findings that it is the management of the reminiscing process that is responsible for the level of well-being exhibited by elderly persons.

The linkages between old age and intensive preoccupation with the past, as well as the relationship between reminiscing activity and mental states, have therefore been established. The factors that impinge upon the reminiscing process to produce positive or negative psychic responses are less well known. Lewis and Butler (1974) have shown that under therapeutic conditions it is possible to intervene in the life review process to alleviate depression and create a more peaceful acceptance of the past and contentment in the present. Therapy aside, however, little is known about what factors enable older persons to manage their memories in such a way as to experience psycho-moral health rather than the lack of it. Most old people are not in therapy, and other studies so far have largely stayed within the psychological realm with results that are difficult to interpret in terms of the relationship between reminiscing activity and the direction of psychic responses.

This study represents an exploratory step into the "natural" social environment as a source of discovering factors that assist aging persons to experience well-being in old age, given the preoccupation with the past. In the following pages, we attempt a reconceptualization of the social-networks approach to identify some specific social ties, and the mechanisms through which they operate, that will allow the older person to assess the past life in a more positive light and therefore enjoy psycho-moral health in the later years. The theoretical approach outlined below led to the formulation of some tentative hypotheses, which were then tested with data collected from a relatively small, but carefully chosen, sample of older persons. The first part of the theoretical framework addresses the sources of the independent variables of the study; the second part relates to psycho-moral health as defined for the dependent variable.

Predicting Psycho-Moral Health: A Social-Network-Embeddedness Approach

Since complex societies such as our own offer a very wide range of possible life options, accepting the one life that has been lived with equanimity appears difficult to achieve. At the start of our search for factors in the social environment potentially predictive of levels of well-being in later life ranging from high to low, we discovered only gloom and doom messages. Relevant work in social gerontology often accentuates status loss and obsolescence as the inevitable fate of most older people in modern society (Cowgill & Holmes, 1972; Rosow, 1974), thus suggesting tremendous barriers against perceiving the past life as worthwhile. The older person is, in fact, being told that anything he or she was or did is no longer of any social significance. Such theories suggest that, in contrast to more traditional social orders, the very organization of modern society provides no social support for the production of psycho-moral health in old age. A similar perspective was developed much earlier by Max Weber (1919) in his speculations concerning the impact of modernization on finding meaning in one's life. Traditional societies, in his view, provided more integrated social constraints with detailed role prescriptions for individuals, which limited what a given individual could reasonably aspire to. Therefore, life itself could be fully lived out, allowing the individual to face death with a sense of completion, indeed one of satiation. By contrast, modern societies propagate achievement and social mobility as values, tempting individuals with prospects of near unlimited opportunities for experience. In addition, they require the performance of many roles located in different sectors of society, making the essentially human task of constructing a comprehensive meaning for the whole of one's life extremely difficult. Modernity, then, has made of life an "infinite possibility thing" (Bellah, 1964). Since the human life span is actually very finite indeed, modern society also promotes a self-conscious awareness of the necessity of selecting only a few from a large number of alternative modes of meaningful existence. This means living with the knowledge that other options have had to be sacrificed.

From this point of view, modernity poses a far greater problem for the last stage of life than could ever be faced by people living in more circumscribed traditional orders. Prospects for perceiving one's past life as unfulfilled and devoid of real meaning, then, appear overwhelming in societies such as our own. But these prospects for a depressed mental state in later life, in part, may be laid to an over-individualized conception of the individual. Weber placed the burden of constructing meaning in life entirely on individuals, asserting, for example, that modern persons have to choose their own ultimate values, essentially unaided by such institutions as church and state. Here the work of Durkheim (1897) provides a useful counterperspective. His empirically grounded study of suicide showed nothing less than the fact that human life terminates if there are no social constraints on the individual. In modern societies, with complexity in organization and compartmentalization of experience, such constraints may operate through the individual's membership in subgroups. But they must be present.

Thus it follows that Weber's over-individualized image of the individual is untenable (Parsons, 1937). People do not just "play" roles, but their social role engagements form an essential part of their sense of self. People become committed to them in binding ways, and therefore social constraints are exercised, making the person behave as a group member rather than simply an individual.

It is a short step from what Durkheim suggested, in our view, to a social-networks approach relating group ties to psycho-moral health in old age. The social networks approach has, in some instances, sought to link ties to individuals, groups, and the larger community to sources of social support that assist persons in coping with stress (Lin & Simeone, 1979). While existing studies tend to show that high levels of social support mediate the effects of stress (and therefore produce better mental health), there is as yet no firm agreement as to the precise definition of social support nor any very complete understanding of the factors and mechanisms through which it operates (Biegel, Naparstek, & Khan, 1980). Nevertheless, recent efforts, and the apparent fruitfulness of such efforts, are creating an impressive literature. Our own exploratory study focuses on the aged as a population group with particular reference to an age-specific, potentially stressful experience. We hope, however, that the ways we have conceptualized and tested the approach to be presented below can contribute to thinking about social support in a more general frame of reference.

Durkheim postulated that elements of the sense of community associated with traditional societies are also present in the complex industrial society and offer a buffer between the individual and the demands for individual achievement and personal responsibility for one's actions that Weber found so productive, in the larger society, of a sense of isolation and meaninglessness. As has been frequently noted, the United States is a highly pluralistic society and the felt needs for such buffers may be unusually prevalent. As Dolgoff and Feldstein have stated, for example, in relation to ethnicity and pluralism:

> . . . It is also possible that identification with an ethnic group serves to counterbalance feelings of alienation brought on in a technological and enlarged society. The growing phenomenon of group identity and its emphasis in American culture as a political and social force also may serve as a means of expression and a means of achieving meaning in people's lives [1980, pp. 299–300].

The notion of social constraints suggests to us that social-network ties to subgroups can shield persons from some of the alienating aspects of our society to the degree to which the person is actually embedded in social subgroups. To be embedded is, for our purposes, conceptually defined as having ties that are perceived as impactful on life experiences, as intra-subjectively binding in the sense that they involve the individual's self-identity; that are, moreover, reinforced by a circle of intimates with similar orientations. The more the person perceives him- or herself to be affiliated and identified with a particular subgroup, the more that subgroup can be a source of social support for the member to find meaning in life by affording a more direct and specific focus of orientation. For the aged person engaged in intensive reminiscing, comparing the life lived with the options and standards available to particular subgroups to which he or she belongs rather than to those of the society at large should lead to a more realistic assessment of that life and hence to a more positive judgment. Accordingly, we developed and operationalized three different mechanisms by which social-network embeddedness could constitute social support in this respect. The first mechanism is called *alternatives reduction*. It was reasoned that the more older persons perceived themselves as influenced in their lifestyles and opportunities by belonging to a particular subgroup, the easier it would be to come to a positive life evaluation. This is because the number of plausible alternatives against which they measure their lives will be reduced and the standards by which the past life is judged can be more realistic. A second mechanism is labeled *responsibility reduction*. As Weber stressed, modern individuals are forced, and far more than premoderns ever were, to assume personal responsibility for their lives. Identification with a particular subgroup, however, should reduce the sense of personal responsibility because of the social constraint exercised on individual choice. Accordingly, the person should arrive at a more positive judgment about the past life when identification is high. Finally, a third mechanism contributing to a positive perspective on the past life should be an ability to rely on significant others to help in reducing perceived life alternatives and personal responsibility. Being closely tied to a circle of intimates who share affiliations and identifications, here labeled *status homophily*, should be related to psycho-moral health by reinforcing the social constraints inherent in membership. The three mechanisms, alternatives reduction, responsibility reduction, and status homophily, constitute the independent variables for this study. Together they represent analytically separable elements of a construct collectively defined as *social-network embeddedness*.

As a general hypothesis to guide the analysis, we postulate: Positive psycho-moral health in later life will be a joint function of (1) the ability to reduce the scope of reasonable alternatives against which the worth of one's life is measured; (2) the ability to reduce personal responsibility for the actual life one has lived; and (3) receiving aid in these two tasks through status homophily in social affiliations and identifications with one's intimates in old age.

Given the framework of this study, the conceptualization and operationalization of the dependent variable—levels of psycho-moral health or well-being—depends heavily on the work of Erikson (1959). This seems appropriate given our focus that preoccupation with the past influences mental states in later life. Briefly stated, Erikson sees the life course as consisting of a series of developmental stages, each of which involves the resolution of a particular dilemma. The dilemma in the last stage of life is that of gaining a sense of integrity about the one and only life one has lived and avoiding a sense of despair with that life, which is no longer significantly revisable. The resolution of the dilemma occurs through the process of reviewing one's past life in view of its inevitable finitude. A sense of integrity is reached when the past life can be viewed as meaningful and worthwhile, given the circumstances that had to be faced. If, in contrast, one's life comes to be judged as permanently flawed, full of needlessly missed opportunities for self-actualization, the result is a sense of despair.

Erikson lays out six dimensions reflecting integrity versus despair outcomes, and we have used these to operationalize the dependent variable, as discussed in the study design section. In Erikson's view, the process of evaluating the past life results in a relatively stable personality trait, a permanent state of psycho-moral health or the lack of it, which persists until the person dies. This does not mean that clinical intervention could not alter that state, but it does suggest in general an enduring and therefore measurable phenomenon.

As yet, we have limited knowledge about exactly when older people develop an intensive preoccupation with the past and how long this preoccupation lasts before the process is essentially completed. Accordingly, it will not be possible to assert that all of the persons interviewed for this study have reached the "permanent state" of which Erikson speaks. Nevertheless, there are studies which show that engaging in intensive reminiscing or life review is associated with a sense of finitude, which in turn is precipitated by such experiences as approaching the age at which one's parents died, loss of a loved one, retirement, or severe illness (Chellam, 1964; Marshall, 1973). It seems reasonable to assume that one or more of these precipitating events lie in the past for most people by the time they are in their sixties. Accordingly, levels of psycho-moral well-being for persons beyond that age should reflect significant progress toward, if not final resolution of, the integrity–despair dilemma by the age range of our sample.

Study Design

The "Sample"

Subjecting the general hypothesis to empirical testing requires recruiting respondents who have presumably undergone scrutiny of the past life. Best available estimates from research and clinical experience, although not yet completely confirmed, suggest that passage through a life-review process has been essentially completed and become a part of life by about age seventy. We therefore set homogeneity in age, ranging from sixty-eight to seventy-two years, as one requirement for our respondents. Age homogeneity was stipulated so that, given the complexity of the design, age itself need not be introduced as a variable. Similarly, the respondents were in self-perceived good health. Physical health therefore was not a variable that could contaminate the hypothesized relationships. Aside from these two factors, however, our hypothesis is a general one, intended to apply to older people across demographic characteristics in this society. To obtain heterogeneity in this respect, we quota sampled for sex, social class, and ethnicity among the elderly, trusting that sufficient variety in religious orientation would be obtained simultaneously. The sample was obtained by assigning each of four mature, well-trained, and experienced interviewers the task of finding his or her quota of respondents in the prescribed age bracket from one of four ethnic groups: Blacks, Jews, Southeastern Europeans, and Northwestern Europeans. The sample was obtained from the city of Pittsburgh, an area of high ethnic diversity. Within each ethnic group, the persons interviewed were to be composed of equal numbers of males and females and equal numbers of middle- and working-class respondents. The interviewers, each of whom recruited respondents from ethnic groups closest to their own backgrounds, were highly successful in obtaining the stipulated diversity, and the refusal rate was low (less than 20 percent of all contacts). The interviewers were also able to obtain full and complete information in detailed, in-depth, face-to-face interviews of approximately two to two-and-one-half hours' duration. A total of 106 elderly persons were interviewed. This number constitutes a sufficient sample to test the general hypothesis. It is inadequate for subdividing the sample by different social characteristics to examine particular subgroup differences. For this exploratory study, however, the intention was only to test the potential fruitfulness of the approach with a diversified sample.

Measurement of Dependent and Independent Variables

Since this research was taking place in largely uncharted territory, the measurement problems were substantial. We had to develop measures for five of the seven psycho-moral health-related variables, as well as for all of our nine predictor variables concerning social-network embeddedness. Following the usual survey approach in such a situation, we subjected the respondents to a barrage of questions, each with face validity for a given variable, and relied on inter-item correlations as the reliability criterion for subsequent retention. When the data had been collected, several problems emerged. In some cases, individual items showed so little variability in responses that they had to be dropped from a particular variable; in other cases, item-to-item correlations were so weak that additional items had to be eliminated. As a result, the range of scores for some variables was more limited than had been anticipated and, to preserve what we could, the items retained for a given variable did not always lead to item-to-item correlations at the "good" reliability level of .75 set forth by Shaw and Wright (1967). Given the exploratory nature of our work and an interest in the existence of relationships between social-network-embeddedness variables and levels of psycho-moral health rather than the strength of those relationships, the modest reliability that was at a minimum achieved across all variables suffices for our purposes.* We now turn to a brief description of the variables, each of which is a composite of multiple quantitatively scored interval items, combined in an additive fashion.

Starting with the integrity–despair dilemma that characterizes the extremes of psycho-moral health or its opposite, Erikson conceived of six interrelated dimensions as constitutive of the phenomenon. It was possible to find two existing measures for the sixth dimension, but new measures had to be developed for the other five. Except for one dimension, guilt, high values on the variables to be described indicate a sense of integrity or well-being, while low values indicate a sense of despair or a depressed mental state.

The first dimension concerns an accrued sense of meaning. Using a forced-choice question format, we asked respondents whether their lives had been good and fulfilling or more on the bad and empty side. The second dimension addresses the acceptance of one's past and only life by use of an imaginary format of "starting life all over again" and asking whether the same or different choices in specific life areas would be made. Erikson's third dimension, sensed relativity of values and commitment to one's own, was operationalized by combining answers to questions relating to the strength of selected beliefs of the respondents and the degree of tolerance for other people's preferences. The fourth dimension concerns a stress on inner conflict and defense. Here a guilt variable was developed. Open-ended and forced-choice questions were organized around an attempt to ascertain the bad times the respondent had undergone in life and the degree to which he or she blamed self or forces beyond his or her control for those bad times. This is one of the two variables for which we ended up with relatively modest inter-item correlations. Guilt is not only a classic psychoanalytic concept, it is also a classic theological one at least in the Judeo-Christian tradition. The survey approach therefore may be an inherently limited tool to tap this Eriksonian dimension. For the fifth dimension, sense of completion with life, a variable called reminiscences was developed. Using an open-ended question format, we asked our respondents for a mini-life review of their passage through three life stages, including one "over sixty years

---

*Data pertaining to the measurement of all study variables, including specification of the items in each, are available from the authors upon request.

of age." Content-analyzing the answers facilitated quantitative scoring of the degree to which a respondent gave positive evaluations of these passages. That degree then serves as the measure of perceived satisfaction or completion with the life lived or, at the low or negative end, the degree of perceived "unfinished business in life." The sixth and last of Erikson's dimensions covers a direct conception of a sense of integrity coupled with general trustingness. Two extant measures were used but were not combined with one another for reasons to be presented later. For integrity, Rosenberg's self-esteem scale (1965) was used. For trustingness, we adapted a trust in people scale (Robinson and colleagues, 1973) for our purpose. For ease of identification both in tables and text, we refer to this set of dependent variables as follows: meaning, acceptance, relativity/commitment, guilt, reminiscences, trust in people, and self-esteem.

Turning to the independent variables, we considered subgroup identifications and affiliations in society that might be used to experience social-network embeddedness as we have defined it. Those that seemed highly likely to operate in this fashion were religion, social class, and ethnicity. Because these social statuses tend to be fixed or ascribed at birth in our society or, in the case of social class, at least at a relatively early point in the life course (Neugarten & Hagestad, 1976, p. 44), individuals can perceive them as constraints on their lives. Of course, it is possible for persons to deny their heritage or, in the case of social class, to attempt to alter it through mobility. Given the ideology of an "open" society, we would expect that to happen to some extent, and that is why it is also possible to assume that there will be sufficient variability in perception of the status constraints to afford a test of the study hypothesis. For those who do accept the notion that heritage has placed limits on their lives, however, such constraints can be used to rule out other alternatives to the life one has lived and, also, because the constraints are attributed to heritage rather than any actions on the part of the individual, to reduce a sense of responsibility for that life. If one also has a circle of intimates who share the same statuses, the sense that life had realistic limitations and that individual control was curtailed can be verified and reinforced as memories are revived and shared.

Accordingly, three different sets of social-network-embeddedness variables were developed, one set each for religion, social class, and ethnicity. The first set, alternatives-reduction variables, measures the degree to which respondents used such affiliations to reduce alternatives in taking the measure of their lives. Referring to both family of origin in terms of religious, class, and ethnic background and respondent's later self-placement in these statuses as separate possible sources of constraint, respondents were asked to rate their influence on such things as the neighborhood lived in, the occupation one had, the friends one made. A forced-choice format was utilized to gauge perceived influence or constraint on one's life, which ranged from very important to not important at all. The second set, responsibility-reduction variables, measured the degree of the respondent's identification with particular religious, social-class, and ethnic groupings. Respondents were assessed on the strength of their own identification, the perceived impact of that identification on choice of a marriage partner (or not marrying), the degree of importance attached to children's identification in these respects (hypothetical where necessary), and the perceived impact of identification on views on national political issues and on community issues. It should be mentioned that, although our interview schedule, by harking back to family roots, attempted to find hyphenated identities, such as "Irish-American" or "Black-American," some respondents (31 percent) insisted that they were just "plain Americans." Anticipating this, we allowed that option as an "ethnic identity," and the relevant questions were slightly altered to fit this option. Social-class-responsibility reduction was the other variable in our total battery for which less than satisfactory inter-item correlations occurred. We have not as yet come up with any particular explanation for this outcome. For our third set, status-homophily variables, respondents were asked about five close associates in their lives and whether these persons shared with them an identical religious, social-class, and ethnic status. Scores were then assigned reflecting the degree to which these significant others shared each status with the respondents. There are, then, nine independent variables in all. They serve to measure the degree to which religion, social class, and ethnicity influence the level of psycho-moral health through mechanisms of alternatives reduction, responsibility reduction, and status homophily.

Results

The extent of structure in the Eriksonian dimensions that a survey approach such as this one reveals is not nearly as strong as his reasoning suggested. Erikson envisioned the six dimensions as closely related, but the configuration that emerged in this study is rather weak, as is evident in Table 4.1. For our respondents, who presumably had been engaged in the life-review process but without the aid of therapy, only meaning, acceptance, and reminiscences are positively correlated with one another. In contrast, relativity/commitment is unexpectedly negatively correlated with two of these variables, and the remaining correlations are

TABLE 4.1. Structure of Psycho-Moral Health Dimensions (Zero-Order Pearson Coefficients)

	Meaning	Acceptance	Reminiscences	Relativity/Commitment	Guilt	Trust in People	Self-esteem
Meaning	-	.51*	.34*	-.23*	.00	.00	.29
Acceptance		-	.32*	-.34*	-.12	.22*	.11
Reminiscences			-	-.18	-.06	-.04	-.14
Relativity/ commitment				-	.03	-.09	.14
Guilt					-	-.12	.00
Trust in people						-	.18
Self-esteem							-

where * = p = .05 or less

either too low to register with statistical significance or erratic. In the table, we have reordered the dimensions slightly so that the configuration we found is reflected more clearly. The lack of the anticipated coherence cannot be attributed to inadequate measurement, as seemingly suggested by the unrelatedness of guilt. Trust in people and self-esteem, although measured by scales with proven reliability in other research, also do not relate to one another or to other variables as would have been expected according to Eriksonian theory. In fact, trust in people and self-esteem should have been significantly positively related to each other as two aspects of the same dimension, but this is not what happens in our data. If our own approach is correct, that attaining meaning and acceptance and fulfillment in life comes about by social-network embeddedness in societal subgroups, then it probably also entails some cost in generalized trust in people. Similarly, since relativity/commitment as measured in this study measures two things simultaneously, tolerance for all values and commitment to one's own, the negative correlations between this dimension and the first three in the table come as no great surprise. The reasoning in this study would suggest that social-network embeddedness would not be productive of tolerance for all values, and in this Eriksonian dimension such tolerance is confounded with commitment to one's own values, which would be more commensurate with our theory.

Because guilt emerged as unrelated to other variables, instead of showing negative correlations as expected, we made some revisions around our own hypothesis with respect to religion. Religion, as previously mentioned, bears some relation to guilt in the Judeo-Christian tradition, since personal responsibility for one's own life is emphasized. Religion therefore may have a potential for producing rather than reducing "bad" reminiscences and guilt. Accordingly, we have revised our general hypothesis that social-network embeddedness, through the mechanisms outlined, will operate to produce psycho-moral health. No prediction about the relationships between religious mechanisms and psycho-moral health is made at this juncture. We also refrain from making any predictions about relationships between relativity/commitment and any of the independent variables because of the confounding elements mentioned above. Trust in people, on the other hand, could show a negative relationship to the social-class and ethnicity variables. In short, we exempt religion, relativity/commitment, and trust in people from our general hypothesis about relationships between independent and dependent variables.

It might be argued that the three coherent dimensions of well-being found in the data from this sample—meaning, acceptance, and reminiscences—are sufficiently reflective of a positive life evaluation and therefore of integrity in Erikson's terms. However, because we are interested in exploring further both how our own approach "works," and the apparent lack of fit with some of the Eriksonian dimensions, we will retain all seven dependent variables in the analysis of the results.

In the results shown below, statistical significance tests are one-tailed for predicted relationships and two-tailed where we do not predict the direction of the relationships or discover relations contrary to the modified hypothesis discussed above. Table 4.2 shows zero-order correlations between social-network-embeddedness variables and psycho-moral health dimensions. Briefly summarized, the results show that the prediction ratio is fairly high, especially with the first three dependent variables where structure was found among dimensions. For meaning, acceptance, and reminiscences, ethnicity and social class produce fairly consistent positive results, especially where responsibility reduction and status homophily are operating. For the other dimensions, there is little to report except that social class does produce self-esteem via responsibility reduction, and both social class and ethnicity produce trust in people via status homophily. The results for religion are less consistent. With alternatives reduction, religion produces meaning and acceptance but also a negative relationship to relativity/commitment (but this is true for social class and ethnicity with the same mechanism, suggesting again the problematic nature of this dimension). Religion, as we had anticipated in earlier discussion, operates most negatively around responsibility reduction, showing a negative correlation with reminiscences and a higher guilt score, as well as lowered self-esteem. The only positive finding is the relationship to trust in people. Religious status homophily leads to more positive results, producing meaning, acceptance, and good reminiscences, as well as trust in people, but at some cost in self-esteem. It is interesting that status homophily across all three factors does produce trust in people, suggesting that embeddedness in an intimate circle of one's own kind makes trust in people generally viable.

Zero-order correlations, then, do indicate promise for the social-constraint or social-network-embeddedness approach to the life-review work of modern men and women. The results, however, need clarification, especially around the rather ambiguous role of religion. There are too many variables and too few respondents in this study to afford an opportunity to apply more than limited controls. We cannot control both for the influence of the three status groups and the mechanisms through which they operate. Given the fact that ethnic and religious self-identification and group affiliations are very much interrelated in reality in many cases, attempting to separate these influences from one another in

TABLE 4.2. Predicting Psycho-Moral Health (Zero-Order Pearson Coefficients)

Network Embeddedness Variables		Meaning	Acceptance	Reminiscences	Relativity/ Commitment	Guilt	Trust in People	Self-esteem
ALTERNATIVES REDUCTION	Religion	.27*	.40*	.08	-.38*	.03	-.04	-.07
	Social class	.28*	.18*	.07	-.31*	-.26*	-.15	.15
	Ethnicity	.15	.11	.27*	-.44*	-.16	-.17*	.04
RESPONSIBILITY REDUCTION	Religion	.09	.14	-.19*	-.10	.22*	.17*	-.25*
	Social class	.16*	.41*	.27*	.03	.05	-.14	.25*
	Ethnicity	.28*	.16*	.40*	-.03	-.15	-.02	.13
STATUS HOMOPHILY	Religion	.33*	.28*	.25*	.01	.04	.36*	-.16*
	Social class	.21*	.33*	.32*	-.04	-.13	.20*	-.01
	Ethnicity	.25*	.29*	.34*	-.12	.04	.17*	-.02

where * = p = .05 or less

68

a study of this size seemed a fruitless task. Accordingly, it was decided instead to control for mechanisms.

The next question, then, becomes: Are there really separate mechanisms by which the social constraints, whatever their nature, operate, and can some division of labor for their use in life-review work be discerned? Table 4.3 provides some answers. First, it will be noticed that controlling for the other mechanisms within each social constraint set leads to better prediction across the whole table. Religion now emerges as having the strongest influence on psycho-moral health, as the first three rows in the table show. It also seems clear that religion operates positively through the mechanisms of alternatives reduction and status homophily for the most part, although the former mechanism does relate negatively to relativity/commitment and trust in people. In the responsibility-reduction set, however, religion produces a negative impact on meaning, acceptance, and reminiscences. It does relate positively to trust in people, but also enhances guilt and lowers self-esteem. Moving down the table to the social-class set, the number of correlations are fewer, although generally positive. There is some reduction in trust in people except with status homophily, but also some lessening of guilt in relation to alternatives reduction and an increase in self-esteem with both the responsibility and alternatives variables. Finally, in the third set, ethnicity shows the weakest impact on psycho-moral health when the mechanisms are controlled for one another. Disregarding relativity/commitment where the results across all tables are very difficult to interpret, ethnicity yields effects primarily through status homophily, producing acceptance, good memories, and trust in people.

Overall, the results suggest that religion has the most influence on psycho-moral health, but that this influence can lead to integrity or to despair depending on which mechanisms are operating. Social class and ethnicity are generally more benign but, as far as the data from this exploratory study can determine, less influential on psycho-moral health in old age. Perhaps part of the weakness of social class as a determinant can be laid to the fact that some of our respondents were upwardly mobile and thus had some ambivalence or marginality in their identifications. Also some of our respondents saw themselves as "plain Americans" rather than as belonging to ethnic hyphenated subgroups. Unfortunately, the size of our sample and the number of variables included did not permit excluding this group from analysis. A larger sample where additional subgroupings could reasonably be made among respondents might help to sort out these possibilities. There is evidence that there is some division of labor by mechanism. Among the three mechanisms, the independent effects of homophily produce the most overall positive results. Homophily contributes to acceptance and good reminis-

TABLE 4.3. Relative Efficacy of Network Embeddedness Mechanisms for Psycho-Moral Health (Partial Pearson Coefficients)

Network Embeddedness Factor	Network Embeddedness Mechanism Independent Effect of	Controlled by	Meaning	Acceptance	Reminiscences	Relativity/ Commitment	Guilt	Trust in People	Self-esteem
RELIGION	Alternatives	Responsibility Homophily	.29*	.42*	.27*	-.40*	-.14	-.20*	.11
	Responsibility	Alternatives Homophily	-.18*	-.22*	-.39*	.16	.25*	.18*	-.23*
	Homophily	Alternatives Responsibility	.33*	.27*	.33*	.06	-.03	.34*	-.09
SOCIAL CLASS	Alternatives	Responsibility Homophily	.26*	.13	.02	-.30*	-.25*	-.19*	.16*
	Responsibility	Alternatives Homophily	.11	.34*	.19*	.05	.10	-.22*	.27*
	Homophily	Alternatives Responsibility	.13	.22*	.26*	.00	-.12	.29*	-.12
ETHNICITY	Alternatives	Responsibility Homophily	.03	.04	.11	-.48*	-.10	-.19*	-.02
	Responsibility	Alternatives Homophily	.15	-.06	.16*	.22*	-.10	-.13	.16*
	Homophily	Alternatives Responsibility	.10	.29*	.21*	-.08	.06	.33*	-.10

where * = p = .05 or less

cences in the areas of social class and ethnicity, and in addition enhances meaning in the religious area. This is accomplished at no apparent cost to other areas, and with the enhancement of trust in people.

Discussion and
Implications for Practice

In this study an attempt was made to conceptualize mechanisms of social-network embeddedness for subgroups in society and relate them to psycho-moral health in old age. Psycho-moral health was defined by the six dimensions related to integrity and despair, which Erikson posited as polar outcomes of reviewing one's life, or intensive reminiscing, when life is perceived as approaching its end and no longer significantly revisable. The study results did not demonstrate as cohesive a structure between the six dimensions of psycho-moral health as formulated by Erikson. For future research, it seems evident that certain dimensions need rethinking and reformulation if a more consistent structure is to be achieved. Specifically, we refer to the two dimensions where relativity is combined with commitment and self-esteem with generalized trust in people. In the latter case, it was possible to demonstrate that the two validated measures used did not cohere, as would have been expected if they indeed represent two facets of the same dimension. Also, we feel confident that the guilt dimension is theoretically relevant, but that the measurement of such a concept needs to be improved. Rough as our measurement of guilt undoubtedly was, a significant correlation did occur in the religious area through the responsibility-reduction mechanism, which made theoretical sense. Despite these problems, however, three of the dimensions, meaning, acceptance, and life fulfillment (reminiscences in our variable list), did form a coherent structure, and it was to those dimensions, also, that our independent variables tended to be most frequently significantly related.

Taking zero-order and partial correlations together, we come to the conclusion that social homophily, or being embedded in a close circle of intimates "of one's own kind" has the most potent positive influence on well-being, whether it operates through ethnicity, religion, or social class. Religion emerged as the major source of psycho-moral health or the lack of it across all three areas. Through one mechanism, however, and that one only, the impact was negative. A strong religious commitment did not reduce personal responsibility but rather increased it, making it difficult to find meaning and acceptance in life, and producing bad memories, guilt, and lowered self-esteem. These findings indicate the fruitfulness of our research approach, although further conceptual and empirical work needs to be done to improve the measurements and to identify some of the possible sources of the relatively weak influence found in the areas of ethnicity and social class.

The results from this preliminary study do, however, have some implications for practice. First, it seems fairly evident that the natural social environment can provide a resource for bringing people together in relationships that help older persons to think about their lives in a more positive light and therefore to feel better about themselves and more contented with the present. Life-review therapy is frequently practiced by professionals, but the notion of finding "peer partners" along ethnic, class, and religious lines does not seem to have been discussed. Our study shows that many older persons find significant others who share their affiliations and identifications without assistance, but the network-oriented professional could make an effort to discover relevant groups or associations in communities and neighborhoods and link older people, who are isolated in this respect, to them. This type of intervention might be especially beneficial for more vulnerable, high-risk elderly who are less capable of developing their own peer network. Additionally, where communities and neighborhoods lack relevant network resources, professionals could be instrumental in attempting to develop them as appropriate. At the more formal level, both individual and group-work practice with older people might well be enhanced by linking the persons involved according to similarities in backgrounds, which would help to emphasize the shared experiences and orientations we have found to be beneficial.

In the area of religion, however, the sharing element is more complex. Religion, in this study, proved to be the most powerful element in relation to stress generated by preoccupation with the past. At the same time, it seems to be clear that religious identification can evoke painful moral dilemmas in terms of how the person has managed the past life. Therefore, while the religiously embedded person may be able to take comfort from using religious constraints to reduce life alternatives and from sharing memories with intimate others of the same religious background, care needs to be taken to work in a more sophisticated fashion around religious beliefs. It has been noted that more involvement of the clergy in community and neighborhood networks is rather urgently needed (Biegel & Sherman, 1979), but this study more specifically points out the assistance that pastoral care could provide in discussing religious issues with older people, and perhaps helping them to emphasize more the religious themes of human frailty and divine forgiveness. Although the religious person is often faced with the doctrine of assuming personal responsibility for the life lived, these ameliorating messages are also prominent in Judeo-Christian tradition.

5

Neighborhood as a Support System for Euro-American Elderly

David Guttmann

While the United States is undergoing a resurgence of ethnic revival, and a heightened sense of cultural pluralism (Levine & Herman, 1971; Novak, 1973; Giordano, 1976), empirical research on older Americans of European origin is noticeably outnumbered by data on the "official minorities," namely, Blacks, Hispanics, Asians, and Native Americans. Scholars have given little serious consideration to ethnicity in general and to ethnic neighborhoods in particular nor to the effect these two concepts have on the lives of individuals sixty years old and older—the elderly.

Despite some research on the importance of the family as a key support system for the ethnic elderly (Rosenmayr, 1977; Cantor, 1978; Shanas, 1978; Sussman, 1978), significant gaps remain in theory, knowledge, and methodology in approaching the needs of Euro-American elderly in a culturally meaningful way. In many large-scale studies, "ethnic groups" refers to the above-mentioned "official minorities" only, while groups of European origin are generally classified under the category of "white," "non-minority," or "other," thus ignoring an entire area of unique resources and support systems meaningful to a substantial segment of the total elderly population.

Family, relatives, friends and neighbors, fraternal organizations, the parish, and the ethnic neighborhood itself as a self-contained living environment were recognized by the President's Commission on Mental Health (1978b) to be of critical importance for well-being of the population in general and for the ethnic elderly in particular. The specific role

73

of the ethnic neighborhood for the elderly as a major factor in maintaining values, traditions, and symbolic meanings that affect personal equilibrium throughout life is, therefore, the subject of this chapter. Central to such endeavor is the need to be cognizant of the prevailing perceptions of the ethnic neighborhood by the elderly themselves. Both of these dimensions—the neighborhood and ethnicity—were investigated by Guttmann and colleagues (1979) in a study on the effect of the formal and informal support systems in the lives of the elderly in eight ethnic groups: Estonians, Latvians, Lithuanians, Poles, Hungarians, Greeks, Italians, and Jews in the Baltimore–Washington metropolitan areas. Our focus will be upon findings of this study pertaining to use of support systems in general and the role of the ethnic neighborhood as a support system in particular for Euro-American elderly. First however, some theoretical definitions of the main concepts will be explored.

Theoretical Framework

Three major concepts, employed throughout this discussion and used as variables in the above-mentioned study, are ethnicity, neighborhood, and support systems.

Ethnicity is an inclusive, broad term not easily defined. Most commonly, ethnicity is identified with the cultural uniqueness of a societal subgroup originating from another historical society. In the New World, these subgroups are understood as being derived from immigrant groups, while in the Old World they mainly consist of territorial groups, usually settled for centuries in a given area (Kolm, 1977).

The emphasis on historical derivation implies that cultural uniqueness has existed over several generations and that it has been supported by social structures and processes that make intergenerational transmission of unique cultural patterns possible. These structures and processes pertain mainly to the family and community life of the groups and to such phenomena as language, values, traditions, and customs. Unique cultural patterns and social structures in an ethnic group imply also the existence of some distinct personality developments and models. According to Kolm, ethnicity can be defined as that part of the culture which pertains to its unique, most durable and essential elements and which also constitutes the basis of the group's cultural bond and its cultural identity. In general, then, ethnicity can also be called the core of a culture.

Trela and Sokolovsky (1979) state that ethnicity can be judged by three separate dimensions: (1) cultural distinctiveness—or its distinction in terms of its cultural values and norms; (2) identity—both as a feeling of solidarity with fellow ethnics and as a reflection of the personal subjective salience of ethnicity; and (3) system of stratification as it is related to "life chance" including education, life expectancy, income, and other social desirables.

Neighborhood is an important social milieu. Among the many available definitions, two are particularly relevant for this presentation. The first refers to "neighborhood" in terms of geography and social interaction. Thus, a neighborhood is a specifiable geographic area in which a relatively homogeneous population resides (e.g., "Little Italy" in Baltimore) and in which there are many opportunities for primary-group relationships. The second defines the "neighborhood" solely by its physical properties—size, location, boundaries. McCready (1976) states that not all neighborhoods are ethnic communities and not all "ethnics" live in neighborhoods. Nevertheless, as Greeley (1971) notes:

> When neighborhood loyalty, already something quite primordial, is reinforced by a common religion and sense of common ethnic origins, the commitment to the neighborhood can become fierce and passionate indeed [p. 100].

Warren (1971) has delineated five major functional roles for the neighborhood:

1. As a center for interpersonal influence.
2. As a source of mutual aid.
3. As a base for formal and informal organizations.
4. As a reference group and social context.
5. As a status arena.

To these functions we can add the more emotional, almost unconscious, elements that make the neighborhood so unique. These are summed up by Greeley when he states that:

> Its streets, its markets, its meeting places, its friendships, its accepted patterns of behavior, its customs, its divisions, even its factional feuds provide a context for life that many of its citizens are most reluctant to give up [1971, p. 100].

Closely related to the above is the concept of *support systems* as used in the ethnic neighborhood. Support systems for our purposes can be broadly defined as encompassing the informal and formal activities as well as personal support services required by the elderly to maintain independent functioning in the neighborhood (Cantor, 1979; Guttmann, 1979). The informal supports are provided mainly by the family, by friends, and by neighbors, while the formal supports are offered by governmental and voluntary organizations including churches. Among the critical formal supports provided by the government are such basic services as income and health maintenance, housing, and transportation. The family, on the other hand, provides emotional supports as well as personal assistance, care in times of illness, help with various chores of daily living, and opportunities for participation in group and neighborhood activities.

Informal supports should not be seen as a "one-way street," that is, a nonreciprocal series of supportive actions originating from the family, friends, and neighbors and directed to the elderly. Rather, they are mutually exchanged, as attested to by many studies (Shanas, 1978; Sussman, 1978; Cantor, 1979; Guttmann, 1979). Cantor notes that the informal support system is distinguishable from the formal or organizational component by virtue of its individualistic and nonbureaucratic nature and by the fact that members of the informal network are selected by the elderly principally from among kin, friends, and neighbors.

Study Design

Using the theoretical framework delineated above, the overall study was concerned with four major questions:

1. What are the particular problems and needs of the elderly in different ethnic groups?
2. What are the ethnic support systems that meet these needs?
3. What is the relationship of the services provided by the general community and society to these particular ethnic support systems?
4. How can ethnic support systems be utilized and reinforced within the existing framework of assistance provided by society?

To address these issues, the following methodology was employed. Using the ethnographic survey as a model for the research design, a specially constructed questionnaire was applied to 720 elderly from eight Euro-American groups. (As Cuellar [1974] points out, the ethnographic survey technique enables the researcher to gain knowledge, not by selecting a representative sample, but rather by studying specific populations more intensively.) In addition to the elderly, ethnic leaders or spokespersons, selected through a "snowballing" technique, representing each ethnic group were interviewed with the intent to ascertain their perceptions and actual knowledge about the needs and status of the elderly members in the ethnic communities/neighborhoods investigated. A total of 180 such spokespersons were interviewed. Finally, an Advisory Council consisting of representatives from each participating ethnic group was established and actively involved in the development of the instruments and sampling procedures, as well as the translation of the questionnaire into all seven languages (Estonian, Latvian, Lithuanian, Hungarian, Italian, Greek, and Polish). Recognizing the value of idiomatic expressions and of the native tongue, particularly in the case of ethnic elderly, interviewers were chosen on the basis of their knowledge of both the ethnic language and the study neighborhoods.

Findings and Discussion

Respondent Characteristics

As a combined group, almost five-sixths of the elderly respondents were between sixty and seventy-nine years of age, while one-sixth were eighty years old or older. The Latvian and Lithuanian population tended to have more of the "old old," with over 20 percent of the respondents in these groups over the age of eighty. Italians, on the other hand had only 6 percent over age eighty. Clearly, the old elderly have different needs than the younger elderly, and policy interventions must take into account both ethnic and age differences among the elderly.

Half (50 percent) of the respondents were married while 40 percent were widowed with small numbers having never been married (5.8 percent) or separated/divorced (3.8 percent). Over one-quarter (27.5 percent) of the total sample lived alone and two-thirds (64.9 percent) lived with family members. There was considerable variation in living alone among ethnic groups, with 41.3 percent of the Jewish group living alone as compared to only 16.3 percent of the Italians.

Close to one-third (31.3 percent) of the total respondents were born in the United States. Here again there was tremendous variance among the ethnic groups with three-quarters (75 percent) of the Polish Baltimore group being born in the U.S., while all of the Estonians and Latvians were foreign born. Old immigrants, those who came to this country prior to World War II, constituted approximately one-fourth of the sample; the rest were the "new," post-World War II immigrants. Respondents were considered as Euro-Americans contingent on their own identification as such regardless of the place of birth. Therefore, both second- and third-generation Euro-Americans were included in the study.

Use of Formal and Informal Supports

Respondents relied almost exclusively upon informal support systems, especially the family, to meet their daily needs. There was little use of formal support systems and services. A disturbing finding is the significant minority of the respondents who seemed to have no one to turn to for help and support.

Interviewees were asked whether there was anyone in particular that they confided in or talked to about their problems. Almost all respondents (89.9 percent of total sample) had a confidant. Over four-fifths of each ethnic group reported having a confidant, with the notable exception of the Hungarians, only one-quarter of whom reported that they had a confidant. When asked who this confidant was, respondents overwhelmingly cited a family member, with only 6 percent of the total sample citing anyone outside of the family (i.e., friend). These findings were fairly consistent among all the interview groups.

When asked to whom they would turn for help outside the family, almost one-fifth of the total sample (17.5 percent) replied no one. Over one-third (37.5 percent), however, would turn to friends, and a smaller number (9 percent) would turn to informal organizations. There were considerable differences among ethnic groups, however. For example, only 11.3 percent of the Polish–Washington group would not go outside the family for help, while 27.5 percent of the Jewish group would not do so. Similarly, only 27.5 percent of the Polish–Baltimore group would turn to friends, while 50.1 percent of the Italians would do so.

Respondents were also asked the general question of whether they had anyone who could help them. Again, a disturbing percentage of the total respondents (18.5 percent) said no. Those responding negatively ranged from 35 percent of the Hungarians to 8.7 percent of the Latvians and Polish–Baltimore group. Of those who responded affirmatively, most cited only a family member, while a small number of respondents (6.8 percent) cited a neighbor or friend.

Thus, as we can see, while there is extensive use of the family as a source of support for most of the elderly, a significant and consistent proportion of respondents (approximately one-fifth of the total sample) had no one to turn to in a crisis. It is hypothesized that these respondents are usually old immigrants (those who came to the U.S. prior to World War II) who either are separated from their families or did not establish families of their own. Also included in this group would be the older widows who live in poverty and relative obscurity and those who are homebound because of functional impairments that prevent their mobility and active involvement in the life of the neighborhood. These are the elderly most "at risk," upon whom program and policy initiatives should be focused.

When asked which were the most important problems they needed help with, respondents overwhelmingly cited no problems. Responses were fairly consistent among the eight ethnic groups. For those few who did cite problems, however, health and transportation were ranked the highest. These figures indicate perhaps an unwillingness of respondents to talk about their personal needs, which is not unexpected given experiences of other researchers in trying to reach ethnic populations.

Respondents were then asked a series of questions regarding use of formal support systems. First, they were asked if they had recently used any of ten different formal services. Findings show that few formal services were utilized. Only the church was utilized by more than 10 percent of the total sample. Even Senior Centers, usually located in neighborhoods and often connected with churches, were utilized by less than 10 percent of the total sample. There were differences among the ethnic groups, however, with Estonians and Latvians using police and health clinics, respectively, at twice the rates of the overall sample. Also, the Jewish group made extensive use of known Centers and Greeks and Italians made significant use of the Church. Of the total sample, over half (57.9 percent) made no use of any of the ten services, one-quarter (27.9 percent) used one service, and only 13.7 percent used more than one service.

Interviewees were then asked if they were utilizing Medicaid, food stamps, Meals-on-Wheels, hot lunch program, or housing subsidies. Four-fifths of the entire sample (82.5 percent) used none of these services; of the services utilized, Medicaid was by far the most frequent, utilized by 16.3 percent of the total sample. No other service was used by more than 4 percent of the total sample. Differences among the groups were minimal due to the extreme ranges of the total.

Despite the availability of the formal supports—for example, government and churches—it is mainly the family and ethnic friends in the neighborhood to whom elderly people turn in case of need, and their life satisfaction is closely connected with family relationships. When asked what makes them happy, respondents indicated that having a good family life is most important. It is not astounding, therefore, that half of the sample did not prepare financially for an illness requiring long-term care, indicating that in case of such a crisis they expect to turn to their families for help. This finding is supported by Kulys and Tobin (1980), who found that lack of concern about the future among the elderly was associated with the presence of interpersonal supports.

Neighborhood Attachment

Slightly less than half (46.4 percent) of the total sample lived in the urban city while the rest lived in the suburbs. There was considerable variance among the ethnic groups on this dimension, however. For example, only one-fourth (26.3 percent) of the Latvians and Greeks lived in the city whereas over three-quarters (77.5 percent) of the Polish–Baltimore group lived in the city. Respondents displayed considerable residential stability, with almost three-quarters (73.9 percent) of the total sample residing in their neighborhoods for from six to twenty years, while an additional 11.7 percent lived there for more than twenty years. Although all ethnic groups exhibited strong evidences of residential stability, there were once again variances among the groups, with almost one-third (31.3 percent) of the Jewish group having lived in their neighborhoods for five years or less as compared to only 2.6 percent of the Italians.

Almost all (91.7 percent) respondents indicated that they liked their neighborhoods and felt safe in them. This finding was highly consistent among the various ethnic groups. One reason for these findings, perhaps, is the high degree of home ownership among the sample, with over two-thirds of the sample owning their own homes. Only a small proportion (13.3 percent) indicated that they would like to live in another neighborhood. Attachment to the neighborhoods in which elderly Euro-Americans live is a well-known fact. For example, Biegel and Sherman (1979) found that over three-quarters of the residents they interviewed in southeast Baltimore City, Maryland, and in the south side of Milwaukee, Wisconsin, expressed satisfaction with their neighborhood, with 35 percent being very satisfied. They also found that over half of the interviewees saw their neighborhood as a place where they really belonged.

Attachment to the neighborhood as shown in our study (Guttmann et al., 1979) is even more significant when considered in the light of the finding that nine out of ten elderly respondents lived in ethnically mixed neighborhoods, and only one in six expressed a preference to live in an ethnically homogeneous environment. The Euro-American elderly sample in our study certainly exhibited positive identification with their neighborhoods, as evidenced by their high level of satisfaction with living arrangements, feelings of safety, and involvement in neighborhood life through participation in various formal and informal organizations. There were significant differences among the eight ethnic groups in terms of belonging to neighborhood-based ethnic organizations, ranging from a high of about 90 percent for Jewish, Estonian, and Polish elderly to a low of 35 percent for Italians ($F = 50.838$, df $= 8$, $p = \leq .0001$). These differences in belonging and participation in voluntary associations were compensated for in all groups by the very high degree of pride in ethnic background and a very strong feeling of closeness to the ethnic group and to the neighborhood. Furthermore, all ethnic elderly were quite actively involved in the religious life of their neighborhoods, as demonstrated by membership in religious congregations (a "high" of 97 percent of the Poles to a "low" of 55 percent for the Jewish subjects) and by frequent attendance at religious services.

There was no evidence, however, that these strong ethnic reference orientations automatically indicated an aloofness from, and disinterest in, the larger society. On the contrary, the Euro-American respondents were considerably involved in the broader context, as shown by their membership in nonethnic organizations and, most significantly, by their voting behavior. While only a small percentage claimed intense involvement in national political activities, voting levels averaged 75 percent, thus exceeding the national average of 62 percent for the elderly in general.

Closely tied to the neighborhood as a special support system for Euro-American elderly are their preferences in regard to associations with others—their friendship patterns. As previously indicated, the neighborhood is a veritable stage for acting out life's drama of daily living and survival in a rapidly changing industrialized society. Availability of trusted friends is, therefore, not only a matter of necessity for mental health, as Lowenthal and Robinson (1976) pointed out, but a measure of one's emotional and social standing in the neighborhood as well. For elderly Euro-Americans, regardless of their immigrational status, ethnic friends provide the opportunity to communicate in the native language and are clearly preferred for association over other, nonethnic friends by a ratio of two to one ($F = 56.086$, $p \leq .0001$). Moreover, second only to the family, they are the "responsible others" (Kulys & Tobin, 1980) to whom the elderly turn with confidence for assistance in case of need. Besides the family, friendships and voluntary associations in the neighborhood are important integrative mechanisms. Such informal involvements may be crucial to the well-being of those who, for varying reasons, do not have family support.

Perception of Treatment in
Society and the Neighborhood

The question of role and relevance of the neighborhood for the ethnic elderly was further examined through a series of questions focused upon respondents' perceptions of treatment of the elderly in society at large and in their own ethnic groups in particular. The following questions are asked of all interviewees:

1. What do you think of the way the elderly are treated in America?
2. What do you think of the way the elderly are treated in your ethnic community?
3. Do you believe that your ethnic group treats its elderly differently than the general American population treats its elderly? If yes, how?

Findings show that only one-quarter (29 percent) of the total sample felt that they were treated well by the general community, one-quarter (25.6 percent) felt that they were badly treated, one-fifth (19.9 percent) felt that they were treated neither well nor badly, and one-fifth (21.5 percent) refused to answer the question properly. Although the findings were fairly consistent across the ethnic groups, there were some differences in perceptions among particular groups. The largest differences were between the Italian and Hungarian elderly. Almost twice as many Italian elderly (40 percent) as compared to Hungarian elderly (21 percent) thought they were treated well by society.

Turning to how the elderly perceive the treatment afforded them in their own ethnic community, the results are quite different. Over half (53.9 percent) of the total sample felt they were treated well by their ethnic community, while very few (2.2 percent) felt that they were treated badly. A few respondents (11.8 percent) felt that they were treated neither well nor badly, and one-quarter (25.2 percent) refused to answer the question properly.

Reinforcing the positive attitude of the elderly toward treatment by their own ethnic community, over one-half of the total sample and approximately one-half of each ethnic group except for the Hungarian group rated the treatment of the elderly by their own ethnic groups as better than that of the society at large. It should be noted that one-fifth of the total sample refused to properly respond to questions concerning perceived treatment by the general community and their own ethnic community. It is our feeling that such refusals stem from the unwillingness of many ethnic group members to discuss their attitudes and views with outsiders. This was especially the case with the Hungarian sample, who seemed particularly reluctant to respond to these questions.

The fact that respondents find more support in their own neighborhoods than in society at large may have its basis in the lack of assertiveness that elderly Euro-Americans seem to show in their nonethnic interactions. In their neighborhood and within their own ethnic groups they feel more secure and more accepted than "out there" in the American society. As Kolm (1980, p. 10) has stated:

> Two centuries of assimilationist and melting pot indoctrination has intimidated them and undermined their belief in the legitimacy and value of their "ethnic behaviors," and consequently their self-confidence has been weakened. As a result, some of the Euro-ethnic groups never joined the mainstream of society and do not feel fully a part of the larger social system and the dominant culture.

There are, of course, factors that may color an individual's perception of his or her treatment by society and by the ethnic neighborhood. The ability to make friends and to maintain friendship patterns, which is a significant factor in mental health of the aging, has been noted by researchers (Cantor, 1979). Adaptability to the inevitable losses of old age (death of spouse and friends, retirement) varies with individual experience and personality characteristics. Since many Euro-American elderly will not admit dependence even though they may live alone in or near poverty and are restricted in their mobility due to chronic illnesses—approximately 15 percent of the total sample—their subjective sense of well-being may be an important variable in perception of the treatment accorded them by society and by the ethnic neighborhood.

Implications

We have seen that the ethnic family and the neighborhood provide especially strong support for the ethnic elderly in light of the little use of formal services by this group. We have also seen that almost one-fifth of our sample seems to be lacking any social supports and are thus at risk for developing problems related to physical and emotional health. Finally, we have seen that although there were definite consistencies in the data among the various ethnic groups, there were also significant group differences. There are a number of implications stemming from these findings.

First, the extensive use of family supports and strong satisfaction with and attachment to neighborhoods are positive strengths that should be taken into account and utilized in the design of services. Policy and services should build upon and strengthen informal networks. Despite the fact that neither the informal networks nor the formal service delivery systems by themselves are adequate to meet human needs, professional services often undermine, by intention or accident, informal systems of support. Instead, partnerships are needed which create linkages between informal and formal systems. Such partnerships might operate in a number of ways. Neighborhood organizations and professional agencies might co-sponsor a program or service as a way of reducing stigma and increasing accessibility. Or a professional agency might contract with a neighborhood organization for assistance in the planning, delivery, and evaluation of services. Such a relationship would be based on the expertise and accessibility of the neighborhood organization to its residents' needs and wants. A partnership might also be based upon professionals assisting neighborhood organizations to deliver their own services, for instance, an ethnic group developing its own senior center. Finally, partnerships might involve neighborhood leaders providing training for and consultation with professionals about their community— its values, traditions, strengths, and needs—so that more appropriate services can be designed and delivered.

There is often a tendency by many to romanticize informal supports and to denigrate professional care. Both are needed and important, and both may at times be harmful as well as helpful. A continuum of community/professional care is required which builds upon individual and neighborhood strengths and which provides services in a culturally acceptable manner.

Second, nothing is static. Support systems do not operate in isolation from the demographic, social, and economic forces of society. Such trends as movement of ethnic population to the suburbs, geographic disbursement of families, increasing divorce rates, larger numbers of elderly living alone, and the growing numbers of better educated ethnics of higher social classes all will affect support systems of the ethnic elderly in the future. For example Gelfand and Fandetti (1980) indicate that middle-class Italians in suburban Maryland are much less likely to want their dependent parents living with them than are working-class Italians in Baltimore. For the upper-middle-class Italian, the nursing home is a preferred setting for their aged parents, while working-class Italians would rather have their parents living with them. Thus, as Gelfand and Gelfand note in Chapter 11, family and neighborhood support may need to be augmented by professionally created support mechanisms, such as senior centers. Therefore, not only do policies need to be directed toward what is now, but planning needs to begin for what might happen in the future.

Third, although it is useful to aggregate Euro-American elderly into one group for comparison purposes with other population groups, there is no Euro-American ethnic experience. Instead, there are a variety of experiences of Poles, Greeks, Latvians, Jews, and so on. This means that policy has to take into account, not only the cultural factor in general, but the specific cultural experiences of many groups. However, in practice, it may be impossible for service planners and deliverers to be knowledgeable of the varying cultural experiences of large numbers of different immigrant groups found in the typical city. This points all the more to the need to establish linkages with the informal community leadership, who have such knowledge.

Finally, there is a need to focus attention on the "at-risk" group of elderly who appear to have no or few supports. Our study report (Guttmann et al., 1979) documents that ethnic leaders, or spokespersons, were often unaware of who these at-risk individuals were and what their needs are. As a first step, the ethnic community itself must become more aware of which subgroups of elderly in their population need the most assistance. Then, they should test and evaluate the means and resources the ethnic neighborhood has available to it to address these problems. Finally, appropriate partnerships with professionals should be developed, but only after the community itself has more of a "handle" on identifying and defining the problem.

A further step toward increasing the ability of the ethnic community to care for its own would entail providing ethnic families, especially those who have elderly members in their households, with accurate information about existing services and community supports. The importance of the family with regard to the decision-making process concerning resource utilization has been noted by Guttmann and colleagues (1977), who found that the children and relatives of the elderly play a very important role with regard to the information they make available to their elderly members. Our study revealed that one of the most urgent needs of many ethnic elderly was the translation of various documents from English to the native language, as well as an explanation of the procedures by which a certain sevice may be obtained.

In summation, the role of the ethnic neighborhood as a support system, for which we have presented preliminary findings, needs to be investigated further. Such research concerning the ability of a neighborhood to meet the needs of older persons should be studied both through objective measures, such as the physical condition and density of housing, and by subjective measures, such as perceived satisfaction with the fulfillment of needs (Toseland & Rasch, 1978), with special emphasis upon the unique cultural orientations that are involved in aging.

6

Primary Prevention in the '80s: The Interface with Community Support Systems

Thomas Plaut

There is now increasing realization that treatment efforts alone cannot significantly reduce rates of illness/disability or death. A number of writers, including Dubos (1959), cite evidence that most significant progress in improving peoples' health is the result of broad societal changes rather than specific medical interventions. In the mental health field, it is clear that treatment approaches over the last fifty years have not led to any reduction in rates of mental illness. Recently, prevention activities in the mental health/mental illness field have been receiving increased attention. This chapter summarizes these recent developments; presents principal objectives of prevention/promotion programs; discusses different "levels" of intervention; analyzes the interface with community support systems; and describes some barriers to the future growth of prevention activities.

The concept of "primary prevention" originated in the public health field. It refers to activities directed at reducing the occurrence or the rate of new cases of an illness or disease. Generally, the term *secondary prevention* refers to early case-finding and treatment. *Tertiary prevention* relates to continuing treatment and activities directed at disability limitation. In the mental illness field it often is difficult to draw sharp distinctions between persons who are "ill" and those who are "not ill." There are not the clear-cut distinctions associated with infectious diseases. In this chapter *primary prevention* refers to those activities di-

Views expressed herein are those of the author and do not necessarily reflect the opinions, official policies, or positions of the National Institute of Mental Health.

86

rected at persons and groups of persons who do not exhibit any identifiable psychiatric symptoms, who would not be diagnosed as psychiatrically ill by current criteria. Reference here is to the primary prevention of *mental* disorders. Some of the issues discussed are unique to this area. Others apply equally well to the prevention of *physical* disorders. *Community support systems,* as used in this chapter, refers to: (1) natural helping networks to which people belong, (2) worksite relationships, (3) religious groups, and (4) self-help or mutual aid groups (President's Commission on Mental Health, 1978b, Vol. II, p. 144).

Recent Developments

The recently increased interest in prevention in the mental health field is paralleled and reinforced by analogous developments in the health and medical care field. The latter has been stimulated both by skyrocketing costs of medical care and by accumulating evidence that factors other than the quantity and quality of medical care are related to substantial differences in rates of morbidity (illness) and mortality (death). In 1974, the Canadian Ministry of Health issued a major report which emphasizes that persons' health status is highly correlated with their life-styles and that changes in these life-styles could lead to significant improvements in health (Lalonde, 1974). "Life-styles" includes nutrition, exercise, and other health-related behavior such as smoking, drug and alcohol use, driving, use of firearms, and management of stress. Adverse consequences of poor coping with stress are often seen in impaired physical as well as mental health (Lazarus, 1966; Klerman, 1974; Glass, 1977). In the U.S., impetus for preventive activities has been provided by the more recent report of the Surgeon General of the Public Health Services (*Healthy People,* 1979). This document suggests strategies for improving the health of Americans and particularly emphasizes the importance of behavioral approaches.

In the late 1970s, there was an upsurge of interest in the area of stress. Many conferences, workshops, and courses were offered under a variety of auspices. Some approaches to stress management have had solid research underpinning, particularly biofeedback methods (Shapiro, Tursky, & Gershon, 1969; Sargent, Green, & Walter, 1973) and relaxation (Benson, Rosner, Marzetta, & Kleinchuk, 1974). Other approaches, including aspects of "holistic medicine," while apparently effective for some persons, have not yet been systematically evaluated (Pelletier, 1977).

Related to the area of stress management is renewed interest in personal responsibility for one's health. Emphasis on the "activated" patient (or consumer), which is an integral aspect of a life-style approach to health, is highly congruent with a key theme of support groups, that is, the ability of persons to help one another and in that very process to help themselves. It involves a radical departure from the classical notion of physician–patient relationships in which the doctor is the technical expert who prescribes for the relatively passive patient.

In the mental health field there is a striking contrast between the reports of the two major study commissions (*Action for Mental Health*, 1961, and President's Commission on Mental Health, 1978a) in terms of emphasis on prevention. The first report downplayed the importance of this area, the second devoted one of its eight major sections to it. In addition, another separate section of the recent report deals with the role of social support groups. The Alcohol, Drug Abuse and Mental Health Administration of the U.S. Department of Health, Education, and Welfare (now Department of Health and Human Services) organized a major conference on prevention in the fall of 1979 (*Proceedings*, 1980). At approximately the same time, the National Institute of Mental Health established an Office of Prevention to coordinate and provide leadership for the federal mental health agencies' efforts in the mental health prevention/promotion area. A *Journal of Prevention*, with an editorial board of nationally known mental health experts has been established (first issue, fall 1980).

The Report of the Task Panel on Prevention of the President's Commission on Mental Health (Vol. IV, 1978b) presents a generally optimistic review of current knowledge regarding prevention efforts. This point of view is also reflected in an earlier NIMH publication (Klein & Goldston, 1977). There is not, however, agreement among mental health specialists regarding the effectiveness of currently utilized prevention activities (Eisenberg, 1977; Lamb & Zusman, 1979). Part of this disagreement can be traced to the particular standards being used to assess the adequacy of the knowledge base for the undertaking of preventive/promotion efforts. Many treatment efforts in the mental health field, particularly those of a psychosocial nature, are widely utilized and well-supported financially, even in the absence of definitive evidence regarding their effectiveness. Many critics of prevention programs appear to be applying a double standard, that is, requiring greater scientific evidence for effectiveness for preventive activity than for treatment activities. For example, the White House Office on Science and Technology has recently estimated that no more than 15 percent of generally accepted medical technology (surgery, pharmacological therapy, etc.) has been evaluated and found to be effective (Klerman, 1979). Yet such "treatments" continue to be used. Current resource-allocation decisions in the health and mental health fields almost always seem to favor clinical services over prevention/promotion activities. At times of funding shortages, existing prevention/promotion activities are likely to be the first casualties and new prevention thrusts will have great difficulty in being initiated.

Objectives of Prevention/Promotion Programs

Some of the current controversy and confusion regarding mental health preventive activities relates to failure to specify what is being prevented. Prevention efforts can be directed at various target populations and can have different objectives. The targets may include individuals and groups who are (1) at "high risk" for major mental illness (schizophrenia and manic–depressive disorders)—program example: counseling, supportive, and other activities directed at the children of mentally ill patients; (2) vulnerable to other clearly defined mental disorders as specified, for example, in the *Diagnostic and Statistical Manual of Mental Disorders* of the American Psychiatric Association—program example: counseling, supportive, and other activities directed at young children whose parents have died; (3) suffering from moderate anxiety or depression (but not clearly "ill" in terms of current psychiatric usage)—program example: mutual-aid groups for single parents; and (4) children with blockage in normal development. Eisenberg and Perron (1979, p. 148) refer to this as the prevention of development attrition ("a sequential and cumulative failure to attain levels of cognitive and affective development sufficient for personal and social competence")—program example: home-based infant stimulation for babies in multiproblem families. A broader, and more difficult to measure, objective of prevention programs is the promotion of mental health, for example, improving coping and enabling people to realize their full potentialities.

Some approaches are not targeted at any single "at risk population" or directed at the prevention of any particular class of disorders or problems. The work of several behavioral scientists (Cassel, 1976; Jessor & Jessor, 1977; Bloom, 1979) highlights life circumstances and life events (crises) that may increase vulnerability to a broad range of mental and physical disorders. The emphasis here is on interventions that can have nonspecific preventive consequences. Such intervention strategies, of course, represent a radical departure from medical model theories, which generally stress the role of identifiable factors in the etiology of a single disease or illness.

"Levels" of Intervention

Preventive programs and activities can also vary greatly in the nature of the systems they are seeking to have impact upon or influence. Interventions may be focused on individual, group, community, or institutional levels. For example, while the ultimate impact of mental health promotion programs is generally phrased in terms of changing or helping individuals, many efforts do this indirectly, through intermediate mechanisms or structures such as changing the policies and practices of various social institutions.

Some mental illness preventive interventions are directly focused on individuals, for example, teaching people better ways of coping with stress, improving cognitive problem-solving skills, teaching relaxation skills, and anticipatory guidance to parents of seriously ill children. Other preventive approaches focus on small (generally face-to-face) groups, including, but not restricted to, the family. Many support systems fit into this category. They include particularly mutual-aid, self-help groups like Parents Without Partners, Alcoholics Anonymous, and Widow-to-Widow groups. Mental health preventive efforts can also be focused at the neighborhood or community level. An example is strengthening the role of "natural helpers" and increasing their utilization through improved communication (information exchange) and various approaches to legitimation of their roles. In neighborhoods or in communities, a range of activities can be organized to strengthen informal "helping" networks and overcome the sense of alienation and isolation. Thus, an important mental health spinoff from a community-wide clean-up campaign or neighborhood-sponsored little league teams is the breaking down of communication barriers between neighbors. Under many circumstances this can increase the likelihood that informal support (helping) networks will be established that will be available to persons when they are under stress or in crisis.

Institutional changes, at both micro and macro levels, constitute the last level of preventive interventions. *Micro systems*, as used here, refers to local school systems, correctional systems, medical and health care institutions, day-care centers, and the like. The objective is to bring about changes in the ways in which these organizations operate (policies and practices) so that they are more likely to promote mental health and less likely to be deleterious to the psychological health of the individuals and families who are their natural clientele. For example, for years parents of young children were allowed only very brief visiting periods on the pediatric wards of hospitals. The rationale was that children would be upset and tearful when their parents left—and this was difficult for hospital staff to deal with. In recent years it has been increasingly recognized that for most youngsters there is less of a sense of desertion and abandonment when parents visit regularly and for more than the very brief periods that were the case under prior policies.

Macro institutional change refers to modifications in the larger society: reduction of racism or sexism, income redistribution, modification of attitudes toward death, or drug and alcohol use. Bringing about such large-scale societal changes, while very well carrying promise of a "mentally healthier" society, is not generally viewed as the responsibility of mental health agencies and professionals. As preventive interventions become invested in more complex systems, systematic evaluation of results becomes more difficult and perplexing.

Interface with Community Support Systems

Community support systems relate to mental health promotion/mental illness prevention objectives in two major ways. First, these support systems have the potential to increase opportunities for maximal personal psychosocial and emotional growth and development. Second, they can function as critical supports for persons and families at times of crisis or stress and thus reduce the likelihood of negative psychological effects.

Increasingly, there is emphasis on shifting attention away from mental illness prevention toward mental health promotion. For example:

> Promoting mental health means enhancing the competencies and well-being of individuals, groups, and communities through the application of multiple person-centered and system change efforts. Whereas traditional clinical interventions are aimed at changing psychological or psychosocial factors in an identified patient or client system, mental health promotion strategies are aimed at: (1) improving the well-being and strengths of normal and at-risk populations through competence-training strategies; and (2) modifying social policies, social systems, and environmental factors which impede the mental health and well-being of groups in the community [Ketterer, Bader, & Levy, 1980, p. 264].

Competence-building programs are one major strategy in mental health promotion. They cover a broad spectrum of activities, ranging from the teaching of social and interpersonal cognitive problem-solving skills, to affective education for school-age children. While such programs generally involve some elements of a teacher–student, expert–trainee relationship, peer learning also usually is critical to the success of such efforts. This "one-student-teaching-another-student" element has many of the characteristics and dynamics of support systems. Similarly, stress management programs (which seek to improve persons' abilities to cope with the pressures in their daily lives) are generally conducted more along the lines of traditional educational programs. Many are work-site based, but some have focused on quite different populations. Tableman (1980, p. 252) describes a stress-reduction program organized specifically for AFDC (welfare) mothers. She asserts that the "support system" characteristics of these classes were an important factor in their success in modifying and improving the coping abilities of the partici-pants. It is reasonable to assume, therefore, that another group of AFDC mothers, coming together for manifestly different purposes, such as improving their children's nutrition, might end up learning from one another stress-management skills very similar to those explicitly focused on in Tableman's formally organized course.

Social isolation and feelings of alienation are generally viewed as fertile ground for the development of emotional disorders. Thus, workers interested in the prevention of mental illness believe it is cru-cial to help people become parts of significant social networks, to be identified with some "community." Encouraging people to utilize nat-ural help networks or deliberately organized mutual-aid groups is the top priority of the recently established Office of Prevention in the Cali-fornia State Department of Mental Hygiene (Roeppel, 1980). In 1980, this newly established office committed a large part of its budget to the development of a mass-media campaign directed at facilitating persons' use of various support systems and at encouraging people to form mu-tual-aid groups.

The objectives of such programs are to "legitimize" for the public the use of social support groups and to alert persons to the fact that reliance on such groups can be particularly helpful at times of loss or other life crises. An increasing number of federally supported commu-nity mental health centers, primarily as part of consultation and educa-tion programs, have sought to support and encourage the development and growth of self-help groups in their communities. Frequently, the groups are organized around shared life events such as bereavement, illness of a child, or marital disruption. In many communities, churches and other religious organizations have also assisted in the development of such self-help groups, especially those for single parents. The public educational campaigns of some mental health organizations (professional as well as citizens') have recently begun to emphasize the role of support networks for individuals' mental health. They may, for example, as in the case of Roeppel's California campaign, stress that people pay atten-tion to the condition of their networks so that they can be sure support will be available when it is urgently needed at times of crisis.

Only recently have mental health professionals begun to realize the important preventive potential of work-site based support networks. The work setting provides a continuing source of potentially significant social relationships second only to the family. An interesting spinoff of women's liberation—and of the increasing number of women in higher-paid jobs—is the greater comfort of many men to turn to co-workers (male as well as female) for support and assistance at times of crisis in their lives. Women have traditionally been more comfortable in using work settings for social support, sharing their feelings and concerns among their co-workers. With the growth of numbers of women managers, this behavior has become acceptable for males as well. In this sense, men have begun to be liberated from the total separation of their world of work from their personal lives. The rise in divorce rates—and the greater willingness to talk with work colleagues about the feelings associated with this often distressing life event—has also broken down some of the past barriers to any personal discussions in the workplace. Labor, management, and employee health and assistance programs can all serve as vehicles for support and encouragement of work-site helping networks.

Another type of mental health promotion/mental illness prevention program focuses on institutional changes. These include efforts to "humanize" (through changes in policies, practices, and personnnel) organizations such as hospitals, day-care centers, homes for the aged, nursing homes, and public housing projects. It is believed that creating less stressful, more humane environments will have a beneficial impact on persons and families significantly affected by these settings. For example, at times mutual-aid groups, i.e., parents of seriously ill children, have undertaken to change hospital policies that they felt were detrimental to the mental health of their sons and daughters. Similarly, parents' organizations have sought to modify practices in the public schools that they considered psychologically unhealthy (including proponents of both more and less sex education!). Finally, to the extent that a better, more equitable society would be a more mentally healthy society, a broad range of mutual-aid self-help groups that have moved into the arena of social action can be viewed as functioning in the mental health promotion/mental illness prevention arena.

Barriers to the Development of Prevention and Community Support System Initiatives

The absence of an adequate knowledge base—derived from research studies—as a major reason for not undertaking preventive programs has already been referred to. This may, however, represent more of an ideological statement than an objective assessment of scientific evidence; that is, some persons deeply committed to clinical approaches present arguments about effectiveness of prevention activities rather than confronting directly their own basic commitment to direct treatment approaches.

A barrier of a different nature is the orientation of most current mental health professionals. Generally, psychiatrists, social workers, psychologists, and psychiatric nurses in the United States are attracted to work in the mental health field because of clinical (patient-care) interests, and it is these aspects that are emphasized in professional training programs. The generally indirect and often delayed evidence of success of preventive or promotion activities contrasts with the direct personal experience of actually helping people that most clinicians have when they are working with patients. In addition, it appears that mental health workers, even more so than other health professionals, have been reluctant to utilize community support systems, to encourage their clients or patients to use such groups. The reason may be that these professionals view social-psychological support as the core of their own specialized skills and thus they are unlikely to acknowledge that others—especially nonprofessionals—also have something of great value to contribute in making people's lives more bearable and satisfactory.

Finally, there are two broader characteristics of contemporary American society which make more difficult the development of prevention and community support system initiatives. First, there is the crisis-oriented nature of American society. This is reflected in our health care system, which places so little emphasis on prevention. For example, most proposed national health insurance plans provide no funds for preventive activities. It is also seen in the reluctance to make short- and long-range planning a central part of social policy determination. Second, there continues to be a separation of the world of action, productivity, and achievement from the world of affect, emotion, and personal experience. The Protestant work ethic can lead to a denial of the importance of feelings, to their suppression. An apparently permanent impact of the 1960s has been a greater valuation of this side of men's and women's natures. Women's and men's liberation movements are also playing an important part in breaking down some of these past barriers. However, the widespread continuing separation of these two aspects of human nature makes the wider development and utilization of community support systems as means to prevent mental illness and promote mental health more difficult.

Some Issues for the Future

Community support systems clearly can play an important role in preventive mental health programs. One of the challenges for the future is how to utilize these support systems maximally and how to strengthen them and increase their availability to and use by those persons who need them.

While most attention—in both physical and mental health areas—has been directed at groups focusing on particular illnesses or "life conditions," the greatest mental health potential may rest with those neighborhood (or community) support groups that are of a more "generic" nature, that is, that are available to assist persons through a variety of life crises. What kinds of deliberate efforts by existing organizations or institutions can be most effective in building such broad-based support groups?

Historically, many religious groups have sought to provide this kind of support for their membership. Recently, a number of church groups have begun to make conscious efforts to encourage the growth of mutual-aid self-help groups among their members. In the past, much of this "support" role of the church has focused on the personal relationship to the priest, minister, or rabbi. How can such religious, organization-based efforts be strengthened and expanded? Perhaps local mental health programs (through the efforts of either professional staff or citizens) can encourage and assist churches and synagogues to move in this direction.

What are appropriate roles for various human services (including health/medical care, mental health, and social service) organizations in supporting the role of mutual-aid self-help groups as an important component of a community's preventive mental health activities? A number of authors (for example, Gartner & Riessman, 1977; Silverman, 1978) have emphasized the danger of professionals or professionally dominated agencies "taking over" or co-opting mutual-aid groups. Key roles of these formal structures may lie in advice-giving to leaders as groups are being organized—particularly in relation to administrative and organizational matters and the direct provision of "services" such as meeting space, phone answering service, or duplicating facilities.

While youth-run alternate services, such as "hot lines," have become an important type of mutual-aid system in many communities, there appear to have been few deliberate efforts within the structure of the public educational system to develop support groups among children themselves. Classroom groups or subgroups appear to contain within them remarkable potential for providing the kind of psychological-social assistance that is at the heart of self-help systems. Few teachers are aware of this potential, are comfortable in these roles, or are supported by their structures to utilize their classroom groups in this way.

Probably the most untapped locus—and one presenting major resistances—is the work setting. The emphasis on dealing with affective (social-emotional) types of problem-solving is alien to virtually all work settings. The emphasis "at work" generally is on production and efficiency. Despite evidence of considerable sharing of concerns among co-workers, some types of personal problems are unlikely to be discussed with fellow workers. This is particularly the case, of course, among men—and the world of work continues to be dominated by men. The recently increasing interest in reducing stress at the workplace may provide an opening for the further development of support systems (formal or informal) in this setting. As some of the barriers between familial worlds and work worlds begin to break down (flex-time, work-based child-care centers, increased opportunities for part-time work, etc.), this may also encourage the development of social support groups in the work-site.

As has been mentioned previously, there are two major mental health impacts of community support groups. The first involves assisting persons to cope more effectively with crises, with difficult life events, and with continuing problems (chronic conditions or illnesses). The second involves changing or modifying social systems or institutions, making them more "humane." Most continuing social support groups have been in the first category and there may be some intrinsic conflict between helping people to cope better with the stresses in their lives and organizing people for social action to change a school system, a medical care system, a social welfare agency, the administration of a public housing project, or the like. Support groups help people to be less dependent on medical and other technically skilled professional specialists. They help persons to take more responsibility for their own health (physical and mental) and welfare. However, there is some danger that such an emphasis on "individual responsibility" will be accompanied by less attention to societal and institutional factors that can have major impact on persons' mental health. Ryan (1971) refers to this essentially conservative characteristic of self-help groups as "blaming the victim."

The full potential of community support systems as a major element of preventive mental health work remains unexplored. This will continue to be the case as long as professional training in the mental health disciplines emphasizes clinical work and promotes the notion that mental health specialists are experts who "prescribe" to patients. As the United States gradually moves toward some form of national health insurance, care will be needed to ensure that barriers are not created to block the further growth of the social support system movement. Fortunately, the medical care field is increasingly interested in the social and behavioral components of health. The accompanying emphasis on modifying life-styles as a preventive approach is likely to be accompanied by an increasing realization of the potential contribution of community support systems. We can only hope that the mental health field will move along similar lines.

7

Self-help and Mutual-support Groups: A Synthesis of the Recent Literature

David Spiegel

Depending on the eye of the beholder, the term *self-help* may conjure up an image of sturdy Jacksonian self-reliance or antiprofessional amateurism, of pulling oneself up by one's bootstraps or religiously oriented zealotry, of mobilization of community support or professional neglect. There is a growing and generally sympathetic, if not entirely systematic, professional literature regarding the ever-expanding self-help movement. Recent interest in this area has been sparked by the development of the community mental health movement in the United States with its sobering attempt to provide population-oriented mental health care. Self-help is a natural component of the social-psychological perspective, which emphasizes the importance of the social milieu in influencing an individual's psychological state. Some anthropologists speculate that the family itself is the primordial model of a self-help group and that incest taboos themselves were established as a way of expanding, through marriage, networks of mutual support for physical protection from other families. Many now formidable social, political, and economic organizations had modest beginnings as mutual-support organizations, dedicated to improving the lot of their members with common problems (Tax, 1976)—for example, many labor unions, and the International Harvester Corporation, which began as a utopian farming cooperative.

Clearly, however, the term *self-help* can be overapplied to the point

The author gratefully acknowledges the assistance of Marie Killilea in planning and reviewing the manuscript and of Dyhanne Warner, Ph.D., and Phillip Berghausen, Ph.D., in assisting in the literature search.

of meaninglessness, and for the purposes of this review, self-help and mutual support groups comprise those voluntary associations of individuals with a common problem, stigma, or life situation which involves no professional control, although there may be professional involvement of a consultative kind, and in which there is no financial profit. Such groups usually engage in a combination of mutual help to members and to the public and political activity.

This chapter presents a review and synthesis of the burgeoning recent literature on self-help and mutual-support groups. Such an examination is timely because of both the growth of self-help as a more recognized and accepted phenomenon in our society and evidence provided by recent research of the importance of self-help in health and mental health service delivery. The chapter will highlight previous reviews, discuss self-help in a historical context, relate self-help to deviance theory, analyze relationships between self-help groups and professionals, examine typologies of self-help groups, explore recent approaches to research, and then focus specifically on the role of self-help groups in mental health problems and life transitions. The role of self-help groups with medical care, though an important issue, is beyond the scope of this chapter and will not be reviewed.

One important issue to be examined in this review is the balance of cooperation versus competition between various professional support systems in the health and mental health areas and self-help groups. While many professionals remain skeptical about the efficacy of self-help approaches, much support on a theoretical basis has come from professional circles. For example, the effectiveness of milieu and therapeutic community approaches within psychiatry (Moline, 1977) lends credence to the idea that a thoughtfully structured association of individuals with common problems can provide genuine mutual help, given certain very real limitations.

There is growing interest on the part of the federal government in self-help groups. A section of the recent report of the President's Commission on Mental Health (1978b) was devoted to community support systems in general and self-help groups in particular. The report cites an estimate that there exist more than half a million self-help groups, noting, for example, that Alcoholics Anonymous has a worldwide membership in excess of 750,000 and that the National Association for Retarded Citizens has more than 1,300 local units with a membership of more than 130,000. Also, Gussow and Tracy (1976) have observed that there is a self-help group for nearly every major disease listed by the World Health Organization. The Mental Health Commission's report concludes with recommendations that community mental health centers should provide information about available mutual-help groups; that clearing houses on mutual-help groups be assembled by region to facilitate communication among self-help groups and with professionals; and that training on community support systems and mutual-help groups be included in all training programs in the social, behavioral, educational, and medical sciences. In addition, the report recommends that federal financial support be available through state mental health associations to develop further peer-oriented supportive networks and to improve referral to existing networks and that a national conference of volunteer programs in the health, mental health, educational, and social welfare areas be convened to improve relationships among natural and professional support systems.

Previous Reviews

Killilea (1976) provides a clear historical and theoretical review of mutual-help groups. She develops the concept of the support system as articulated by Caplan (1974, 1976b): those attachments which improve adaptive competence at times of life stress. Self-help groups are analyzed in the framework of a social movement that represents attempts by various constituencies to provide an acceptable cognitive structure for their problem and their relationship to broader society. In addition, such social forces as a search for spiritual guidelines in a fundamentally secular society, an expression of the democratic ideal via consumer participation in health care delivery, a shift in the economic structure of the society from the industrial revolution to the service revolution, and a modification of folk healing systems in contrast to professional health care systems all provide an important impetus for the self-help movement.

Killilea notes that self-help groups provide community settings that span a broad spectrum with respect to intensity and duration of involvement. These range from total institutions (Goffman, 1961) of the Synanon type, to subculture organizations such as Alcoholics Anonymous, to supplementary communities such as Parents Without Partners, to life-transition communities such as ex-patient organizations. Another distinguishing issue among self-help groups is their approach to the definition of deviance (Katz & Bender, 1976a). Self-help organizations range from groups like Alcoholics Anonymous, which have provided mutual support for those who accept a deviant label, to those like the homophile and gay rights groups which have successfully fought in the political arena to have the label "homosexual" removed from the American Psychiatric

Association's list of psychiatric diagnoses. The therapeutic effectiveness of self-help is variously attributed to communality of experience, mutual support, receiving help through giving it—the helper-therapy principle (Riessman, 1965)—differential association, collective willpower, sharing of information, and constructive activity toward agreed-upon goals. Self-help groups are contrasted with traditional psychotherapy according to the relative importance of insight, the role of finances, the importance of treating symptoms versus understanding causes, and the role of a judgmental attitude about behavior.

Killilea calls for more systematic exploration of the use and usefulness of self-help groups, historical patterns in the development of such groups, the role of professionals in them, and referral patterns among mutual-aid organizations and between them and formal delivery systems. As of now, this call has been only partially heeded. Descriptions of self-help groups abound—with literally hundreds of articles—and some specific historical questions have been addressed. Several descriptive reports of the importance of professional noncontrol and the relationship with professionals have been provided. However, little has been done regarding referral patterns. Several studies have attempted to address the difficult issue of effectiveness (Bailey, 1965; Wagonfield & Wolowitz, 1968; Stunkard, Levine, & Fox, 1970; Stunkard, 1972; McCall, 1973, 1974; Garb & Stunkard, 1974; Levitz & Stunkard, 1974; Lieberman & Bond, 1976, 1978; Hughes, 1977; McCall, Siderits, & Fadden, 1977; Henry & Robinson, 1978; Lieberman & Borman, 1979).

Gartner and Riessman (1977) provide an excellent survey of the self-help movement, notable especially for its dialectical analysis of the role of self-help within the broader political context and for its useful directory of self-help groups. They emphasize the "consumer-intensive" aspects of self-help, in which increased use is made of the active and informed participation of consumers as contrasted with that in professional caregiving systems. They note that this fact creates conflicting possibilities: on the one hand, more informed consumers come to demand more responsive professional services; on the other hand, those who provide better for their own needs may receive even less attention from formal service delivery systems. The authors' dialectical approach is particularly useful here—both can occur, and they argue against disengagement from the struggle with service bureaucracies despite the risks involved in developing a potentially adversarial relationship.

The political context of self-help groups noted by Gartner and Riessman above was discussed by Riessman in an important earlier work in which he asserted the capacity of self-help groups to be sources of community empowerment. He states:

The power of self-help mutual aid groups derives from the fact that they combine a number of very important properties: These include the helper-therapy principle, the aprofessional dimension, consumer intensivity [*sic*], the use of indigenous or peer support, and the implicit demand that the individual can do something for him or herself. . . . In essence, one of the most significant characteristics of mutual aid groups is the fact that they are *empowering* and thus potentially delineating. They enable their members to feel and use their own strengths and their own power and to have control over their own lives [Riessman, 1965, pp. 98–99].

New Historical Perspectives: Profession versus Confession

Recent authors trace the roots of self-help back through the centuries. Back and Taylor (1976) begin with St. Ignatius of Loyola, describing his progression through a personal medical crisis to the establishment of a mutual-support group, the Jesuit Order, which became a social move-ment as part of the Counterreformation. Interestingly, this order was a forerunner of various kinds of professionalism and has traditionally placed a great emphasis on formal training and academic values.

Hurvitz (1976) starts after the Reformation, noting that the word *religion* derives from the Latin root *ligare* ("to tie") and that many early religious practices involved public group confession. A number of Pro-testant groups emerged emphasizing the importance of group confession as a prerequisite for change. One of these, the Oxford Group, while too exclusive to include alcoholics, became a model for Alcoholics Anony-mous. As other authors have done (Dumont, 1974; Killilea, 1976), Hur-vitz ties the self-help movement to a synthesis of the Judeo-Christian heritage with American pragmatism and social conscience. Personal change or growth is tested in fact, not in theory, by self-help groups. The current self-help movement is related to the secular unions and friendly societies of the late eighteenth and early nineteenth centuries in England by Katz and Bender (1976a,b). These guild and union relation-ships were formed to establish standards of work and pay and to provide support for members who became ill or died. They were related to such working-class support systems in the United States as the Pan-Hellenic Union and the Polish National Alliance.

A personal crisis resulted in Clifford Beers' *A Mind That Found Itself* (1948) and the eventual founding of the Mental Health Association (Back & Taylor, 1976). It is interesting to note that William James, the most prominent psychologist of his day, and Adolf Meyer, the most prominent psychiatrist, both provided endorsements for Beers' book.

The pattern of one individual going through a personal, physical or spiritual crisis, then making a public declaration of his crisis and its resolution, and gathering around him a group of followers, is a common one, from the time of St. Ignatius to the era of Clifford Beers. American mutual-support customs such as barn raisings and volunteer fire brigades have been described as forerunners of self-help (Tax, 1976). More recently, the self-help movement has been extolled as fulfilling part of the democratic ideal and as being anti-authoritarian (Vattano, 1972; Dumont, 1974; Steinman & Traunstein, 1976).

Deviance Theory and Self-help

The problem of deviance is hardly confined to the self-help movement and yet is quite relevant to it. Most groups insist on having deviants and create them should none volunteer (Dentler & Erickson, 1959). The tremendous social burden of bearing a deviant label is eloquently described by Goffman (1974). Some authors maintain that deviance redefinition is the primary work of self-help groups. Steinman and Traunstein (1976) argue that self-help groups are the response of the disadvantaged to labeling and control by professional bureaucrats. Shatan (1973) considers political activism inseparable from the self-help process, a position supported by other authors (Wittenberg, 1948; Alinsky, 1967; Katz & Bender, 1976b; Smith, 1976). Others state that rather than redefining deviance, self-help groups emerge after the common problem or stigma has been somewhat "detoxified" (Lieberman & Borman, 1976).

There seems to be agreement that at the least, self-help groups may provide disadvantaged people with clearer access to a caregiving system than the somewhat distant and abstruse professional system (Tyler, 1976). Formal caregiving networks can be rigid and by their absence of responsiveness may stimulate the growth of alternative grass roots organizations (Borman, 1975; Tracy & Gussow, 1976). Piven and Cloward (1976) suggest that the formal welfare system itself is largely responsible for the development of the National Welfare Rights Organization, which vigorously challenges it. It is interesting to note that Recovery, Inc., a self-help group for psychiatric patients well-described by Wechsler (1960a,b, 1976) and Lee (1976), developed during a time when psychoanalysis was at its zenith in the United States. The psychoanalytic emphasis on insight before action was countered by Recovery's emphasis on changing behavior and dealing with symptoms rather than causes.

Self-help groups at the least provide a small supportive community for the sharing of an attribute that is stigmatized in the broader community. Step by step, the self-help member can "go public" with his stigma, first privately with a relatively supportive group from which he later derives courage for public revelation often leading to public action (Spiegel, 1976).

Relationships with Professionals

The common expectation of conflict between professionals and self-help groups is only rarely confirmed. More often, despite areas of disagreement, professionals and self-help groups are publicly quite supportive of one another. Lieberman and Borman (1979) support this argument in a recent book based upon studies of a variety of self-help groups. The authors conclude:

> Self-help groups are often erroneously believed to be anti-professional. The findings reported in this volume indicate not only that seasoned professionals have been involved in the founding and support of more self-help groups but also that most participants utilize professional help to a greater extent than do non-members of self-help groups and, in a number of cases (CR groups, NAIM, & Mended Hearts), indicate fairly high satisfaction in their experience with professionals [Lieberman & Borman, 1979, p. 407].

Exceptions often involve some inevitable criticism of the way professionals work (Borman, 1975). For example, in the "big book" of AA, the organization's manual for members, instances are cited of a professional's not being able to meet the needs of a patient who was subsequently helped by AA (Alcoholics Anonymous, 1955, pp. 18, 26, 400).

Some writers are outspokenly antiprofessional (Hurvitz, 1970; Steinman & Traunstein, 1976). They note the lack of consumer control over professional service delivery. Further, they observe that while a severe symptom may be merely troublesome to a professional, it constitutes a challenge and an opportunity for evidence of dramatic change by self-help groups. While this is something of an artificial distinction, Hurvitz makes an interesting point in stating that a new member of a self-help group is encouraged by being likely to encounter successful converts, as the unsuccessful usually drop out.

As a rule, self-help and mutual-support groups seem to flourish in areas which are of lesser interest to professionals or which involve large numbers of clients who lack access to professionals (Tracy & Gussow, 1976). A classic example is the development of the Ostomy Clubs, which work quite effectively with an aspect of post-surgical care that had often been neglected by health professionals in the past. Conflict does emerge when professionals attempt to maintain or establish control of a self-help operation (Kleinman, Mantell, & Alexander, 1976).

While advocating greater cooperation between professionals and self-help groups, Durman (1976) contrasts their differing approaches as "problemizing vs. normalizing needs" (p. 436). The former creates the expectation that intensive and extensive intervention is necessary. Nuttal, Nuttal, Polit, and Clark (1977) points out that the availability of self-help groups adds to the total array of services and makes it more likely that an intervention can be found that is appropriate to the severity of the helpees' situation rather than meeting the needs or interests of the helper.

Katz (1965, 1970, 1972) observes that there is far better integration of self-help concepts and volunteer principles in European social service systems than in America. He relates this to the tradition of the "friendly societies" in Great Britain and in various trade union medical programs, which were forerunners of national health services. He is critical of professional isolationism in social work, but at the same time notes that many self-help groups become professionalized as they grow. He argues that the upper-class tradition of volunteering for social service in this country might well be expanded to include self-help volunteers from all social groups.

Spiegel (1977) analyzes the usefulness of professionals as consultants to self-help groups. Professionals as consultants can share expertise and encouragement, which are often critical in the early development of a self-help group. The professionals do not share power or control over the direction of the organization, however, and this is an unaccustomed role for many. Such a supportive consultative relationship is described in the development of a group working toward the prevention of burn injuries. The group used consultation in development and obtaining foundation support and is currently quite effective in education and legislation regarding burn prevention. Public professional support is not lacking for self-help groups, as evidenced by a conference report in a major community psychiatry journal (Huey, 1977a), which cites a number of prominent professionals offering unequivocal support for the effectiveness and importance of the self-help approach. Other authors encourage professionals to make more use of the self-help concept (Powell, 1973).

Adler and Hammett (1973) incorporate psychotherapy and psychoanalysis within the framework of self-help. They note that any social contact may have a therapeutic effect, given the pervasiveness of the placebo effect and of social structure in human life. They describe the self-help group as a manageable model of the socialization process with healing aspects. In their social model of psychological dysfunction, they present three stages: crisis, a period of social disruption; conversion, the introduction into a new social system; and cult formation, in which a new hierarchy and ideology are cemented. They include the therapeutic community and even psychoanalysis within this self-help model, arguing that what may be of therapeutic importance in psychoanalysis is the gradual integration of the patient into an alternative social structure with a rather elaborate and well-defined ideology.

In an interesting contribution to the literature on the imparting of meaning to a stigmatized experience or attribute, Borkman (1976) discusses the role of experiential knowledge in self-help groups as contrasted with professional knowledge. Both types of knowing are ontologically equal, coexisting as religious truth does with the scientific variety. She distinguishes experiential knowledge as being pragmatic rather than theoretical; oriented in the here and now and holistic rather than segmented. Thus, possession of it confers a status of equality. For example, the experience of being an alcoholic in AA confers a similar kind of equality on its members as the collegial relationship does among professionals. This approach is particularly useful in clarifying the fact that these two types of knowledge can be useful and valid in appropriate contexts, and while they may be in conflict, they need not be.

Opportunities for various types of collaboration between professionals and self-help groups abound. As an example, Yalom and colleagues (1978), in a systematic study of group psychotherapy with alcoholics, noted that AA was clearly a partner, not an adversary:

> From the outset, we viewed the therapy groups for alcoholics as complementary, not antagonistic, to AA. Many of the patients derived considerable support from concurrent AA membership; indeed, we very much doubt whether several patients could have maintained sobriety without AA support. When AA and psychotherapy seemed to be working at cross purposes we learned that invariably the patient at these times used AA as a form of resistance. Patients working well in therapy soon learned how to draw strength from each mode of help available to them [Yalom et al., 1978, p. 425].

Typologies of Self-help Groups

New attempts to categorize self-help groups constitute variations on the theme of mutual support versus political activism (Katz & Bender, 1976a). This distinction has been well-described by Tracy and Gussow (1976), who divide health focused self-help groups into Type I and Type II groups. Type I groups provide direct services to patients and relatives, including education, coping skills, and peer support in helping individuals deal with medical problems. Examples of Type I organizations include Emphysema Anonymous, United Ostomy Club, AA, and Overeaters Anonymous. Type II groups, on the other hand, focus not on specific individuals with medical problems but instead on the class of individuals afflicted with particular medical problems. Activities include emphasis on promoting biomedical research, public education, fund raising, and lobbying activities. Examples of Type II organizations include the National Heart Association and the American Diabetes Association.

Individual members of groups and self-help groups themselves have been noted to progress from a stance of secrecy regarding a stigmatized attribute to broader public and political involvement (Spiegel, 1976). As another example, the Center for Independent Living in Berkeley, a self-help program for physically handicapped individuals with federal, state, and private funding, is described as having undergone dramatic development from individual mutual support to political and social action (Kirshbaum, Harveston, & Katz, 1976). CIL members in wheelchairs have blockaded streets to support their demand for adequate public transportation for the handicapped, and a former CIL director with a serious physical handicap has served as director of rehabilitation for the State of California. There is similar activism among the geriatric population (Beverly, 1976; Taietz, 1976; Anderson & Anderson, 1978). On the other hand, this transition from mutual support to political involvement may not always be smooth, and tensions may arise over conflicting goals (Davis, 1977).

This bipartite distinction is also employed by Jacques and Patterson (1974), who divide self-help groups into those which focus on coping, largely consisting of individuals with problems, and those which focus on social advocacy, often composed of family and friends of individuals with given problems. They emphasize the fact that status is defined from within, based on common problems and behavior, rather than from outside the group, and that any individual who attempts to import his status from the outside society into the group is likely to meet with considerable difficulty.

Durman (1976) proposes a tripartite typology based on the relationship between the self-help group and public funding. The first type consists of groups like AA, which work in an area that already has attracted public interest and funding. The second type consists of groups in areas of potential but not current interest to the public sector, for example, food cooperatives. The third type, typified by Parents Without Partners, contains those groups which work in areas of little real or potential interest to public agencies. He thus deemphasizes the importance of the mutual-help versus public-activity distinction.

Others (Levy, 1976; Katz & Bender, 1976a), by contrast, focus on the kind of problem addressed and present a four-part typology. In Levy's first type, the focus is on behavioral control and the paradigm is Alcoholics Anonymous. His second type of self-help group involves itself with a stressful predicament or life problem, an example being Parents Without Partners. Those groups which concern themselves with problems of survival are the third type, examples being consciousness raising and gay pride groups. The last type involves personal growth, for example "integrity" groups and the sensitivity-training movement. For the first two types in Levy's scheme, Katz and Bender substitute social advocacy and "outcast haven" groups. The difficulty in classifying such groups is compounded by Levy's observation that there is wide variability among the meetings of the same group, which is not surprising given the observation of others (Dumont, 1974; Steinman & Traunstein, 1976) that there is an anti-bureaucratic and unregimented quality that is especially important to the nature of self-help groups.

In a particularly interesting article, Antze (1976) proposes that there is an important relationship between the cluster of symptoms addressed by a self-help group and the structure and ideology of the group. In this sense the variety of self-help groups provides a kind of natural laboratory for testing ideologies that may be specifically helpful to individuals with common characteristics or problems. He emphasizes the importance of self-help groups in providing support to maintain a conversion, adding that the process of persuading others about a conversion can be a powerful means of persuading oneself. This is consistent with Festinger's observation (1957) that individuals faced with a logical incongruity may support their belief and their particular solution to the problem by actively recruiting others to their belief. Using an approach reminiscent of the structural anthropologist, he contrasts the ideology of Alcoholics Anonymous with that of Recovery, Inc. The emphasis on submission to a higher power and on one's allergy to alcohol which characterizes AA is described as countering the grandiosity and false sense of control over drinking typical of many alcoholics. Bean's thorough study of AA supports this observation (1975a,b). She notes that the atmosphere of interest in the public statement by members of having "hit bottom" is particularly encouraging to the chronically self-deprecating alcoholic. Recovery, Inc., on the other hand, emphasizes the importance of willpower and choice, which is an antidote to the enforced passivity and neurotic helplessness that characterize many of Recovery's members. Synanon's practice of gaming, which stimulates intense emotional reaction, and the emphasis on performing concrete tasks within the community confront the addict's common tendency to distance himself from emotions and responsibility for behavior. This approach would seem to be a fertile one for future exploration and classification of self-help groups, and it may provide clues to professional caregivers as well.

New Approaches to Research

Despite the previously noted call for more systematic research in the area of self-help (Killilea, 1976), there have been few scientific research studies of self-help in comparison with the large variety of descriptive reports. There have been, however, a number of studies of self-help groups devoted to the treatment of obesity. Particularly notable has been the work of Stunkard and his colleagues in studying TOPS (Take Off Pounds Sensibly). This problem lends itself to objective research since outcome can be measured quickly and easily: the number of pounds lost. Wagonfield and Wolowitz (1968) noted that less than 1 percent of TOPS members they studied had consulted any mental health resource, suggesting that this group does not attract individuals who would otherwise seek psychiatric help. They found a large dropout rate at the beginning, nearly 50 percent of new members leaving within the first six months. A later study of TOPS by Garb and Stunkard (1974) demonstrated a greater dropout rate in chapters where the weight loss was the least, while confirming the earlier finding with dropout rates of 47 percent at one year and 70 percent at two. They demonstrated that membership in the organization consisted of a relatively small group of long-term members and a much larger group of newly enlisted members, and that the chapters with the highest dropout rates were also the most active in recruiting new members. They found a strong association between a greater degree of overweight and longer membership and also found that those members who lost the most weight tended to stay longer. They were unable, however, to answer the question of cause and effect in this association.

They also found considerable variation among the TOPS chapters in terms of effectiveness. Earlier reports by Stunkard and his group (Stunkard et al., 1970; Stunkard, 1972) were quite enthusiastic and reported that weight loss in TOPS groups was at least comparable to, and in some instances better than, that in various professionally run weight-loss groups. Later papers were more temperate (Garb & Stunkard, 1974; Levitz & Stunkard, 1974), reporting that professionals utilizing behavior modification techniques were more effective in producing weight loss than TOPS groups. They also reported that the implementation of behavior modification principles by TOPS leaders enhanced their effectiveness and reduced dropout rates. In this study, unlike previous studies, they reported that TOPS members gained weight rather than losing. They recommended that the self-help group be used as a screening device for selecting the most appropriate candidates for professional behavior modification approaches.

In a study of TOPS utilizing MMPI measures, McCall (1973, 1974) reported MMPI differences between weight losers and nonlosers and "normalization" of MMPI profiles after sixteen weeks of group treatment. Using interactional observations of TOPS, McCall and colleagues (1977) studied differences between relatively successful and unsuccessful TOPS chapters. They found that such interpersonal and attitudinal variables as emotional concern and enthusiasm were related to relative success, whereas content and procedure were less important. Their data emphasize the importance of the leader as a role model and of the leader's sympathetic concern with the group. The members' attitude toward the TOPS program was also positively related to weight loss. This process/content distinction is an important one in psychotherapy outcome research (Strupp, 1973) and so is a likely candidate for importance in self-help groups as well. Such observations conflict with Antze's speculations (1976) that it is the structure and ideology of the group that are uniquely important, although the data are insufficiently precise to eliminate the possibility that both factors are important. In addition, Wagonfield and Wolowitz (1968) observed the sanctioning of a considerable amount of verbal aggression in TOPS groups, and they speculated that this may be significant in the work of groups of individuals dealing with oral conflicts.

A survey questionnaire approach is employed by Cutler (1976) in gerontological research. He relates a self-report of satisfaction with life and participation in a variety of voluntary associations, including fraternal groups, service clubs, veterans groups, discussion groups, professional societies, church-affiliated groups, and other groups. Presumably, self-help groups were included in this survey sample among 438 individuals over age sixty-five, although no specific mention is made. The study is included to point out that group association goes considerably beyond self-help, and a number of factors in social group membership may be of importance. Cutler found that only membership in church-affiliated groups was associated with psychological well-being. He speculates that religious organizations frequently sponsor special programs for the elderly and, thus, the religious groups may consist of individuals with more similar and age-related problems and interests, a finding certainly consistent with the theme of commonality and identification which permeates the self-help literature. This speculation is supported by Trela's finding (1976) of a positive relationship between social class and membership in age-graded associations.

Using the well-standardized Profile of Mood States Scale, Hughes (1977) performed a study of the adolescent children of drinking parents, controlled for membership in Alateen. He found that Alateen members suffered less emotional and social disturbance than peers who did not belong to the group. Bailey (1965) also notes that there is a relationship, although not necessarily a causal one, between a spouse's membership in Al-Anon (1975) and the probability of a husband's joining AA. Members of Al-Anon were more inclined to view alcoholism as a combined physical and mental illness, as opposed to nonmembers, who viewed it as just a psychological problem. This study indicates that the ideology of the self-help group is clearly absorbed and believed by the members.

In an excellent article, Henry and Robinson (1978) summarize a recent national survey in England of Alcoholics Anonymous. They emphasize the importance of active involvement and not merely attendance at meetings and cite some extremely useful statistics. They note that members attended an average of 2.1 meetings per week and that 60 percent of those who had been members for more than ten years still attended more than one meeting a week. Less than 2 percent had never talked at a meeting and almost two-thirds spoke regularly about their experiences. They found that half the membership had sponsored a newer member, and that over time sponsoring someone was associated with a decreased likelihood of dropping out of AA. More than one-third of members met informally in social activities, and three-quarters of the members surveyed reported having made new friends in AA, while less than one-third reported continuing to see the majority of friends they had had before they joined AA. These data support the idea that AA helps its members find new social networks that are supportive of new behavior.

Further research with self-help in the health area was conducted by Lieberman, Borman, and associates over a number of years. In a recently edited book (Lieberman & Borman, 1979), they report the results of their research concerning how self-help groups are started and structured, who participates, how self-help groups work, and the degree of success of these groups in meeting their goals. Among their general conclusions based upon this significant body of research is the fact that while their studies show that in specific ways self-help groups can provide important benefits to specific members, there is little evidence of harm done to individuals as a result of self-help group participation. Thus self-help is "safer" than psychotherapy and encounter groups, according to the authors. They see self-help groups along with professional assistance as part of a continuum of mixed care and not as a replacement for society's responsibility to those in need.

Often the perceived needs of the community in mental health terms differ among professional and community groups. In a study of adolescent mental health needs, Nuttal and co-workers (1977) discovered that community members rated alcohol abuse and employment counseling as being the primary needs, whereas mental health officials emphasized serious emotional problems and school disturbances as being of primary importance. Their observation is that professionals tend to rate as most important those problems with which they are trained to cope. This disjunction among perceived needs reinforces the idea that self-help groups can provide a means of communication by which the community makes clear its determination to seek further help with problems not addressed by professionals.

Some authors are skeptical of using client satisfaction regarding the target complaint as an outcome measurement (Lieberman & Bond, 1978). In an extensive questionnaire study, they found that as compared to controls entering group psychotherapy, members of consciousness-raising groups had differences in goals regarding internal feeling states that could not be accounted for by more objective data regarding differences between these two populations (Lieberman & Bond, 1976). They also found a lack of change in such symptoms as anxiety and depression, and argue that the differences in goals among seekers of self-help approaches versus seekers of traditional psychotherapy approaches are not great enough to justify using goals as a criterion. They recommend the utilization of data beyond even systematic questionnairies administered to participants regarding their subjective change or satisfaction. In particular, they express interest in measures of social role performance relevant to the self-help group involved and the ideology of that group. They cite as an example data that marital stress and strain and less adequate coping strategies were associated with participation in consciousness-raising groups. Unfortunately, few self-help groups provide us with the opportunity for the simplicity of evaluation of those which deal with obesity. Given the social nature of the self-help process, social variables such as role functioning will add richness to the pool of outcome data, although given the democratic and anti-authoritarian spirit of many self-help groups, richness would be lost if client satisfaction were overlooked.

Self-help and Mental Health Problems

In the realm of identified mental illness, the relationship between the self-help movement and professional caregivers is especially problematic. The two approaches are often conceived of as competitive, and professional mental health interventions are inherently expansive (Dinitz & Beran, 1971), which can create territorial conflict.

Wechsler's early and important work in describing various expatient organizations (1960a,b, 1976) deserves mention. He described a variety of professionally run and independent aftercare organizations for psychiatric patients and noted their slow growth in comparison to the membership of AA. He was particularly intrigued by Recovery, Inc., a self-help group founded by a psychiatrist, the late Abraham Low, in 1937. Wechsler observed that the method seems to work, in part, by ordering the members' psychological structure and thereby reducing anxiety. He emphasizes the importance of confession in a sheltered social environment. In an unusually balanced discussion, he notes that there are obvious rigidities in the Recovery method and that it may foster regression and an absence of psychological insight. Nonetheless, he sees the organization as being supportive and available to a group often deprived of social resources. Recovery meetings have been incorporated into the inpatient program of at least one state psychiatric hospital (Lee, 1976) and were reportedly quite helpful, although the median number of meetings attended by a patient was two, with only 37.1 percent attending three or more times.

The connection between the development of a more recent self-help organization, Integrity Groups, and dissaffection with traditional psychiatry is explicit. Mowrer (Mowrer & Vattano, 1976) describes his disaffection with psychoanalysis on the one hand, and the profound positive influence of Harry Stack Sullivan on the other, with developing his interest in interpersonal process as starting points for his development of Integrity Groups. His focus is on interpersonal directness and honesty, the hallmark being "honesty, responsibility, and mutual concern and involvement." Leadership is shared among the group members and the groups focus on encouraging honesty and honoring commitments. The success of such groups is described by Madison (1972), who emphasizes the importance of developing and maintaining a group culture in the face of expansion, a problem for many self-help groups.

In a study of 1,700 women members of consciousness-raising groups (Lieberman & Bond, 1976; Bond & Lieberman, 1979), the authors report that while interest in women's issues was the reason most often

stated for joining such a group, seeking help and the desire to fulfill
social needs were the next two most frequently cited factors in the
decision to join, ahead of political motivation or the desire to explore
sexual awareness. Many of the members had had previous therapy experiences and viewed their consciousness raising as an addition rather
than an alternative to therapy. Interestingly, they found that the most
significant processes resulting in help were group sharing of common
problems, feelings and fears, sense of involvement, and risk-taking
about secrets. The development of insight and role analysis were considerably less important. Members were at least equally inclined to discuss
their own problems in dealing with society as they were to discuss
society's problem in dealing with them, and mutual support rather than
shared politics seemed to be the major operating factor. On the other
hand, several descriptive articles emphasize the importance of political
content in women's groups (Norman, 1976; Davis, 1977). There are
other reports in the literature of self-help approaches to a variety of
psychiatric problems (Weiss & Bergen, 1968), including social withdrawal (Takahashi, 1975) agoraphobia (Hardy, 1976), life upset (Silverman & Murrow, 1976), former drug abuse (Brown, 1971), and child
abuse (Bandoli, 1977).

It is worth noting that there is considerable overlap between the
factors helpful in various kinds of self-help psychotherapy groups and
those described as being useful in more traditional psychotherapy.
Yalom (1975) lists factors in the curative process of group therapy as the
installation of hope, universality, imparting of information, altruism, a
corrective recapitulation of the primary family group, a development of
socializing techniques, imitative behavior, interpersonal learning, group
cohesiveness, catharsis, and existential factors. All of these factors with
the possible exception of a corrective recapitulation of the primary
family group have been mentioned in the self-help literature as being
useful (Katz, 1965; Killilea, 1976; Back & Taylor, 1976; Levy, 1976;
Lieberman & Borman, 1976). Clearly, a combination of inspiration,
learning, helping, and a sense of community are critical to the functioning of a variety of self-help groups as well as psychotherapy groups. As
mentioned earlier, the interaction between self-help groups and mental
health professionals has been a problematic area. At best, competition is
described or predicted at least as often as cooperation. Dean argues that
a group such as Recovery, Inc., is "not a substitute for psychiatry, but a
self directed program that may be used to supplement psychiatry, or
alone in certain cases where psychiatric treatment is not available or
mandatory" (Dean, 1971, p. 75). He notes that Recovery can be a useful
aftercare device for discharged psychiatric patients. On the other hand,

some formal mental health systems have attempted to incorporate self-help principles (Hallowitz & Riessman, 1967; Spiegel & Keith-Spiegel, 1973) into their services.

Self-help and the
Task of Transition

Hirschowitz defines the task of transition as "detachment from a former role and the structuring of roles appropriate to a new situation" (Hirschowitz, 1976, p. 1972). Recent attention in the popular and professional literature has underscored the fact that such a process is a normal concomitant of human development. Should help be required for every individual going through a life transition, it becomes obvious that mental health professionals, even were they the best to handle such transitions, would not be able to take on the task. A variety of self-help groups have emerged which concern themselves with life transition from birth—the La Leche League helping new mothers learn to nurse—to death—the Widow to Widow program, which helps women deal with losses.

Silverman and Murrow (1976) describe the role transition help offered nursing mothers by the La Leche League, an organization with more than a thousand groups, each consisting of ten to thirty mothers. They note that the League helps mothers who feel guilty about their ambivalence toward their new baby and members feel that they can be more empathic as mothers themselves than physicians can. They help prepare new mothers for delivery, give them support in insisting on their rights while in the hospital, provide understanding and "normalization" of postpartum fatigue, provide concrete advice regarding physical preparation for nursing and the baby's behavior, and, in general, provide support for the difficult transition to motherhood. The authors describe a self-help process with stages of impact, recoil, and recovery reminiscent of Adler and Hammett's (1973) description of crisis, conversion, and cult formation. Silverman and Murrow's recoil theory sounds like a preconversion searching period in Adler and Hammett's terms, but the overall concept of seeking a new cognitive framework for a life crisis is quite parallel.

Weiss (1969, 1976) describes the usefulness of Parents Without Partners, an organization that addresses a variety of life-transition needs with varying degrees of success. He notes in particular that while the desperate need for intimacy felt by many members is not often met, other kinds of social contact are provided which are helpful, if not entirely fulfilling. Silverman (1970, 1972, 1976) describes an interesting preventive intervention organized by a mental health professional but employing mutual-support concepts to help widows through their bereavement. Widows who had worked through their own grief sufficiently made phone calls and home visits to more recently bereaved women. They found an almost immediate presumption by the new widows that the visiting widow could understand the suffering of the newly bereaved. Abrahams (1972, 1976) did an analysis of the notes taken at the widows' service line, the phone component of the Widow to Widow Program, and noted that loneliness, either wanting someone to talk to or wanting to meet other people, was by far the most common need expressed by callers, especially those recently bereaved, and that requests for specific information were important but less common. The aides in this program often made referrals to professional agencies when they felt the caller was seriously disturbed.

A similar process is described in groups that attempt to help young homosexuals undergo the transition from private to public expression of their sexual preference (Humphreys, 1972; Devall, 1973). Enright and Parsons (1976) report on a program in which a nonhomosexual professional provided support for nonprofessional homosexual counselors in cooperation with the Metropolitan Community Church. They attempted to assess outcome by noting a drop in emergency room visits and reported suicide attempts by identified homosexuals, at the same time that there was an increase in the use of the telephone crisis line by members of the gay community. These few examples serve to make it clear that the self-help model is being effectively employed in various stressful life transitions and crises. This is potentially an area of rapid growth for self-help in view of social recognition of the stress brought about by these life transitions and the comparative ease with which people can recognize and are willing to seek nonprofessional assistance for these stresses.

Conclusion

This review has focused on the recent descriptive and evaluative professional literature regarding self-help and mutual support and has not attempted to summarize the vast literature produced by the variety of self-help groups themselves. The professional literature abounds with descriptions of self-help approaches and is rarely critical of the overall value of self-help groups. There are occasional criticisms of professionals for refusing to recognize the importance of the self-help approach or for attempting to interfere with it by insisting on professional control of self-help organizations. Although several authors have lost some of their early enthusiasm for the self-help approach, there is general consensus that self-help is an important complementary approach to traditional health and mental health services. Self-help approaches are more flexible, less bureaucratic, and often more responsive to the individual problems of their clients than are professional systems. They are clearly cost effective and offer both concrete help to newcomers and an enhancement in self-esteem to those who turn their experience into a valuable asset to be shared with others.

There can be little doubt that transformation of the meaning of having a stigmatized attribute or problem is of critical importance in the self-help process. Having hit "rock bottom," being stigmatized in the broader society, can become a ticket of admission to a self-help group. The shared stigma provides evidence to other group members of sincerity and knowledge about the common problem. Once a member in a self-help group has taken the step of admitting he needs some sort of help by joining the organization, he experiences a new kind of pride and shifts from the role of penitent to that of teacher, a role transition not available to the traditional patient.

The more formal outcome studies are few in number, but promising. As in any developing scientific field, description is followed by more systematic study. There are bits of evidence on the basis of pencil and paper tests and outcome measures such as client satisfaction and weight loss that self-help groups are effective, if not always as effective as they claim, or if not always providing exactly the type of help members seek.

DeToqueville called America a "nation of joiners." Our political and intellectual heritage is rich in the protection of diversity and the resentment of autocracy. The self-help approach has provided a fertile social laboratory for testing alternative approaches to treatment and placing control of treatment and support in the hands of consumers. It has most often complemented and enriched professional therapy rather than competed with it. Many individuals partake of both in the course of their lives. More research is needed and facilitation of self-help approaches is welcome in a number of areas. Self-help has been with us since the inception of social organization. The challenge for professionals is to use it wisely, aware of both limitations and potential, and to be unafraid to share the position of helper with those who are helped.

Part II

Programmatic Interventions

Community support systems are varied and broad ranging. Interventions with such support systems necessarily, therefore, are diverse. In this part of the book we shall examine a number of program strategies utilizing community support system approaches. In doing so, we will also continue the effort at conceptualizing support systems begun in Part I.

Comer and Hamilton-Lee argue that support systems in the black community have been perceived by the larger community as being deficient. In a circular fashion, such perceptions have led policymakers to undermine and weaken such systems. Presenting a historical review of the family, church, and school as key and important social bonds of blacks in the United States, the chapter focuses upon an innovative school project in New Haven, Connecticut, aimed at improving education levels of black school children by increasing parent involvement with the school and developing collaborative relationships between parents and staff. Periodic evaluations of the project have shown positive results, and the intervention is receiving both commuity-wide attention in New Haven and national recognition. Comer and Hamilton-Lee feel that the real success of the New Haven project is due to its building on the strengths of existing community support systems, a theme upheld in many other chapters throughout this book.

Pancoast and Chapman discuss findings of a recently completed research project funded by the Office of Human Development Services, DHHS, aimed at analyzing variations both among types of informal care and among interventions with informal support systems. They studied thirty mental health and human service agencies which work with informal services. On the basis of their collected data, they conceptualized informal helping as consisting of six types—family and friends, neighbors, natural helpers, role-related helpers, people with similar problems, and volunteers—presenting case examples of different ways of intervening with each of these helper types. This study contributes to the notion of the great variety and diversity within informal support systems and the need for the formal sector to understand this in designing effective interventions and linkages with the informal system. Knowledge of

119

how informal support systems operate is still at a fairly primitive level, and the authors argue that more research is needed in this area.

Pargament feels that religious support systems and their relationship to mental health have been too little understood and appreciated. He notes that religion and mental health have been incorrectly perceived as independent concepts and that instead they should be examined as related and intertwined since each carries meaning for the other. One of the unique roles of religion cited by Pargament is its opportunity to affect others throughout the life span through religious rituals, educational and counseling programs, and community-service activities. He presents examples of a wide range of religious support programs and the ways in which they assist individuals and groups in dealing with life crises and problems in living. Unfortunately, the interface between religious and mental health communities is too often based upon miscommunication and mistrust. Pargament explores the reasons for this and suggests appropriate remedies.

Gelfand and Gelfand's chapter, like those of Baum and Baum and of Guttmann in Part I, focuses upon the elderly. The authors, concerned about the limitations of informal networks due to the changing characteristics and circumstances of the future population of elderly, argue that the multipurpose senior center can serve a number of support system functions. They discuss present and future trends among the elderly affecting support systems, including increasing geographic distances between elderly parents and their children; larger numbers of elderly living alone; and a large number of elderly living in the suburbs. Thus, as they say, families in the future may provide "intimacy at a distance," and there may be limitations also in the ability of friends and neighbors to provide assistance that requires a "long-term commitment." They see the senior center as helping to strengthen informal support systems of the elderly by providing a place for informal contact, opportunities for the establishment of confidant relationships, and the provision of consultation and support to informal "leaders" and groups.

Platman's concluding chapter discusses support systems for the chronically mentally ill. He documents both the severe problems facing this population group and the strong stigma felt toward them by the general public. Deinstitutionalization problems of the 1960s and 1970s are well known, and Platman discusses a number of "innovative" model programs that have been developed recently. While he believes that these programs have achieved some successes, they are in large part "provider" dominated and tend to increase the dependency of the mentally ill. In addition, they provide little support to the needs of families of the mentally ill. Platman feels that professionals need to encourage the development of self-help programs for the mentally ill and cites the positive experience of both Fountain House and the Fairweather Lodge model. He warns that self-help groups should not be anti-professional but rather should utilize professional assistance where appropriate and helpful.

8

Support Systems in the Black Community

James P. Comer and
Muriel E. Hamilton-Lee

Black communities in America have always had unique social support systems to meet the needs of their members. Although generally misunderstood, ignored, or belittled by the larger community, these support systems have played an essential role in the lives of black Americans from the earliest days of slavery to the present time. They have assisted a wide range of blacks from rural sharecropper families to urban ghetto residents and the poorest members of the "underclass" to the most successful corporate lawyers, physicians, or businessmen.

As noted by Scherer (1972), a sense of community is a natural and fundamental part of human life.

> A basic requirement of existence has been the social bonds that unite each man to others, the most intimate being those of the family and close kin groups. But other, wider, social bonds have been needed to link men to more extensive social arrangements [p. xi].

Black communities are no exception.

This chapter will present a brief historical overview to outline the most significant forms of social bonds that have existed among black people in this country: the family, the church, and the school. Such a review is important not only to help clarify continuing misconceptions about the lives and cultural patterns of black people, but also to point the way toward strengthening black communities through the continued development of those institutions that have sustained us in the past.

Black Americans today continue to face an ongoing struggle to sustain their personal and community strengths in the face of economic, political, educational, psychological, and legal obstacles created by the white-controlled society. To illustrate some of the dynamics of this struggle and the concurrent positive potentials for overcoming the barriers, a detailed description of a research/action project in New Haven, Connecticut, will be presented. This project, drawing upon family and church support systems, has successfully developed a public school-based system of social supports for a number of low- and low-middle-income black families. Based upon lessons learned through the project, the chapter will conclude with implications for strengthening black community support systems.

Traditional Support Systems among Black People

The Family

Until recently there was a general assumption that black Americans had somehow existed in this country without the benefit of strong or reliable family units. Perpetuation of such a myth has been based on both a political need to denigrate black people in order to justify ongoing policies of control and discrimination and a carefully developed American naiveté born out of a fundamental need to deny the harsh realities of history experienced by black people in order to preserve a positive majority group and national image. During the slavery period, it was beneficial and guilt-relieving for white America to accept the theory that Africans were somehow less than true human beings. Since the end of slavery, theories of so-called family or cultural weakness and dysfunction serve the same purpose and relieve the society of primary responsibility for the social, economic, and psychological problems among black people.

Research by Blassingame (1979), Genovese (1974), Gutman (1976), and Abzug (1971) have helped to destroy some of these myths about black families. While not dismissing the horrors of slave conditions and the dehumanization inherent in such a social-economic system, recent documentation has shown that most slaves did in fact live in family units; that most maintained a powerful support unit against seemingly insurmountable odds. As stated by Blassingame (1979):

> The love the slaves had for their parents reveals clearly the importance of the family. Although it was weak, although it was frequently broken, the slave family provided an important buffer, a refuge from the rigors of slavery. . . . The family was, in short, an important survival mechanism [p. 191].

In order to reconcile their African cultural roots and their new condition of servitude in America, black families created many adaptive coping mechanisms. Although slaves were not allowed to enter into "legal" or "official" marriages, strong and lasting monogamous bonds were the rule, not the exception among adult slaves. Many plantation owners in fact encouraged the development of strong family units in order to create a more stable slave population. The love and loyalty among family members could then be used to coerce the slaves into cooperative behavior. When families were broken by the sale of one or more members, the community of slaves on a plantation would create a secondary support system of relatives and neighbors to serve as an extended family. Child-rearing, economic cooperation, emotional supports, and other traditional family functions were readily shared by various kinfolk and friends so that the basic family was not allowed to fail.

Another type of family survival mechanism grew out of the total lack of power or authority held by the slave father to physically protect his wife and children. The absence of this important familial function, along with the concurrent absence of economic independence or security, prevented slave fathers from fulfilling a prescribed role expectation that was important not only in the African cultures from which the slaves had come but also in the American culture by which they were now being judged. The result was a predictable loss of prestige, respect, self-respect, and general psychological good health experienced by black males thus emasculated by social norms.

Faced with this reality of powerlessness, black men and women were forced to develop new ways of defining family roles and new standards by which to judge the success of any particular family unit. Black adults had to become resourceful to find ways of maintaining a minimal level of authority for the husband and father within his family while at the same time not posing a threat to the slave master. Black men often put great energy into cultural or religious activities, which were generally tolerated by their white masters. According to Blassingame (1979), "Having a distinctive culture helped the slaves to develop a strong sense of group solidarity. They united to protect themselves from the most oppressive features of slavery and to preserve their self-esteem" (p. 147).

The post-slavery periods of Reconstruction and black migration to the North saw some minor improvements in the social, economic, political, and psychological experiences of black families in America. As documented by Abzug (1971):

> When freedom came, slaves implemented the dreams of family life which
> previously had had such marginal reality. It was, indeed, the creative ten-
> sion betwen the marginal reality and the idealization of family that provided
> the true heritage of slavery in terms of the family [p. 27].

Families that had been separated during slavery were often reunited.
The possibility of at least minimal job opportunities gave new hope to
many families—particularly in terms of black males gaining a small
amount of economic success and political recognition.

Yet the continuing realities of economic oppression, political powerlessness, and physical-psychological insecurity put tremendous pressures on late-nineteenth-century black people and required enormous
strength within families to sustain their members. As discussed by
Comer (1972), the post–Civil War period was one of danger and despair
for blacks in both the South and the North.

> Attempts to organize for group advancement were frequently met with
> violence. "Freedom" was a cruel joke. . . . For even the most determined
> family man, working at the lowest level of the job market made it hard to
> support a family. Getting ahead was hardly in the realm of possibility [pp.
> 99, 169].

Thus, shared child-rearing among black relatives and friends, shared
housing, income, and services, and strong emotional mutual support
systems—most often church based—were as necessary after as during
slavery.

To some extent, all families serve the above functions. But the black
family was doing so without the support of the institutions of the larger
society—judicial, economic, and so on. Indeed, a major role of the black
family was to teach its members how to survive and thrive in spite of the
hostility and abuse expressed by white individuals and institutions.

Early sociological descriptions of black families (DuBois, 1899; Frazier, 1939) emphasized the problems faced by such families. Numerous
stereotypes promoted in scholarly journals and the mass media alike
implied that these problems reflected group inadequacies rather than
societal ills. It has now been clearly demonstrated that the great majority of black families have been able to overcome the numerous problems
by sheer determination and unique coping abilities born out of basic
survival needs (Billingsley, 1968; Hill, 1971; Stack, 1974). The solid
support system provided by the family—both nuclear and extended—is
at the heart of the black community's continued vitality today.

On the other hand, the black family and community are probably
under more stress today than at any time since slavery. The progress of

more fortunate blacks and the societal need to ignore racist and detrimental policies and practices serve to prevent our society from fully facing up to the severe problems facing the majority of blacks. Current helping programs—economic or educational—are not only not enough, they are not based on the adaptive mechanisms blacks have utilized over time. Any effort to improve the living conditions and future potential of black communities in this country must begin with a fundamental commitment to understand, respect, and strengthen the institution of the black family.

The Church

Works by a number of sociologists and historians have recounted the history of the Christian religion among black Americans—from its early roots as a sanctioned emotional escape from the tyranny of slavery to its sophisticated institutionalization among urban middle-class blacks of the 1970s (Woodson, 1921; Frazier, 1963; Comer, 1972; Meier & Rudwick, 1976). All such studies acknowledge the importance of the black church as a vital support system within black communities of all types.

Among African slaves, religious worship was not only an attempt to hold onto cultural and spiritual beliefs brought from the homeland, but also an essential form of social cohesion and emotional communion in an otherwise hostile world. Missionaries sent into the South by northern Anglican, Methodist, and Baptist churches to help "civilize" the slaves were able to make use of an already-existing system of religious activity within black communities.

In spite of its subtle and not-so-subtle anti-black beliefs and practices, the Christian church grew rapidly among both slave and free blacks during the late eighteenth and nineteenth centuries. What typically began as separate black components of white Protestant congregations would gradually break away to form quasi-independent black churches of the same denomination. Thus, for example, in Philadelphia a group of black Methodists, led by Richard Allen, developed the Free African Society and the African Methodist Episcopal (AME) Church in the 1780s. In New York, the AME Zion Church was organized in 1821. In Newport, Rhode Island, the African Union Society and Church were also created in the 1820s.

Both during and after slavery, the black church was more than a church. It was a "substitute society" (Comer, 1972)—a source of value-setting, direction-giving, judgmental activities to bind the black community together in spite of the uncertainties of secular family, political, or economic life. It was the primary reference point of the black commu-

nity. It was to blacks what the city council, employers, and other powerful individuals and institutions were to whites. Indeed the local black
minister was to his congregation what the mayor was to whites. The
black church had such power because it fulfilled social and psychological
needs that could not be met in the larger society.

The church became an agent of social control: to recognize and
reward monogamous marriages, to stress the importance of strong,
male-headed families, to censure unconventional or immoral sexual behavior. But it also had the power to lead the community in efforts first to
survive and then to overcome racial oppression. Religious services provided crucial emotional catharsis for people who were being constantly
bombarded with dehumanization and frustration in all other settings. It
was an important place to obtain and express skills and talents that could
not be obtained or expressed in the larger society—organization, planning and implementation skills, oratorical, musical, and other expressions. As described by Comer (1972):

> The church was the place to discharge frustration and hostility so that one
> could face injustice and hardship the rest of the week.

> The black church had another important function: it was a place for partici-
> pation and belonging. . . . There was a little bit of respect for everybody
> [pp. 16–17].

Church congregations also served as a base for economic cooperation, mutual-aid societies, schools, social or fraternal clubs, and communications. In his detailed sociological studies of Phiadelphia and the
country as a whole, DuBois (1899, 1903) shows clearly the extensive
network of social and economic supports provided by religious-oriented
groups, suggesting that the black church served as a vital and lively
institution in every black community.

Today's black churches continue to serve as important support systems. The need for a sanctuary from the tensions, frustrations, and
anger created by the hostile larger society still exists for most black
Americans. The church's functions of cooperative economics and mutual
assistance continue to meet an important need for members of most
black religious groups.

Yet the black church today, like the black family, is under enormous
stress. The reliance on science and technology to address human problems has decreased the power of all churches and church leaders. The
development of social services that are not black-church based or supported has reduced the intensity of the emotional tie of blacks to the
institutions. At the same time, many blacks still do not receive a strong
message of belonging from the political, economic, and service-giving

institutions of the society. Thus they have lost the motivating, direction-giving effect of the church without gaining the same from the larger society.

The School

Schools as social support institutions in black communities have had a less definite role than families or churches. According to Lightfoot (1978):

> The historical and contemporary relationship between American blacks and public schooling has been passionate and ambivalent. Schools have always held out the promise and hope of liberation and enlightenment at the same time as they have been recognized as social and economic vehicles of oppression and denial [p. 125].

During the early years of black life in America, formal education was by and large an offshoot of religious activity by missionaries who recognized the benefits of exposing their new members to the Bible as part of their persuasion away from African spiritual forms. Yet to teach a slave how to read was also seen as a dangerous, potentially revolutionary act and for this reason was actually outlawed in all southern states by the 1830s. Illiteracy was to serve as an important social control of the black population.

What education did take place was done secretly, within families or close-knit community groups, in the desperate hope that the younger generation could look forward to a time of greater opportunity in American society. Research by Bond (1934), Woodson (1968), and Genovese (1974) documents the early struggles of black families to educate themselves and their children in spite of tremendous odds against their success.

The determination and optimism held by a majority of black families about the potential of education as a vehicle for overall social improvement were increased by activities of the Freedman's Bureau during the Reconstruction period. White philanthropists and religious groups from nothern states became actively involved in the effort to bring former slaves closer to the American mainstream culture by exposing them to basic skills—although there was clearly still no enthusiasm for developing a comprehensive, high-quality educational system for blacks. Actual participation in formal education was extremely slow to become an accepted pattern for black children or adults. Census records indicate that by 1870 only 9.9 percent of the black population was enrolled in schools, as compared to 54.4 percent of the white (Comer, 1972). Not until the mid-twentieth century did a significant number of black children become part of the public education system in this country.

More recent records indicate that the inequities in educational opportunity have continued. To cite several examples, as late as the 1930s, the nine states containing some 90 percent of the black population allocated an average of three times more per pupil for white students ($49) than for black pupils ($15). In 1955, the fifty-two segregated land-grant colleges across the South for whites received 25.7 percent of their benefits from federal funds, while the 17 land-grant colleges for blacks received only 3.1 percent. The 1964-1965 endowments for all 106 black colleges in this country were only about half that of Harvard University alone (Comer, 1972).

As black Americans have moved in large numbers from the rural South to northern urban communities from the Reconstruction era to the present time, they have consistently encountered mediocre, often crowded education systems designed to provide only a minimum of skills. Urban schools in general have consistently failed to truly educate black students. Problems of inadequate staff preparation, inappropriate attitudes, and inadequate supports from parents, who are themselves undereducated and overwhelmed by sheer survival problems, create an inevitable syndrome of student underachievement and failure. Too often education in black schools takes a back seat to violence, antagonism, apathy, and hopelessness.

Nevertheless, most black Americans continue to hold high hopes that education can be a door to better living conditions and economic/political opportunities for their children. As recently as the 1960s, one of the most promising components of the federal government's War on Poverty was the emphasis on a general commitment to improving educational services across the board—whether in urban ghettos, migrant labor camps, isolated rural areas, or senior citizen communities.

Unfortunately, it soon became clear that these efforts to bring about fundamental improvements in the education of black children were based on shallow assumptions that failed to take the historical–systemic realities of black oppression and white racism into account. Teachers, school administrators, and educational policy planners seemed to believe that black families could overcome years of economic denial and resultant psychological damage and immediately provide home environments of stability and support to stimulate their children's education achievements. Black parents, on the other hand, seemed to believe that the educational system could immediately modify its traditional patterns to accommodate the effects of a different historical experience and different life-styles and meet the educational needs of their children.

The resulting misunderstandings and conflict between black communities of the 1970s and the educational systems attempting to serve them have made it very difficult for public schools to play the role of supportive institutions for those communities. Comer and Schraft (1980) and Lightfoot (1978) describe these frictions in some detail, but also point to ways of overcoming the myriad of problems through systematic, realistic approaches for working with black families to create the positive social support systems that schools *can be*.

New Haven Project—An Overview

The Baldwin–King School Project, begun in 1968 in New Haven, is one such approach. Through the application of theoretical constructs to a real-life situation, we have been able to demonstrate the feasibility of creating a new level of educational opportunity for urban black children, many of whom would be written off as failures in traditional school situations. We have also seen how such an approach can serve as a broad support system to address the problems and needs of black parents as well.

After the initial five-year grant period, the Baldwin School parents and staff chose to return to a more traditional, strict disciplinary program for their children. The project description which follows therefore focuses attention on the King School, which has been involved in project activities since the outset.

Martin Luther King Elementary School serves a 99 percent black population. More than 50 percent of the children are from families receiving Aid for Families with Dependent Children. It ranks among the lowest of all schools on the poverty index utilized by the city. In 1969, the reading and math scores on standardized achievement tests of its fourth grade students were eighteen to nineteen months behind grade level. There were serious attendance and behavior problems. The relationship between home and school was difficult. Today, despite additional economic and social deterioration in the neighborhood, by the fourth grade the students are at grade level in language arts and less than two months behind in reading and math on the Iowa Test of Basic Skills. Daily attendance is among the best in the city. There have been no serious behavior problems in the past five years. Parents are positively and intimately involved in the work of the school.

Co-sponsored by the Yale Child Study Center and the New Haven Public Schools, the School Project is based on four specific assumptions: (1) schools function better when parents and staff work as a collaborative team; (2) parents who are poor and/or politically powerless cannot play active roles in their children's education until the barriers between them and white middle-class society are greatly reduced, until a climate of trust and mutual respect is created; (3) educational intervention must take place at both an individual and a system or institutional level; and (4) when schools function smoothly, all children can learn at a reasonable level. Our experience over the past twelve years supports the validity of these assumptions.

In addition, a fifth basic premise has been derived from the program: Parents who become actively involved in their children's schooling often become generally mobilized and involved with other institutions of their community. This also appears to improve the functioning of their families. Thus, comprehensive parent participation in schools can serve as a stepping stone to a more positive way of coping with family needs and the larger society.

To operationalize our program concepts, we had to address numerous problems. Because open access to mainstream societal institutions is denied, many black families achieve social and psychological survival through techniques of avoidance, being passive, playing "Uncle Tom" roles, being super cool or super tough, or "ripping off" the system in whatever way possible. Unfortunately, such behavior patterns often lead to troublesome family and child-rearing conditions. Children from such environments are more likely to participate in antisocial activities at an early age. Because of the marginal social status of the black poor, even children who enjoy a desirable developmental experience often do not learn skills needed to cope in the social mainstream and often have low aspiration levels.

A vicious cycle develops in school. Low-income black children, with talents and skills that are of value outside of school but inappropriate or marginally useful in school, often respond to the foreign expectations of the school with acting-out or withdrawal behavior. School staff, prepared to respond only to the "cultural average" often respond to low-income minority children as if they are "bad" or deficient in intelligence and incapable of desirable social conduct. This leads to a pattern of excessive punishment, low expectations, and remedial activities. Because such activities do not meet the needs of healthy, active youngsters, they, in turn, heighten the acting-out behavior to the point that many schools become disrupted.

Teachers and administrators become frustrated and angry and blame the students and their parents for school problems. Parents and community often accuse schools of willfully failing to educate their children. When the staff is predominantly white, they are often accused of racism. The students soon give up on schools or develop patterns of behavior and academic performance that take a generally downhill course even though they remain in school.

The primary objective of our project intervention team (a psychiatrist, a social worker, a psychologist-evaluator, and a helping teacher) and the school staff is to interrupt the forces contributing to this cycle of staff, parent, and student failure and to replace it with insights and practices that lead to success at King School. Because schools are a symbolic and real manifestation of the larger society from which many blacks are excluded and of which they are suspicious, a major program strategy is to concentrate first on improving the overall climate of relationship between home and school.

A key element in improving this climate was the development of a Parent Participation Program. This program and a governance-management team made up of administrators, teachers, and parents has facilitated improved student behavior and performance, permitting greater time and energy of the staff to go into improving the Teaching and Curriculum Program. This eventually led to greatly improved student behavior and learning. As parents and the community become involved in supporting the program of the school, the school is able to serve as a support system to the families involved.

Before discussing the parent-school collaboration component of the project, a synopsis of other project components is helpful. With funding by the Ford Foundation and the New Haven Title I Office in 1968 and by the National Institute of Mental Health after 1973, the project has included work with parents, teachers, school administrators, support staff, and mental health specialists.

Teachers. The intervention team suggests positive, creative ways of relating to students and parents based on child-development and mental-health principles. It facilitates the application of these principles to teaching and curriculum development.

School administrators. Principals, with parents and teachers, have created communication and policymaking mechanisms based on human-relations and child-development principles.

Support staff. Reading specialists, nurses, classroom assistants, and other auxiliary staff members have been included in the program planning, resource identification, implementation, evaluation, and modification process.

Mental health specialists. Our Yale Child Study Center Team— primarily through the in-school work of social workers—has played the role of translating child development and group process theories into day-to-day practice in a way that facilitates the work of all other staff and parents.

Program evaluations have been conducted on a continuing basis, using pre- and post-standardized test scores, parent interviews, teacher/administrator interviews, reports of outside observers, and special studies of nonacademic areas of arts, physical education, and pupil personnel services. Findings indicate consistent improvements in relationships, service and performance (Costello, 1973; Comer and Schraft, 1980; Comer, 1980). Parents, teachers, and school administrators who had previously been suspicious and fearful of each other now work together regularly to plan and carry out school-wide activities and to meet individual children's needs. School-sponsored services range from field trips for the students to consumer and health counseling for the parents to curriculum workshops for the teachers. Parent participation has moved from angry confrontations to active, positive involvement of more than forty parents in school functions during the year. We could not use a control group for comparison; however, on the Iowa Test of Basic Skills, children at King have ranked ahead of those at all other Title I schools (a government-funded program for compensatory education in low-income schools) in the city for the past several years.

Most importantly, the project has stimulated the creation of a *climate of achievement* at King School. Nothing is more essential to the success of an educational institution, whether it serves wealthy, middle-class, or poor children.

Parent and School Collaboration in the New Haven Project

We chose to develop a parent participation model that would build on parent and community strengths rather than weaknesses. Given the usual way that mainstream institutions work with low-income, minority people—as if they are deficient—and the distrust and lack of confidence that it engenders, this was not an easy task. We felt that it would take at least five years to improve the climate of parent–school and in-school relationships to the point that academic achievement would greatly improve. As stated by Winters and Schraft (1977), "Involving parents with schools cannot be approached precipitously. It is a delicate and intricate process that requires thoughtful planning, careful execution and a long time commitment" (p. 2).

As is frequently true of new projects, the first year was chaotic. Neither parents nor school staff members were accustomed to truly active parental involvement in school functions or decision making. A two-week summer workshop before the beginning of the second year facilitated the development of the Parent Participation Program. Administrators, parents, and teachers worked together to plan a curriculum for the school. While such a curriculum was not fully developed and implemented until after workshops over the next four years, the initial summer workshop enabled staff and parents to come to appreciate each other as people with a common purpose, common skills, and complementary abilities, and to arrive at a broad consensus about what they expected of the school and the children. This process provided a level of trust and direction needed to begin the school improvement process.

The subsequent workshops exposed parents and staff to what it feels like to be a child in school, to the options in teaching methods and materials, and to parents and staff skill developent opportunities. All of these skills gave the staff, and parents in particular, the skills needed to work cooperatively and collaboratively in the school.

During the second project year the program developed a system of positive contacts between home and school on a regular basis. These included extensive dialogues between parents, teachers, and administrators; structured workshops; social events planned by parents and staff; and a variety of other means to continue to reduce the misperceptions and distrust that had existed in the past. Thus parents are in school for support purposes, and, in turn, being supported, rather than being summoned only for negative reasons or discipline problems.

It is not realistic to expect working parents or parents facing multiple problems to have as much time or energy to participate in school activities as do nonworking, more crisis-free affluent parents. For poor black parents, schools have often been frightening places where they are made to feel unwelcomed or out of place. To permit as many as possible to participate as their time, energy, interest, skills, and comfort would permit, a three-level pattern of participation was eventually elaborated.

At the first level, broad-based participation takes place in activities such as social events to raise money for special occasions, period report card conferences, pot-luck suppers, general meetings, school fairs, and special interest workshops with outside speakers. From 50 to 100 percent of a school's parents can generally take part in one or more of these events during the year. Through these activities the parents can feel at least a minimum of involvement in school functions without making a major commitment of time or talents.

Level Two of the structure involved a smaller number of parents—often betwen 10 and 40 percent—in activities requiring more time and commitment. The core of the parent participation is at this level, primarily through involvement in the Parent–Teacher Power Team. Although similar to traditional PTAs, the PTP Team works closely with school administrators and the Yale Child Study Center mental health specialists to develop new attitudes on sharing responsibility for school operations. A high degree of communication with all parents is emphasized (through fliers, newsletters, phone calls, and/or home visits) to continually stress the willingness of the school to be open to the parents.

At this level parents become directly involved in daily school operations such as planning and assisting with field trips, playground supervision, hobby groups, tutoring, or assisting in the library or cafeteria. These parents receive training through workshops offered by teachers, central office specialists, or consultants.

The workshops include not only specific suggestions for carrying out these school tasks but also general discussions of overall curriculum content, child development and psychology, school management, discipline, and whatever other concerns the parents express as they participate in day-to-day experiences with the children. Often the workshops provide an opportunity to discuss family issues such as budgeting, nutrition, home health care, adult education, jobs, family interactions, behavior problems, or adult emotional challenges. They also provide a frequent forum on community-wide issues such as safe street crossings, adequate playgrounds, police and fire protection, vandalism, improving or restricting neighborhood commercial enterprises, and so forth.

Level Three of parent participation involves a small number of parents who are involved, with teachers and administrators, in making policy decisions for the school. Not more than 1 to 10 percent of the parent body is generally involved at this level, requiring a major investment of time and energy. Parents who participate to this degree have usually come up through the other two levels and have thus received a fair amount of preparation for the complex issues they must deal with—from school budget to staff selection and developing curriculum.

It is important to prepare parents to work at the second and particularly the third level. They do not automatically have the expertise to make meaningful contributions in these areas. Because of this, in many programs most parents drop out after expressing initial interest, or react in disruptive ways. They are then criticized for a lack of sustained interest or not performing "professionally." Such criticism is unfair and counterproductive where no training has been provided. Too often such reactions are an excuse for eliminating all parent participation in meaningful school activities.

While supporting parent-sponsored activities, our project's social worker, teachers, and mental health staff are able to assist parents in developing skills that can be useful not only in the school but in family-management, job, and other activity areas. This, and other program experiences, have led to the development of a program entitled the "Social Skills Curriculum for Inner City Children." The curriculum is designed to provide low-income children with the social skills needed to be successful in mainstream social institutions, including school. Parent participation ensures that this takes place without violating student and community needs and styles.

The curriculum does not require a diminution of time or interest in the teaching of basic skills. It is carried out during what would ordinarily be "free" or elective time. It involves an integration of the teaching of academic subject areas, the arts, and the social skills. Activities are organized around units representing major adult performance areas: politics and government, banking and business, health and nutrition, and spiritual or leisure time; with activities such as elections, a store, banking, food preparation, and a gospel choir. For kindergarteners, a special language/reading preparation program has been utilized for children identified as high risk.

A number of the special units and other activities of the school build on the vitality of the community—church-based parent skills, church choir activities, parent talent, and so on. This makes it easier for parents to be intimately involved in the planning and implementation of the school program. They are helping and receiving help in supporting the school and in promoting the life coping skills of their children and themselves. In providing such help, the school has become a family and community support system. The program of the school has also stimulated a number of parents to undertake personal development activities such as returning to school, finding or upgrading jobs, starting a small business enterprise, and participating in local civic and political work.

Implications

Since the professionalization of helping activities in the 1930s and 1940s, helping agencies and agents have too often attempted to do for people in need rather than to enable them to do for themselves. National social policies, built on the implicit assumption that poor or otherwise needy people are not motivated or able, often contribute to the creation of institutional policies and practices that weaken or eliminate community-based support systems. The demeaning implication—too often reflected in and transmitted by the attitude of the helper—is recognized by those served and often promotes acting-out or dependency behavior.

Blacks—more poor and marginal to the political and economic mainstream than most—have been generally perceived as less able, with deficient skills and support systems. The existence and importance of black community-based support systems have been poorly understood and thus easily weakened. The relationship barriers between the black community—particularly less well-educated blacks—and the institutions of the larger society have always been widely misunderstood or denied, and as a result, little effort is made to address the problems in the organization and management of many service, political, economic, and social-development programs.

The key to the success of the Martin Luther King, Jr., School program is the fact that it has been built on existing support systems—family, church and school, people, skills, and tradition—rather than ignoring or trying to replace these elements. The program recognizes the community, families, and students as unfamiliar and underdeveloped with regard to school or mainstream expectations—not "sick" or incapable—and provides the necessary orientation and supportive development.

The basic program design created in 1968 is still in operation, although it has become more relevant to the needs of the participating children and their parents because of the lessons we have learned by self-assessments and external evaluations. The project has been used as a model for improving the learning environment of two additional schools in New Haven—one elementary and one middle school—and is now contributing to a city-wide school improvement effort. It is receiving national attention as a method for meeting the challenges of urban education.

Initial project budget levels were substantial: over $300,000 per year; however, as the project matured, more and more responsibility has been designated to existing school staff, with less and less input from the Child Study Center specialists. But the project was a research and development effort and replication costs can be significantly less. Schools that have replicated the project in New Haven have been able to do so by allocating part of their Title I funds and assigning existing staff members to the specific areas of activity suggested by our project design, with little or no additional funds necessary.

Future efforts to facilitate the development of the black community—family, neighborhoods, schools, and other institutions—should be based on an appreciation of black community-developed support systems. The King School program suggests that community and mainstream support systems can be linked in a mutually reinforcing relationship—a relationship that reduces the distrust and alienation that interfere with the effectiveness of the mainstream programs in the black community and the participation of many blacks in the American mainstream.

9

Roles for Informal Helpers in the Delivery of Human Services

*Diane L. Pancoast and
Nancy J. Chapman*

Human services and mental health professionals have recognized for some time that the services they provide are only a small portion of the support, problem-solving, crisis-intervention, and caring that occurs in a community. Teachers, medical personnel, police, clergy, and others have been seen as important parts of the overall help that is available to people. But, in an even broader sense, there is a whole world of informal caregiving that deserves a more comprehensive examination than it has received thus far. Surveys of where people find help when they have problems consistently show that family, friends, neighbors, and other personal relationships are the principal source of help for a wide range of problems for most people. (Litwak & Szelenyi, 1969: Gourash, 1978).

Some agencies have begun to realize that a partnership with these informal caregivers can result in a more appropriate response to the needs of clients and communities and have sought ways to form mutually beneficial relationships. While the formal system has always been aware of the informal system and worked with it to some extent, the former has only recently begun to develop explicit techniques for cooperating with and reinforcing that system.

This chapter is based on an investigation of thirty agencies that have developed programs to work with informal helpers and to interweave formal services with the help provided by the informal sector. By informal helping we mean the relatively unorganized, spontaneous, and mu-

This research was supported by Grant #18-P-00088, Office of Human Development Services, DHHS, "Natural Helping Networks and Service Delivery."

tual exchange of help between people in everyday life. It is contrasted with services provided by paid staff under organized auspices. Though similar in philosophy, the programs included in our study are very diverse in their target populations, the agencies in which they are based, and in their specific goals. While only ten of the agencies explicitly used a mental health framework in describing the goals of their program, all fit within a broad definition of positive mental health, that is, all are intended to help people deal with the large and small problems of everyday life by expanding the ability of the informal system to provide material and social support and by creating better ties between the informal and formal helping systems.

The overall purpose of our research is to begin to describe the variations among types of informal care and among the approaches agencies are using as well as to identify problems and issues in this field. This chapter reports on one aspect of that study. It describes the characteristics of six types of informal helpers and gives examples of how agencies are working with each of them to deliver services. Although the concepts of community support and informal helping are becoming common in the human services, in order for these concepts to be embodied in a range of programs that take advantage of the potential for informal exchange we must differentiate among the types of informal helpers and the appropriate ways of working with each. This chapter argues that different types of informal helpers have different characteristics, helping activities, and roles within the informal system. Understanding these differences will contribute to more sensitive and effective supportive interventions by the formal system.

Methodology

A number of criteria were developed as the bases for identifying and choosing programs to be included in the sample. First, a range of target populations were included in order to contrast how approaches to working with informal helping may vary according to different target-population needs. Target populations included were the elderly; children, youth, and families; developmentally disabled and handicapped; psychiatrically disabled; and underserved or disadvantaged communities. Second, a variety of approaches were sampled based on a typology of agency approaches to working with informal helping developed by the researchers (Froland, Pancoast, Chapman, & Kimboko, 1979). Third, agencies were defined as programs operating with paid professional staff engaged in service delivery, or involved in activities applicable to human

service delivery, and currently operational. Fourth, the interaction between agency and helping network was to be characterized by equality
(viewing helpers as colleagues or peers), an emphasis on diffusing help to
a broad group of individuals through identified helpers, and sensitivity to
the cultural norms of the helpers and network. Finally, the helping network itself was expected to involve mutual exchanges directed toward
promoting positive functioning or adjustment and occurring in an indigenous setting.

An inventory of sixty programs was developed from reviews of the
literature, personal contacts and referrals, advertisements in professional
or program media with national circulation, and recommendations of
individuals working in the field. The criteria listed above were used to
select the final sample of thirty programs. Table 9.1 identifies the programs by target population, agency size, and urban–rural location. The
desire for a diverse set of programs and target populations led us to relax
some of our ideal expectations regarding the genesis of informal helping
networks and their relationship with agency staff. Although we expected
to include only agencies that worked with existing informal networks,
we found that particularly for some target populations, informal helping
systems were absent or unable to provide sufficient care. For these
clients, agencies found it necessary to foster new sources of informal
support.

The major source of data regarding each program was a one- to
three-day site visit by one of the research staff. Program staff were
interviewed following a standardized discussion guide, and agency reports and records examined for information about the overall agency,
the program that specifically worked with the informal helping system,
characteristics of the informal helpers, their relationship with the staff,
and the communities or neighborhoods in which the programs were
located. Whenever possible, informal helpers were observed, but the
main information source was data supplied by agency personnel. This
information was integrated and organized in the format of answers to
questions included in the discussions and was also utilized as case
studies of each agency. The wide variation among the programs pre-
cluded a more standardized format.

The informal helping discussed in this chapter is seen through the
eyes of particular agencies and as such is not necessarily representative
of the range of informal caring that exists beyond the purview of the
formal system (cf. Curry & Young, 1978). This perspective, however, is
very likely representative of the types of informal caregiving that are
most relevant and accessible to formal professional caregivers.

The six helper types that are the focus of this chapter are conceptual

TABLE 9.1. Sample Distribution

Problem Focus	Staff Size[a] and Agency Setting						
	Large		Medium		Small		
	Urban	Rural	Urban	Rural	Urban	Rural	Total
Elderly	2	0	3	1	2	1	9
Children, youths, and families	1	0	0	1	3	0	5
Developmentally/ physically disabled	0	0	2	0	2	0	4
Mental health related	3	0	1	1	0	1	6
General community	1	0	1	0	2	2	6
Total	7	0	7	3	9	4	30

[a] key to staff size: Small = 1-5 paid staff; Medium = 6-15 paid staff; Large = 16+ paid staff.

140

types developed by the authors which seemed to best capture the variations among the informal helpers with whom the programs worked. Because the agencies often used a variety of approaches, each of which differed in the types of informal helpers worked with, the units of analysis presented in this chapter are the approaches used by the agency. The approaches were classified into five types (Froland et al., 1979): personal networks, neighborhood helping, volunteer linking, mutual aid, and community empowerment. Within the thirty agencies a total of sixty approaches of these five types were identified, with some programs using only one approach and others several. For each of the sixty program approaches, the staff member making the site visit filled out a detailed rating sheet on the characteristics of the informal helpers involved in that approach. Included were ratings derived from content analysis of types of helping activities, reciprocity of exchange, agency resources used to support helpers, and personal attributes used to select helpers. In most cases, ratings were on a four-point scale ranging from "always" to "never" or from "very typical" to "not at all typical."

Types of Informal Helpers

The six types of informal helping identified in this study are family and friends, neighbors, natural helpers, role-related helpers, people with similar problems, and volunteers. In order to make the helper types concrete each has been portrayed as part of the personal network of a hypothetical elderly widow, Mrs. Jones, in the descriptions to follow. Mrs. Jones' *personal network* consists of all the links she has with others. The ties vary in intimacy and frequency of contact; some of them may involve exchanges of help, or could if the need arose. This more limited set of relationships constitutes her *helping network*. While the network is hypothetical, the specific instances of helping activities are chosen from examples in our study.

Family and friends. The most intimate relationships are usually with family or with friends. Mrs. Jones has a sister who lives several blocks away and with whom she is quite close. Her sister still drives a car and includes her in shopping trips and other jaunts. Mrs. Jones' son and daughter have moved away but call and write frequently and spend Christmas with her. Her daughter came to spend a week with her after Mrs. Jones had hip surgery last year.

Neighbors. Neighbors most intimately involved in helping usually live next door or very close by but, particularly with agency encouragement, they may come from a much larger area. Mrs. Jones knows all the long-time neighbors on her block by name, but would consider asking only two of them for help. They take in each other's mail when one is out of town and check in on each other if the blinds are not up at the usual time.

Natural helper. These are people who seem to help many others, people that many turn to when they have a problem. They may be helpful within a neighborhood context, or they may be actively involved in a wider network. There is one neighbor of Mrs. Jones who has been especially kind to her. This woman also belongs to her church and has a number of elderly friends for whom she performs various services. Each week she drives Mrs. Jones to a meeting at the church and is always willing to stop along the way for other errands.

Role-related helpers. These are people such as storekeepers, bank tellers, mailpersons, or ministers who come into contact with many others and thus have many opportunities to help. Mrs. Jones knows a man at her bank who has become increasingly helpful to her in handling her financial affairs. She always asks his advice when she visits the bank and he makes sure she is served promptly since he knows it is hard for her to stand for long periods since her hip surgery.

People with similar problems. There are ties that are often fostered by an agency or institution that brings together people with similar problems who can help each other based on their shared experiences. When her friend from church suggested that she might be interested in a recently formed widow's group at the senior center, Mrs. Jones was skeptical. She didn't think she would enjoy talking to a group of widows, but since she had been a widow for some time she thought she might be able to offer some support and advice to more recently widowed women. She now attends the group regularly.

Volunteers. Mrs. Jones has such a large and active network that she is not likely to need to be linked to a volunteer. She does eat lunch regularly at a lunch program at the senior center, which is staffed by volunteers.

The six types of helpers vary along a number of dimensions, as shown in Table 9.2. Some are relationships between helper and recipient which occurred spontaneously and are long-standing while others have been created or catalyzed by a formal organization. Some are locality based, the helper and recipient living within the same neighborhood or small community; others involve contacts made in another context. Some involve equality of exchange between the helper and recipient, at least over the long term, while others are more like those with professional helpers in that the exchange is likely to remain unequal. The

TABLE 9.2. Characteristics of the Helper Types

Helper Type	Preexisting Ties	Locality Based	Equality of Exchange	Centrality of Role
Family, friends	x		x	
Neighbors	x	x	x	
Natural helpers	x	x		x
Role related	x	x		
Similar problems			x	
Volunteers				

helping role is a central part of some individuals' activities, while for others it is just part of the exchanges that almost everyone is involved in at one time or another.

The types of helping are best seen as activities or roles rather than types of people. For example, the same woman may be actively involved in supporting an elderly parent (family and friends), part of a cooperative day-care exchange (similar problems), and a volunteer in a socialization program for ex-patients (volunteer). Some helping may result from interest in a particular problem and may take different forms over time. Parents of a retarded child might belong to a support group when their child is an infant, then volunteer in a special preschool program, and later become active in an association advocating the establishment of more group homes for retarded adults as their child's needs change.

Characteristics of Each Type of Helper

The following helper profiles are based on ratings of the research staff of a number of personal attributes of the helpers, their helping activities, and the agencies' interventions. Tables 9.3, 9.4, and 9.5 present the relationship between specific variables and the helper types. These tables show the level of each variable for each of the six helper types. To simplify reading of the tables, the levels are indicated by 0, +, ++, representing low, medium, and high mean scores on that attri-

TABLE 9.3. Helper and Recipient Characteristics

	Family and Friends	Neighbors	Natural Helpers	Role-Related Helpers	People with Similar Problems	Volunteers
n[a]	7	13	4	7	21	8
Sex of Helper (% female) *	41-60	41-60	41-60	21-40	41-60	61-80
Personal Attributes						
Leadership in network *	0	+	++	++	0	0
Helping skills *	+	+	++	+	0	+
Motivation *	++	+	++	++	+	++
Shared experience *	0	0	+	0	++	0
Special knowledge	0	0	0	+	0	+
Target Population						
Elderly	4	5	1	3	6	1
Mental health	2	3	1	1	6	2
Disabled	0	0	0	0	4	3

Families	2	5	0	0	0	1
General community	0	0	3	2	5	0
Status Relationship-- Helper and Recipient						
Helpers higher in SES *	++	0	+	+	+	+
Helpers have same life situation, problems *	0	++	0	+	+	0
Helpers cope better with problems	++	+	+	++	+	++

Note: The notations "0", "+" and "++" indicate the range into which the mean score falls. Specifically, ++ = $M > 3.0$; + = M between 2.0 and 2.9; 0 = $M < 2.0$ on a scale ranging from 4 "very typical" to 1 "not at all typical."

a Numbers indicate the number of approaches out of the total of 60 program approaches.

*Indicates one-way ANOVA, $p < .01$.

145

TABLE 9.4. Helping Activities

	Helper Type					
n[a]	Family and Friends 7	Neighbors 13	Natural Helpers 4	Role-Related Helpers 7	People with Similar Problems 21	Volunteers 8
Kind of Network Worked With						
Individual client (not part of their personal network) *	0	0	0	+	0	++
Personal network of neighbors, friends, family *	++	+	++	0	0	0
Peer group, mutual aid, or common interest *	0	0	+	0	++	0
Locality-based *	0	++	++	+	+	0
Length of Relationship *	Long-term	Moderately long	Long-term	Moderately long	Moderately long	Moderately long
Helping Activities						
Caretaking (material assistance, services, money)	+	+	+	+	0	0
Joint action (cooperative communal activity, organizing, advocacy, planning) *	0	0	+	+	+	0

	one	many	many	many	many	no designated helpers and helpees	several helpers and helpees
Friendship (association, emotional support) *	++	+	+	++	0	++	+
Problem-solving (cognitive guidance, linking)	+	+	+	++	+	+	++
Reciprocity (returns to helper)							
Tangible over short-term	0	0	0	0	0	+	0
Tangible over long-term	+	+	+	+	0	0	0
Pass along to others	+	+	+	+	+	+	0
Expected part of helping role *	0	+	+	+	++	0	0
No expectations of reward	+	++	+	++	+	+	++
Rewards external to relationship needed *	0	+	+	+	+	0	+
Number of People Helped per Helper *	one	many	many	many	many	no designated helpers and helpees	several helpers and helpees

Note: The notations "0", "+" and "++" indicate the range into which the mean score falls. Specifically, ++ = M > 3.0; + = M between 2.0 and 2.9; 0 = M < 2.0 on a scale ranging from 4 "very typical" to 1 = "not at all typical."

[a]Numbers indicate the number of approaches out of the total of 60 program approaches.

*Indicates one-way ANOVA, p < .01.

TABLE 9.5. Agency/Helper Relationships

			Helper Type			
n^a	Family and Friends 7	Neighbors 13	Natural Helpers 4	Role-Related Helpers 7	People with Similar Problems 21	Volunteers 8
Helper Role in Agency						
Turnover rate	+	+	0	+	+	+
Difficulty recruiting	+	+	+	+	0	++
Difficulty identifying	+	+	+	0	+	+
Difficulty retaining	+	+	+	+	+	+
Expected Effect on Network						
Expand ties of existing network	+	++	+	0	+	0
Change content of exchange	+	+	+	+	+	0
Create new connections *	0	0	+	0	++	0
Reinforce existing relations *	++	+	++	+	0	0
Tie informal to formal system	+	++	++	++	+	+

148

Agency Support of Helper

Develop identity as helpers *	+	+	+	+	0	++
Improve helping skills *	0	0	0	0	0	++
Access to helpees *	0	0	+	+	+	++
Associate with other helpers	0	0	0	+	+	+
"Helper therapy"	0	+	+	0	+	+
Training *	0	0	0	0	0	++
Space	0	0	0	0	+	0
Publicity	0	0	+	0	+	0
Technical assistance	0	0	0	+	0	0
Encouragement	++	++	++	++	++	++
Access to formal services	+	++	0	+	+	0

Note: The notations "0", "+" and "++" indicate the range into which the mean score falls. Specifically, ++ = $M > 3.0$; + = M between 2.0 and 2.9; 0 = $M < 2.0$ on a scale ranging from 4 "very typical" to 1 = "not at all typical."

[a] Numbers indicate the number of approaches out of the total of 60 program approaches.

*Indicates one-way ANOVA, $p < .01$.

bute. For each variable, significant differences in actual mean scores among the six helper types based on one-way analyses of variance are shown by an asterisk (*) after the name of the attribute. Since the data are based on indirect measurement of the variables via site visits, staff interviews, and agency records rather than direct contact with the informal helpers, significance levels were used only as indicators of important areas for more refined study. It is interesting to note, however, that the ratings generally confirm the *a priori* differentiation into types.

In Table 9.3, the personal attributes of the helper refer to the attributes that the agency focuses on in identifying or selecting informal helpers. The helping activities (Table 9.4) were identified from content analysis; the four sets of activities shown represent the four factors that emerged from factor analysis of the activities. Agency support of the helper (Table 9.5) refers to the resources or other support that the agency offers the informal helpers. These range from tangible support in the form of space or publicity to such intangibles as developing an individual's awareness of the importance of the helper role to the client. The "helper therapy" principle (Riessman, 1965) states that often the helpers receive as many benefits from their helping activities as do the recipients. The ratings of reciprocity are based on the agencies' reports of what the helpers expect and receive in return for their efforts. In some cases they may receive aid in return, at least over the long term as between parent and child; in others, they simply contribute to the general fund of helping in the community, expecting that "what goes around comes around" (Stack, 1974). The variable "expected effect on network" refers to the effect the agency expects that their intervention will have on the informal helping network.

The following section defines each type with comments, where relevant, from the literature on informal helping. Particularly significant characteristics based on the data summarized in Tables 9.3, 9.4, and 9.5 will be discussed and examples from the case studies included. Since our treatment of these tables is selective rather than exhaustive and since it would be cumbersome to relate each statement to the relevant table, the tables are presented only to provide supportive information and to facilitate comparisons across helper types on the individual variables.

Family and Friends

Despite the fact that family and friends are the most intimate and ubiquitous sources of help for all but the most isolated individuals (Sussman, 1965; Wellman, 1979a), few service agencies have developed conscious, well-thought-out ways of interacting with this form of helping. We found seven programs that were making an effort to identify these helpers and offer various forms of support to them. Four of these programs were for the elderly, one was for families, and two were in the general area of mental health.

In general, we found that programs that work with family and friends focus on what social network analysts call the *personal networks* of identified clients, that is, the total network of ties that one individual, such as Mrs. Jones in the illustration, has with others. The members of a personal network are often tied to each other as well as to the focal person by ties of kinship or friendship. These agencies might be involved with anyone in their client's support system who was providing or might be able to provide assistance. Thus, agencies often worked with an integrated system that might include neighbors, natural helpers, and role-related helpers as well as family and friends.

Among the family and friends, helping was generally based on the individual's commitment and motivation to help rather than on special skills or knowledge. Yet they were offering substantial assistance, ranging from socializing and checking in to see that everything was all right to home maintenance or intensive home nursing care. They were also important sources of advice and information about services.

Identification and recruitment of the helpers was not difficult since they were usually already involved with the client. Generally, the intervention by the agency was short-term and intended to reinforce existing relationships either by helping the individual better perceive or make use of his or her personal network or by helping the members of the network deal with a problem or crisis (e.g., illness, nursing home placement) facing the focal individual. The agency may help the focal individual work out with members of the network a sharing of tasks that will allow the individual to weather a short- or long-term limitation in functioning. For example, a plan might be worked out among several friends for one to do grocery shopping while another provides transportation to medical appointments. This is particularly crucial when one or two members of a network feel overburdened and unable to continue helping; often they are able to continue a positive relationship with the individual if others can be found to take over a few chores. In addition to mobilizing informal services, formal services may be provided with the specific purpose of supporting the informal helpers. For example, respite care, a visiting nurse, or homemaker services may be provided to an adult child caring for a disabled parent in their home. In one case, the program provided training to helpers to make their interactions more supportive to members of their personal network.

Neighbors

The concept of neighbors or neighborhood is often ambiguous because it can refer to several different levels of social organization (Keller, 1968). For a number of people, the neighborhood is seen primarily as their own block; on this block are the people they know personally and with whom they are most likely to exchange help. For planning or political purposes, however, a neighborhood is usually considerably larger and may encompass several square miles. The programs in our sample worked with neighborhoods at both levels of size and complexity.

Those agencies that worked with the smaller-scale neighborhood often used a personal network approach, including neighbors as part of the personal networks of their clients. While some neighbors may come to be defined as friends, in general the relationship combines a high level of knowledge about many aspects of one another's lives with a fairly low level of involvement (Keller, 1968). Unlike with family and friends, there are generally more defined limits on the forms of helping that are appropriate to ask for and offer (Litwak, 1978).

The programs we studied found that people sometimes need a broker to go to neighbors and ask for help. Often simply letting it be known that a neighbor needs help is sufficient to produce offers of assistance. An elderly man, for example, was reluctant to ask new, young neighbors (he described them as "hippies") for help with lawn mowing. A worker was able to make an arrangement whereby a young neighbor was able to borrow the lawn mower in exchange for mowing the elderly man's lawn. Brokerage does not always go so smoothly, of course. One program matched a person who wanted to grow a garden and was willing to share the produce with an elderly neighbor who had a large backyard. The erstwhile gardener managed to plow up the yard but did nothing else, leaving the owner with a yard full of mud and weeds! The agency was able to enlist the help of other neighbors to clean up the mess.

For agencies working with the larger-scale neighborhood, the goal of agency intervention was usually to increase the connections among neighbors. Several programs were able to organize groups to provide home repairs or transportation services to "neighbors" who might not have been previously known to the helpers but did reside in the same, commonly identified neighborhood. In other cases, they supported or helped develop block or neighborhood associations, as well as block watches for crime prevention. Some programs have found that neighborly ties that have weakened over time can be revived. Elderly people in a stable neighborhood, for example, may have associated with many of their neighbors when their children were at home but lost contact once the children grew up and moved away. Often just the provision of any opportunity to interact again is enough to revive these old acquaintances. A more unusual example is a program for deinstitutionalized mental patients and mentally retarded persons that is informally working with a volunteer-run cafe in the community. An important neighborhood gathering spot, the cafe was discovered to be dealing very sensitively with those mental health clients who frequented it, so the program began to develop more ways to integrate its clients into the activities of the cafe's patrons.

Natural Helpers

While we are almost all involved in helping and receiving help from others, there are some people for whom this is a more central role in their lives or who are simply better at it than most of us. They are people turned to by many others for aid and advice, either for general problems or for specific areas in which they are felt to have expertise. These are the people we have termed *natural helpers* or *central figures* (Collins & Pancoast, 1976). For the natural helpers in our sample, helping was less based on the mutuality of neighbors or the obligations of kinship or of long-standing friendship and more on a personal motivation to help others and natural helping skills which earned them the respect and confidence of those with whom they interacted.

Some natural helpers held positions of community leadership. For example, one natural helper in a small New England town was elected president of the Senior Council. In addition to her official duties, this position enabled her to extend her helping activities to more of the town's elderly and to adult children who were primary caregivers for their elderly parents. Others prefer to confine their helping activities to a circle of relatives, friends, and neighbors. One such natural helper provided free car repair services while, at the same time, teaching teenagers how to fix cars. Another provided health and child care advice and services to a number of young mothers in her neighborhood.

While many natural helpers did not feel they were doing anything special, members of their network were usually aware that the helpers were exceptional people. One helper said, "My husband calls me the community mother," but she, like other helpers, denied that she was doing anything extraordinary (see also Snyder, 1976). These helpers tended to have long-term relationships with those they helped and with the agency. They usually were of the same socioeconomic status as those they helped and had similar problems, but they exhibited superior coping abilities.

The agencies working with natural helpers were generally seeking to reinforce the helpers' activities by providing social, emotional, and material resources and by linking appropriate formal services to the informal ones. Agencies in our sample worked with the natural helpers in a variety of roles. Some developed defined roles for them within the agency program, although their manner of working was usually informal and unpaid. These included block workers delivering senior activity calendars to the elderly on their block, lay therapists within a community mental health agency, and housing facilitators who were resources for information about housing rehabilitation within their neighborhoods. Although in these cases not everyone who filled these roles could be classified as a natural helper, the agency's emphasis was on recruiting natural helpers, who were encouraged to continue helping within their own networks. Other agencies worked with natural helpers in a way that recognized their abilities without creating a new role for them by providing them with information about programs, consulting with them about difficult "cases," helping them develop support groups, and accepting referrals of cases that needed professional attention.

Role-related Helpers

While these people may also have the interpersonal skills that are typical of the natural helper, they come to the attention of the agency because of an influential role they hold in the community. Some fill roles such as a minister or public health nurse that are considered helping roles. Others have a position that locates them at a crossroads where they are likely to be turned to for help because of their visibility. These include storekeepers, postmasters, teachers, and managers of residential hotels.

Within our sample, role-related helpers were often active on agency-sponsored task forces, boards, and other committees concerned with improving services or generally upgrading an area. Other examples from our survey included a postmistress in a small town who allowed the post office to become the main social center; a pharmacist who helped older people pay their bills and always had a pot of coffee on; an herbalist in a rural area; and a fundamentalist minister on an Indian reservation who developed a youth center within the church and was one of the primary sources of transportation for an isolated community.

This was the only category of helper in which men were in the majority, perhaps because most of the occupations involved are largely male-dominated. Within their agency-defined helping role, they were less likely to provide friendship and emotional support than advice, referral, and some services.

Some programs have tried to create ongoing links with such helpers to enable the helper to become a source of information and referral; they also often work to make the institutions and businesses involved more responsive to the needs of their clients. For example, pharmacies and restaurants can be encouraged to offer delivery service and banks to have quicker service for the handicapped, who find it difficult to wait in line.

People with Similar Problems

This was the most common type of helping we found in our sample, although it is not the most common form of helping in the general population (Lieberman & Mullan, 1978). A survey in California (Field Research Corporation, 1979) found that while 39 percent of those interviewed confided in a friend in times of emotional stress, only 9 percent sought out others with similar problems. Since our survey was based on informal helpers who were known to and involved with formal services, the relatively large number of mutal-aid activities in the sample probably reflects the greater attention that has been paid to this form of helping than to the other types by professionals.

This is in some ways the most "artifical" form of helping described here in that it was the only form which seldom occurred in the homes of those involved and in which short-term returns were expected by the participants. Helpers with similar problems sometimes helped each other within the context of self-help groups, including groups for abused women, widows, caregivers to the elderly, and parents of young children. Casual drop-in contacts fostered by a senior center or a program providing temporary child care were another basis for mutual aid in the programs we sampled. One-to-one relationships were a third type. Examples include parents of mentally retarded children who were matched with parents who had just found out their child was retarded and who provided support and information on a family-to-family basis. In another case, a physically disabled person who was good at repairing wheelchairs taught the skill to other disabled persons.

Much of the interaction among such groups in our sample involved friendship and the pleasures of associating with similar people as much as the solution of problems. The participants needed to have no prior experience helping others and their ongoing relationships with others were not important to the helping process. While shared experience was the main qualification for helpfulness, a number of the examples in this category involved statuses rather than specific problems. For example, being old or having young children gave people something in common but was not treated as a "problem."

The agencies generally developed a mutual-aid approach in one of three ways. Some were approached by an individual or small groups who had already decided to organize a mutual-aid program and knew that they needed agency resources in order to attract more members and make their effort succeed. For example, mothers who met when their retarded children were enrolled in the same preschool decided they would like to help parents of newly diagnosed retarded children. They asked the Association for Retarded Citizens to help them publicize their program, give them training, and match the new parents to the experienced ones. In other cases, workers in the agency became aware of people with similar problems in the course of other activities and suggested to them that they might be able to help each other. One program became aware of a number of agoraphobics in the community and was able to link them together into a mutual-aid network. Finally, some programs created settings where people with mutual interests could meet one another and form their own friendships. A senior center serving an inner-city population consisting largely of elderly men introduced them to one another in the center and encouraged them to expand the contact into a friendship. The involvement of the agency in ongoing support of mutual-aid groups varied widely, from very minimal support to continued direction of the effort.

Volunteers

Volunteers are probably the most familiar type of informal helper to most professionals. This form of help is usually stranger-to-stranger and channeled through a formal organization. Of all the forms of helping described here, it is the most likely to involve inequality of status between the helper and recipient—both in terms of socioeconomic status and of general coping ability. There is also an unequal exchange relationship, with the volunteer clearly defined as the helper. While a mutual relationship may develop, and indeed is often encouraged by these agencies, it is not usually part of the standard volunteer role. Because there was already a rich body of literature on volunteerism, we chose only examples in which the volunteer was encouraged by the agency to be as "natural" as possible—to use his or her own personal skills and network on behalf of a client or group of clients and to develop a relationship based, as far as possible, on the model of a naturally occurring friendship.

This was the only type of help in which women predominated,

probably reflecting the greater numbers of women who have time for extensive volunteer activities. Motivation in terms of a willingness to help and concern for the problems was a more important personal characteristic than helping skills or ongoing relationships. Problem-solving was the most common helping activity.

This type of helping requires the heaviest input of professional assistance to initiate and sustain. Recruitment of volunteers is a constant effort. In some cases the volunteers received training about the special needs of a particular target population or about formal service that might be useful, but they were expected to carry on their helping activities in their own or the client's territory and with a minimum of supervision. This type of helping was found most often in programs dealing with persons who would be least likely to have flourishing networks of their own: the isolated elderly, child abusers, the developmentally disabled, and the chronically mentally ill. Since work with such populations can be emotionally draining, the volunteers frequently needed rewards external to the helping relationship in order to maintain their motivation. To deal with this problem, many programs set up support groups for the volunteers. In many cases these became a form of mutual aid for the participants, meeting needs that had little to do with the ostensible purpose of the contact.

In the end, the agencies hoped that the volunteers would function rather like the natural network of family, friends, and neighbors that these individuals were lacking. In time, many do become friends and develop relationships that go beyond the original volunteer role.

Conclusion

It is clear from the descriptions of the six helper types that they differ significantly in the personal attributes of the helpers and in the neighborhood context and content of their helping activities. These factors in turn influence the approach an agency can take in working with them. If agencies are aware both of the wide range of informal helpers who can be identified and the unique strengths and limitations of each, they will be better able to develop effective partnerships with the informal system. For example, a program for the elderly based in a neighborhood would do well to consider encouraging neighbors to help out those nearby rather than organizing volunteers to be linked to local elderly that they may not know. The latter requires more staff time devoted to recruiting and supporting the volunteer and does not build on the strength of existing relationships. On the other hand, if the elderly person is fearful of her neighbors, lacks social skills, cannot reciprocate for neighborly services, or has problems such as widowhood not shared by her neighbors, a volunteer or a person with similar problems might be a more appropriate helper.

In designing the study, the six helper types were derived from the interactions of four characteristics assumed by the researchers to be important features of informal helping: preexisting ties, locality-based ties, quality of exchange, and centrality of role (see Table 9.2). Analysis of our findings shows that the above characteristics could be effectively used to distinguish helper types from one another and that these characteristics did affect the way agencies could work with helpers. Thus our initial assumptions proved accurate. We would like to focus now on one of these characteristics in detail because it seemed especially important in terms of its effect on agency–helper relationships.

A critical dimension of informal helping is the origin of the relationship—whether it is preexisting or created by the agency (see Table 9.2). In the first category, which includes family and friends, neighbors, natural helpers, and role-related helpers, the helping relationships are *embedded* in ongoing networks of relationships among people who share other bases for relating—kinship, residential proximity, membership in clubs or churches, patronage of the same stores and institutions. The second category consists of people with similar problems and volunteers whose helping relationships are *created*, usually by a formal agency, to meet a specific need. Examples of working with agency-created ties were included because they were attempts by the agencies to develop an informal helping system for people or problems for whom systems either did not exist or were not effective. These created helping ties are those most commonly recognized by formal service agencies, partly due to the nature of their clients; informal systems that function well have little need of agency intervention.

There are a number of contrasts between the two categories of helpers that are important for professionals to understand if they are to work productively with them. In many ways the strengths of one category of helping are the weaknesses of the other.

Embedded helping relationships are likely to be meeting basic needs—material assistance, health care, protective services—and to be long-term relationships with a heavy investment of time, responsibility, and concern. They require few agency resources to be initiated or maintained. They are highly individualized and sensitive to the preferences of the participants. They are extremely flexible, reflecting what Diana Trilling has called "the endless improvisation of mutuality" (Harlow, 1979, p. 48).

On the other hand, embedded relationships help fewer people per helper. They are dependent on existing relationships and therefore on opportunities for such relationships to develop. Although we found such helpers in every kind of setting from the most rural to the most urban, some would argue that the opportunities for developing and sustaining such relationships are lessening due to mobility, changes in family size, structure, and work roles. The second implication of embeddedness is that the helping relationship is affected by the other relationships in the network and by the values, mores, and knowledge of the participants. Help may be given only to certain favored persons (e.g., of the same race or religion) or heavy conditions may be attached. Because the relationships are highly idiosyncratic, agencies that want to relate to them must be willing to be very flexible and to spend some time at the outset identifying the helpers and understanding the culture of the particular network or neighborhood.

Created relationships present the opportunity for people to develop new helping roles, skills, and values. This makes them especially useful for people who are isolated and do not have flourishing networks. Their initiation can be directed by the agency and hence can be better targeted on the needs and clients the agency is most concerned to serve. They are also more specialized and therefore more compatible with specialized formal services. They are more open and egalitarian than embedded relationships in the sense that a willingness to help or participate is the only requirement for helper status. This type of helping is relatively easy for agencies to link up with since helpers can be recruited by advertisement, by referral, or from the client group.

Created helping relationships also have drawbacks, however. They require a fairly heavy investment of agency resources in order to initiate and sustain them. The helping relationships tend to be shorter in duration than embedded ones and involve fewer basic services and more short-term problem solving. The agency is probably more able to impose a created helping relationship on a recipient. This may have negative consequences for the persons being helped, who may find the relationship less satisfactory than one they have initiated and feel they have either "earned" by past services or can repay at a future time. As R.A. Parker has said, "If one turns to the recipients of tending services it is instructive to consider what kinds of terms they are prepared to accept for *being* helped. In some ways acts of giving are less problematic than acts of receiving" (Parker, 1980, p. 21).

These contrasts are posed to suggest how one dimension of informal helping can suggest guidelines for planning future research and intervention programs rather than to argue that one form of informal helping is better than another. The most common pattern we found among our sample was a mixed model in which agencies were relating to several different types of informal helpers and providing formal services as well. This model seemed to most closely mirror the variety and spontaneity found in informal helping activities. It also permitted a finely calibrated meshing of what services the informal sector could provide and what needed to be provided under formal auspices. Where the agency did not provide formal services directly, they were very active in coordinating the efforts of other formal services and those of the informal helpers.

The list of informal helping patterns we have described is probably incomplete. Human-service and mental-health professionals are just beginning to recognize the value and importance of informal caring for formal services, and as they continue to explore additional ways to provide roles for informal helpers, other patterns of informal helping are likely to emerge as relevant. The task is one of changing our perceptions to broaden our appreciation and awareness of the ways people can and do help each other.

10

The Interface among Religion, Religious Support Systems, and Mental Health

Kenneth I. Pargament

In recent years, mental health professionals and social scientists have attempted to develop a greater understanding of the role social support plays in the enhancement of mental health status. Toward this end, the impact of social support systems such as the family, neighborhoods, work relationships, and self-help groups on the psychological and social well-being of people has been documented. Relatively neglected in these examinations have been the roles of religion and, more specifically, religious support systems in assisting individuals to deal with the events, problems, and crises that arise in daily living.

The importance of religion in today's world is frequently brought to public attention through dramatic events such as the Jonestown tragedy, brainwashing experiences associated with cults, and the rise of Islamic fundamentalism. Less dramatic but more profound are the day-to-day religious involvements and religious experiences of people. A few statistics will help illustrate this point:

- As of 1977, it was estimated that 62 percent of Americans held formal membership in a church or synagogue (Jacquet, 1977).
- A 1978 Gallup Opinion Index indicated that 83 percent of Americans received religious training as children (Gallup, 1978).

The author would like to thank the clergy and students who assisted him in gathering much of the information reported in this chapter. Particular thanks go to Ms. Susan Snyder for her valuable insights and assistance in collecting and organizing this material, to Dr. Paul Schubert from the Psychological Studies and Consultation Program of Detroit for his assistance in locating sources of information, and to Rev. Vaughn Maatman and Rev. Blair Raum for their help in stimulating the development and form of the chapter.

- Sixty percent of Americans pray to God at least once a day; 52 percent of Americans state that religion is very important in their lives (Gallup, 1978).
- Surveys in 1968 indicated that 98 percent of Americans reported that they believe in God, 85 percent believe in heaven, and 73 percent believe in life after death. A later survey indicated that 53 percent of Americans believe in the existence of the devil (Rosten, 1975).

Clearly, religion represents a meaningful personal and social force in the lives of many Americans.

In this chapter, the implications of religion for the psychosocial well-being of people will be examined critically. Particular attention will be paid to the relationship and significance of religiously sponsored support programs to mental health. Specific programs will be presented and discussed not necessarily for their "uniqueness" but as examples utilized to underscore the variety of roles played by religious support systems. In addition, avenues leading to a more productive interface between members of religious, mental health, and social science communities will be explored.

Religion and Mental Health: Definitional Issues

As a prelude to this discussion, it is necessary to consider the meaning of the concepts "religion" and "mental health." Each of these concepts often suggests different meanings to different people. For example, some define religion primarily as a social institutional experience. For others, religion is defined as personal beliefs regarding one's relationship to God, other people, and the unknown. Others define religion more generally as an encompassing framework for approaching all aspects of life, one which involves values, beliefs, and behaviors (Glock & Stark, 1965). Mental health has also been defined in a variety of ways, ranging from the absence of psychopathology, to attitudes, values, and beliefs about oneself, others, and the world, to a set of coping skills for dealing effectively with the events in one's life (Jahoda, 1958; Allport, 1961).

Comparing the concepts, religion focuses on a set of questions regarding the meaning of life, the existence and nature of God, and the mysteries of the world, which fall outside of what is usually considered to be the domain of mental health. Often overlooked, however, are the *common concerns* embodied by both concepts. Defined as individual processes, religion and mental health alike suggest practices of, rules for, and beliefs about the "good life." At the institutional level, both religious and mental-health systems are concerned with activities for stimulating and enhancing these practices, rules, and beliefs. In short, religion and mental health, as concepts and systems, share an interest in the well-being of people.

This discussion suggests that religion and mental health should not be treated as independent concepts. Yet in numerous articles that have examined the contribution of religion or religious systems to individual mental health, mental health has been defined as an entity very much separate from religion. In this process, the efficacy of religion is determined by the degree to which it contributes or fails to contribute to the individual's mental health status. Thus mental health becomes a primary value and religion becomes a secondary value.

Religion and mental health may be viewed more productively as *related* expressions intrinsic to an individual's philosophy and approach to life. From this latter perspective, efforts addressed toward an individual's religious development implicitly carry meaning for his or her mental health status. Similarly, efforts directed at improving the mental health of an individual implicitly carry meaning for his or her religious orientation. More practically, it follows that mental health professionals and members of religious communities have an interest in the programs and activities implemented by each other. How these groups may share their interests in a productive manner will be considered shortly.

The Unique Role of Religion in American Society

Religious institutions are in a unique position to affect the lives of a large proportion of Americans. Haugk (1976) and the Report of the President's Commission on Mental Health's Task Panel on Community Support Systems (1978b) cite a number of factors contributing to the special status of religion. These include the large number of clergy in the United States, many of whom have received specialized training in pastoral and counseling psychology; the large number of congregation members in the United States, representing a significant pool of helpers; the prominence and availability of religious groups and institutions within large and small communities; and the long tradition religious institutions and individuals have of providing human services. Finally, it is important to note that religious systems are able to marshal financial support for their activities. For example, in 1978 the Campaign for Human Development (CHD), sponsored by the United States Catholic Conference, collected over $8 million from local dioceses for its antipoverty programs (Campaign Report, 1978). In 1975, the Council of Jewish Federations provided local Jewish organizations (community centers, educational programs, family and children's services) with $95 million in funds (Council of Jewish Federation Report, 1977). These figures represent contributions from local congregation members and friends only. When one considers the budgets of church agencies receiving private and public monies, the figures become much larger. For example, in 1979 combined budgets of local Diocesan Catholic Charity agencies totaled over $500 million (National Conference on Catholic Charities, 1980).

Underlying the importance of religious institutions as a support system are their inherent accessibility to individuals and groups in need. For example, the right of clergy to reach out and help others is acknowledged by many. Clergy are seen as guiding figures responsive to the concerns of people. In addition, religious institutions are in a unique position to deal with people throughout the life span.

From birth to death, religion offers people a number of opportunities to affect others and to be affected themselves. Few individuals move through their lives without some involvement in religious rituals (e.g., baptism, Bar/Bat Mitzvah, church wedding, last rites). These rituals lend significance to major transitions within the life cycle. Moreover, the teachings implicit in the rituals and the social support accompanying their expression can assist people in preparing for and coping more effectively with significant life changes (Kaplan, 1976).

The Jewish custom of "shivah" illustrates this point. Within Judaism it is customary to visit with a family that has suffered the death of one of its members. During this seven-day period visitors pray with the family and console them in their grief. Talking about the deceased and emotional expression among the family members and visitors is encouraged. This custom serves important purposes. It provides the grieving family with an opportunity to begin the processes of ventilating their emotions, of reconciling themselves to their loss, and of reconstructing their lives. The supportive system in which this process occurs helps maintain the personal integrity of the family members as they experience their loss.

In a similar manner, general involvement in the regular activities of churches and synagogues (e.g., religious services, religious holidays, social/organizational activities) offers people opportunities for interpersonal support, a source of personal identity and meaning in the world, emotional expression, and the development of a set of attitudes and skills for dealing with their lives. From this perspective, churches and synagogues can be viewed, in part, as social support systems (Caplan & Killilea, 1976; Pargament, Tyler, & Steele, 1979).

The resources of religion do not simply duplicate those of the mental health system. Mental health professionals, by and large, do not share the access of clergy and religious groups to many people in need of help. In addition, as Veroff, Douvan, and Kulka (1976) have noted, many Americans state a preference to seek help from clergy rather than from other professionals when faced with problems. Furthermore, they report that there is less stigma in using these services than those offered by other professionals.

To summarize the preceding discussion, the personpower of religious communities, financial resources of religious systems, religions' tradition of helping activities, and natural access of religious institutions to a large population place it in a *unique* position to facilitate personal and social well-being. Toward this end, religion brings to bear a wide range of values, beliefs, and attitudes expressed through numerous programs, rituals, holidays, and involvements in congregational activities. This discussion then has underscored the multifaceted nature and use of religious resources. In the following section, religious support programs will be examined in more detail.

Religious Support Programs

Religiously based support programs, as described in this chapter, encompass institutional activities funded or implemented by religious groups which attempt to enhance the well-being of people. Admittedly, this definition includes many activities, only a sample of which can be reviewed in this chapter. To facilitate our presentation, the scope of religious support programs will be considered within the framework of the following questions: What are the goals of religious support programs? Who implements religious support programs? What are the elements of religious support programs? These questions should highlight some of the important issues raised by these programs and some of the essential differences among them.

Goals of Religious Support Programs

Religiously based support activities have been established to deal with a tremendous variety of problems and concerns experienced by individuals, groups, families, and social institutions. These programs generally address one of three goals: enhanced coping abilities of people facing problems in living, assistance to groups with limited psychosocial resources, and stimulation of social change.

Haugk (1976) has noted that a number of religious programs attempt to enhance the coping abilities of people and prevent the development of serious psychosocial impairment. Throughout the United States, religious institutions from a variety of denominations have developed programs aimed at marital enrichment, parental effectiveness, grief counseling, divorce recovery, coping with aging, and more general problems in living. Bushfield (1970), for example, describes a church-sponsored crisis counseling service in Los Angeles. The service is provided to the general community by trained lay congregation members and clergy through a telephone "Help Line."

Many religious support programs attempt to build the resources of groups with limited psychological, social, and physical assets. For example, religious groups operate a large number of institutions across the country for dependent and neglected children, the retarded, and the aged. Illustrative of other programs are the Kadima and Ezra Schools sponsored by a synagogue in Canada. These schools provide religious education to mentally retarded and learning-disabled students. At the same time, they contribute to the students' sense of personal efficacy and sense of belonging to the Jewish community. FISH, an international organization of Christian people, provides a variety of basic services to groups in need of assistance. Their services include reading to the blind, companionship for the elderly, transportation for shut-ins, and teenage–adult companionship. Pastoral counseling programs also address groups of people returning from institutions to the community and marginal individuals encountering serious problems in living.

Other religiously based programs, sponsored by all major religious denominations, seek broader social change. For example, Dignity, a national organization of gay Catholics, has as its goals the development of a more just theology within the Church, greater social acceptance within society, and an enhanced sense of self-acceptance and personal dignity among gay Catholics. Toward these ends, local chapters of Dignity engage in dialogue with religious and secular groups, provide hotline counseling services to other members, and promote supportive social activities. The Campaign for Human Development (CHD) provides financial support for hundreds of self-help projects that benefit members of the low-income community and attempt to change unfair institutions, laws, or policies (Campaign Report, 1978). For example, groups supported by CHD have engaged in social action efforts to promote better housing conditions, improved city services, and reduced racial tension.

Implementation of Religious Support Programs

Religious support programs have been initiated and sustained by groups at national, regional, and local congregational levels. Nationally based Catholic, Jewish, and Protestant organizations sponsor religiously based support programs, as illustrated by CHD. The major religious denominations also fund in part social services implemented by agencies at the local level. For example, Catholic Social Services, Lutheran Social Services, and Jewish Family Services agencies offer considerable social support, financial support, and mental health assistance to people throughout the country. While the services are physically separated from churches and synagogues and may employ mental health professionals with diverse religious backgrounds, attempts have been made to link some of these services more closely to their associated religious institutions and heritage. Greenberg (1978) states:

> Our Jewish Family and Children's Agencies are more Jewish than we think. But they are not as Jewish as we would like them to be—and we are hard at work exploring ways of enhancing their Jewish dimensions. Most important, we place high value on working cooperatively with all the other Jewish institutions which share our concern for the quality of Jewish communal life [p. 9].

At the local congregational level, many parish clergy are also integrally involved in the development of support activities. They may take on roles of individual counselor, marital and family counselor, group facilitator, and/or social change agent. Dominick (1970), for example, describes a program in which 1,300 clergy and seminarians are provided with some exposure to the problem of alcoholism. A smaller group of these people is trained to recognize and deal clinically with alcoholism among members of the parish and in the general community. Self (1980) discusses a model of pastoral action that facilitates the sense of community among members of local congregations. Pastors working from this approach attempt to enhance the flow of information, build reciprocal patterns of influence among groups within the congregation, and generally coordinate and pace the activities of the congregation. Roman Catholic clergy have been involved in a number of social change activities including prison reform action, advocacy programs for the Spanish-speaking community, and community forums focusing on reducing racism. In 1979, almost 90 percent of local Catholic charity agencies were involved in legislative lobbying (National Conference on Catholic Charities, 1980).

Recently, congregation members have become increasingly a part of religiously based support programs. As with the clergy, the problems members deal with and the roles they take vary. Several programs focus on the development of lay ministers within a congregation. The Stephen Series is one such particularly well-developed program (Haugk, 1978). It involves intense structured training of lay congregation members in areas including communication skills, crisis intervention, and the utilization of community resources, as well as skills in dealing with particular groups such as depressed, lonely, and older persons. These trained congregation members then act as a "caring team" reaching out to others within their church. The process is seen as an enriching one for the lay members themselves and for those they help. Lay people also participate in congregationally based sharing and self-help groups covering a wide variety of issues and concerns—marriage preparation, parental growth, divorce recovery, constructive retirement, and grief recovery (Clinebell, 1977).

A central issue underlying this discussion has to do with who can and cannot legitimately provide religious support services. The onus has fallen for the most part on clergy. As has been noted, clergy have a unique access to people in need. Often overlooked, however, is the unique set of problems clergy face in helping others (Lipman, 1978). For example, as part of the congregation, many clergy rely on those they help for continued employment, promotion, and career advancement. Clergy may also deal with those to whom they provided counseling assistance on a day-to-day basis concerning church matters. This can prove awkward to the clergy. More generally, clergy are faced with the often difficult task of integrating the different roles of teacher, leader, administrator, and counselor. Finally, clergy themselves may lack the support from other clergy and the congregation to sustain themselves and their work.

The growing number of lay members and lay ministers could serve as another pool of resources in the development of religious support programs. As Hester (1976) has noted, however, with the trend toward a growing professionalism in pastoral counseling activities, concerns have been voiced regarding the qualification of lay members and lay ministers to build and implement supportive programs.

Adding complexity to the issue is the question of whether mental health professionals are appropriate providers of support activities sponsored by religious groups. A clear resolution to the problem of who can and cannot provide religious support services has yet to emerge. This discussion, however, has underscored the fact that religious support programs come in all shapes and sizes and require different skills. In addition, potential providers of religious support services have different strengths and weaknesses. Both the nature of the support program and the resources, interests, and needs of the potential providers must be considered in selecting appropriate helpers. Conceivably, helpers from different groups (lay members, clergy, mental health professionals) could pool their resources in implementing particular programs. There are obstacles to this occurring, however, that we will discuss shortly.

Elements of Religious Support Programs

Not to be overlooked in considering religious support programs is the point that these activities are, in fact, religious. To some degree, implicitly or explicitly religiously based programs attempt to convey insights regarding the nature of the human condition, the relationship of people to God and each other, or, more generally, a set of values and practices that will be useful in dealing with life. Programs differ, however, in the elements they incorporate to reach these goals.

In particular, religious support programs vary in the degree to which they incorporate traditional overt religious practices (e.g., Bible reading, prayer, meditation) and consider basic religious questions (e.g., views of God, meaning of life, nature of the soul) in the supportive activities. On the one hand, some pastoral counselors try to separate their roles as pastors and as counselors. When involved in counseling, these individuals choose not to deal with religious doubts and concerns of their clients. In other support programs, formal religious elements are integrated into attempts to enhance the well-being of people. For example, Marriage Encounter, a popular national program in which couples examine their lives together over a weekend with the help of experienced couples and clergy, focuses on the couple's relationship with God as well as with each other. The COME (Congregation Organizing for Mission Endeavor) program, developed by Herbert Mayer in St. Louis, while involving elements of interpersonal support, illustrates a program deeply grounded in formal religious tradition. Based on his religious historical research, Mayer identifies five functions that must be balanced for optimal well-being: worship, nurture, study, witness, and service. Small groups within local congregations are formed and engage in activities designed to promote this balance.

Underlying the differences among these programs appear to be varying views of the essential elements of religious support programs. One position is expressed by Schwartz (1978), who states that involvement by the clergy in mental health services (e.g., psychotherapy, consultation) represents a "rich authentic ministry." Rev. Carl Bickel (1978) takes exception to this perspective, arguing that religious communities have interests, values, and traditions which are unique. Their programs should reflect these resources rather than mimic mental health services. This difference in perspectives has important implications for the interface between members of religious and mental health communities.

Interface between Religious and Mental Health Communities

Relations between members of religious and mental health communities have been characterized by miscommunication and mistrust. At the heart of this schism appear to be questions each group holds about the values and beliefs underlying the activities of the other group. Following Freud, some mental health professionals view religious beliefs as inadequate defenses against personal insecurity and anxiety. From this perspective religion is simply a crutch. Conversely, some members of religious communities view mental health professionals as preoccupied by the value of self-gratification. From this perspective the mental health system simply fosters self-indulgence.

Despite this miscommunication and mistrust, clergy and mental health professionals believe that the values and beliefs underlying various forms of religious expression are congruent with those values and beliefs underlying mental health activities. For instance, Clinebell (1970) maintains that vital churches and temples fulfill their mission by providing individuals with opportunities to develop a number of qualities: a sense of trust, a sense of belonging, a viable philosophy of life, a humanized view of people, experiences of transcendence, and support of individual, family, and societal growth and change. These attributes are consistent with characteristics often linked to positive mental health status (Jahoda, 1958; Smith, 1968). This discussion speaks to the need for an appreciation of areas of convergence as well as points of departure in the approaches of religious and mental health systems to those they serve.

Unfortunately, as Haugk (1976) has noted, many clergy and mental health professionals continue to hold inaccurate perceptions regarding other groups. Perpetuating these stereotypes is the fact that the two groups simply have little contact with each other, contact which might provide the opportunity for personal sharing of concerns and interests (Pargament, Steele, Mitchell, & Schlien, 1979).

Conflict between religious and mental health systems may be further exacerbated by the fact that those interactions that do take place are often unreciprocal. Carson (1976) surveyed approximately eighty community mental health centers regarding collaborative programs between the centers and local clergy. The vast majority of the programs involved use of the expertise of mental health center professionals to enhance the performance of clergy (e.g., education of clergy regarding alcoholism; case consultation; increased clergy awareness of and referrals to available mental health services). Commenting on this pattern of relationship, Bickel (1978) states:

> For decades there have been calls on all sides for a "dialogue between religion and mental health." What has resulted has been to a large extent a monologue in which the clerical and lay members of the religious community have sat at the feet of the mental health professionals. . . . In the struggle for power and recognized competence, the mental health professionals have won hands down [p. 1].

According to Bickel, the nonreciprocal process of interaction only perpetuates the mental health professional's view of the clergy as deficient in sophistication.

Several factors may be crucial to the establishment of mutually beneficial ties between religious and mental health communities. As a basis for entering into these relationships, each group should have some understanding of its own values, resources, and limitations and those of others. Underlying the formation and maintenance of a viable partnership must be a respect for one's own personal/professional integrity and autonomy and that of other groups. At the same time, similarities in values and approach of religious and mental health groups as well as differences need to be recognized.

A number of religiously based support programs have been developed which emphasize collaboration, reciprocal exchange, and the shared concerns of religious and mental health groups. Samaritan Centers, located in the Midwest, represent an innovation illustrative of this approach. The Centers are counseling agencies that focus on enhancing the well-being of the whole person—physical, mental, and spiritual. Housed in churches and accessible to community residents, the Centers are staffed by pastoral counselors and medical and mental health professionals who contribute their special skills as members of a team. Activities at the Centers include marital and family counseling, counseling to people facing life crises and problems in living, and consultation to local clergy. An interesting aspect of the program is the use of in-kind payment (e.g., services to the community) for individuals unable to afford the fee for help received at the Centers.

Religious and mental health professionals have also collaborated in community organization and social action programs. In Baltimore and

Milwaukee, clergy have linked with mental health and social service professionals as a basis for building programs that empower members of the general community (Biegel, 1978). The projects include an advocacy hotline, a neighborhood referral directory, and family communication workshops. In these endeavors, the activities of religious and mental health professionals are coordinated with each other rather than assimilated into each other. Thus, the autonomy of both groups working toward common goals is maintained.

There is considerable room for program development in which religious and mental health groups share their resources for the benefit of the wider community. For example, marginal community members (e.g., returning inmates from penal and mental institutions) represent an underserved group that might benefit from assistance by religious and mental health systems. By working in tandem on select problems, more efficient and more comprehensive supportive programs might be established.

Effectiveness of Religious Support Programs

Often overlooked in discussions of social support programs is a fundamental question: Do they work? As Weiss (1972) has noted, programs, be they mental health, educational, correctional, or religious, once established often develop a life of their own. Whether the program is indeed accomplishing its objectives or whether the program could be improved are questions that have gone unanswered for several reasons. Evaluations of the effectiveness of programs involve time and expense, which are often quite limited. Certain types of evaluations can intrude upon and interfere with the program itself. Finally, the personal sense of ownership and pride, essential to the development of a program, may limit openness to changes in the program once it has been established.

Nevertheless, whether or not support programs are achieving their goals remains an important question. With respect to religious support programs in particular, the question is one that religious groups and social scientists could consider together. In this direction, the critical task becomes one of developing methods of program evaluation that are relatively inexpensive and unobtrusive, yet maximally useful. While this sounds like a near-impossible task, researchers have made methodological advances that make evaluations of this type more feasible than in the past (Kiresuk & Sherman, 1968; Coursey, Specter, Murrell, & Hunt, 1977).

Evaluation researchers and developers of religious support programs could consider several relevant questions. Is the program reaching any or all of its stated goals? Is the program more effective with certain groups of participants than others? Are certain program leaders more effective in general than others? What aspects of the program are people finding most and least useful? What about the program should be modified? What about the program should remain the same? Answers to questions such as these could lead to the development of new religious support programs or useful modifications of ongoing programs. More generally, studies in this area could contribute to a greater understanding of the roles religious support programs play in the lives of people.

A similar set of questions could be raised about support programs established by mental health professionals. Studies of the comparative efficacy of these programs might assist people in selecting activities best suited to their needs. These studies could also point to similarities and differences between support programs developed by clergy and by mental health professionals. Furthermore, leaders of support programs could learn from the experiences of others engaged in supportive activities.

Conclusion

In this chapter, religion has been considered as a multifaceted personal and social force embodying resources that lend it a unique position in American society. Religiously based support programs have been critically examined as a potent form of religious expression, holding significant implications for the well-being of people.

The programs vary along several dimensions, including the problems they address, who implements them, the essential elements they incorporate, their interface with mental health concerns, and, presumably, their effectiveness. Although evaluative information is generally not available, it may be safe to say that religious support programs have an impact on many people. The nature of this impact and the processes by which religious support programs might be improved can be clarified only through systematic study and examination. Research in this area, conceived broadly and pragmatically, should become an integral part of future supportive activities.

Support programs might also be advanced by close ties between religious and mental health communities. As was noted, religious and mental health groups often work independently. At times this is certainly quite appropriate. In other instances, however, opportunities for exchanging unique resources for the ultimate benefit of the general community may be missed. The problems of marginal community members represent a case in point. By linking the skills and knowledge of mental health professionals with resources of the religious community, a more comprehensive and efficacious support system for this group might be developed.

Viable relations between religious and mental health groups must be based upon respect by each group of their own resources as well as the resources of the other. Binding clergy and mental health professionals more closely together is their shared concern for the welfare of people. Working toward this common goal in concert rather than antagonistically is a formidable challenge, but one which holds exciting implications for the well-being of individuals and their communities.

11

Senior Centers and Support Networks

Donald E. Gelfand and
Judy R. Gelfand

Current discussions of mental health and the elderly tend to focus either on formal mental health services or on the positive aspects of informal support networks. It is important, however, to recognize not only the strengths of informal supports but also their limitations. The possibility exists that some social networks may actually be part of the problems facing an older person. A critical examination of the informal-network approach to mental health must therefore include what the networks can be expected to accomplish, what they are unable to accomplish, and to what extent these informal support networks should, or can be, linked to the formal service delivery system.

In some instances the level of assistance required by older persons, especially those over age seventy-five, may place greater demands on the informal support networks than they are able to meet. At the point when the informal support networks falter, community agencies must be able to step into the breach if the older person is to receive the assistance required. Understanding what these agencies can accomplish requires clarity about the mental health needs of the elderly and the orientation of the organizations currently serving the needs of the aged.

After discussing the mental health needs of the elderly and the community support networks' ability to meet these needs, the chapter will concentrate on one service delivery system. Specifically, the focus will be on the development of multipurpose senior centers and our assumption that multipurpose senior centers have the potential to be an important component in meeting the mental health needs of older individuals. The intent of the discussion is to indicate how physical design and programming can help senior centers maximize this potential.

The Elderly and Mental Health

The social-network approach provides a framework for examining the mental health needs of older people. By social networks we mean "those individuals, groups, and parts of formal institutions which have meaning, actually or potentially for a person" (Swenson, 1979, p. 18). The network approach differentiates between weak and strong ties. As characterized by Mitchell (1969) and others, weak ties tend to be low in intensity, wide ranging, and larger in number than strong ties. Strong ties are fewer in number but higher in their intensity. Because they are often extensive, weak ties enable the older individual to maintain contact with others and engage in frequent social interactions. These interactions may help prevent the isolation that can often lead to mental health problems among the elderly. The information provided through weak ties should enable the older adults to ascertain what forms of assistance are available to meet their mental and physical health needs. An extensive number of weak ties may preclude the need for further referrals.

The existence of an extensive network of weak ties provides the elderly with opportunities for socializing and potential resources with which to deal with problems when they occur. Psychologically, the existence of a social network containing weak ties may be critical. Even if it is never mobilized, the existence of the network may foster a feeling of independence. This feeling of independence may stem from the fact that the older persons feel that they have resources they can draw upon, including resources that are not necessarily bound up with their family. Having a network of weak ties that can be activated fosters a continuing feeling of control over the environment, a sense that has been shown to be important to older people both in the community and in institutional settings such as nursing homes. While weak ties may foster a feeling of independence, strong ties are frequently vital for fulfilling the emotional needs of the older individual.

The reciprocal exchanges that often characterize strong ties allow for the development of the intense, primary relationships that Lowenthal (1968) has emphasized in her discussion of the confidant. These confidant relationships, although few in number, are high in intensity. In the confidant form of primary relationships, intimate and emotional content is emphasized rather than instrumental content. Without these strong ties, the "life review" process that Butler and Lewis (1977) have viewed as vital to the successful aging process may not take place. Thus both weak and strong ties are important for the mental health of the aging; moreover, the functional mental health problems that are often assumed to be characteristic of aging are often related to the isolation that characterized the attenuated social networks of many older individuals.

Informal Support Networks for the Aged

At present, the existing community support networks available to the elderly appear to be in a state of transition, in terms of both shape and quantity. The research of Cantor (1979) in New York, Bengtson (1979) in California, and Guttmann (1979) in the Baltimore–Washington area indicates the reliance of white, black, and Hispanic elderly on family members and friends to provide assistance. Assistance is more difficult to provide, however, as people become more geographically distant and live outside of family units. In 1976, 14 percent of the men and 38 percent of the women over age sixty-five were living alone (Glick, 1979), and many of these individuals were living at a substantial distance from their children (Mindel, 1979). While not necessarily resulting in a discontinuation of contact between the older persons and their children, separate residences and geographic distances do mean a reduction in the availability of personal assistance for older persons from family members.

Many older persons choose to live independently. Independent living by older persons is also likely to become more common among many ethnic and minority groups as adult children move to new communities in their quest for social mobility. Independent living for older adults is also a cultural preference among groups such as Mexican-Americans, even if it is not always possible for the aged relative (Crouch, 1972; Cuellar, 1978). Older adults may thus continue to have strong relationships with their adult children, but these relationships may primarily involve "intimacy at a distance" (Jackson, 1971). This pattern of separation between elderly and their children means that community support networks, neighbors, and friends will become increasingly important elements of the older person's life.

While these friends and neighbors can be very supportive, they may not be completely able to replace the assistance provided by family members who are now living at a distance. Friends and neighbors of the older person may also be older individuals who are afflicted with chronic illnesses, low income, and other personal deficits that make it difficult for them to provide assistance to others. Thus, as discussed below, the elderly need elements of both informal and formal support. To be most effective, support systems, informal and formal, should be linked to each other. The senior center provides a unique vehicle to help create such linkages.

Spurred on by funds made available under the Older Americans Act, communities have developed extensive services for the elderly. Older persons still utilize mental health centers in only limited numbers. Fortunately, nutrition programs, legal services, specialized transportation systems, social services, friendly visiting, adult day care, and senior centers appear to have escaped the stigma that many older persons place on mental health programs. A question facing service providers is the relative importance of this formal network of services and the informal networks in the lives of the elderly.

Using Litwak's (1979) approach, we can examine the degree to which informal support networks are capable of meeting the needs of the older person. The primary variables in Litwak's model are proximity, long-term commitment, and the amount of equipment or degree of expertise required to perform the service.

A friend or family member may undertake to escort an older person to a health clinic, even if they live in another neighborhood. This form of aid does not require any long-term commitment, although the friend or family member may drive a considerable distance to escort the person to the appointment. On the other hand, day-to-day assistance in bathing, eating, and dressing requires that the helper live in close proximity to the older person and express a long-term commitment. Neither proximity nor commitment can adequately compensate for the lack of equipment or expertise required to competently carry out the skilled nursing care that may be needed by a seriously ill older adult.

In addition to lack of expertise, other factors may make it difficult for the older person to receive intensive assistance. First, as Litwak notes, there are now fewer individuals in household units available to provide assistance to the older person. Second, members of kinship units outside of the nuclear family are not usually living in the immediate vicinity. Third, neighborhoods are now characterized by individuals whose permanent residence in the area cannot be guaranteed, and this impermanence will affect their willingness to make long-term commitments. Even good friends with a strong attachment to the neighborhood may have limited resources in terms of both time and money and may hesitate in making their commitments open-ended (Litwak, 1979).

In sum, while the neighbors of the older person are best equipped to handle forms of assistance that require proximity, these individuals may hesitate about undertaking assistance that requires long-term commitment or extensive skills. Among family and friends who do not live in the immediate area, proximity, long-term commitment, and skills may all be factors inhibiting the assistance they can provide older friends or relatives. Money management or even nursing care may be undertaken by family members or friends for a limited period, but the "hands on" that is required when an individual needs help with personal care such as bathing may be beyond what neighbors, family, and friends are willing to provide.

Residential Patterns and Informal Support Networks

Much of the research on informal support networks and the elderly has been based on examination of inner-city communities such as Cleveland and New York, where high-density residential areas prevail. As the American population "ages" within the next fifty years, we should expect that older individuals will become a larger component of suburban areas. The suburban population already accounts for two-thirds of the population in metropolitan areas. In 1979, there were already 3,493,000 household heads over age sixty-five living in suburban parts of the fifty largest metropolitan areas of the United States as opposed to 3,774,000 living in the central cities (Gutowski & Feild, 1979).

We thus have two expectations about the living situations of the aged: (1) There will be larger numbers of older people living by themselves, and (2) larger numbers of older individuals will be living in suburban communities. It is also important to recognize that, not only will these future elderly be living in different ecological arrangements than their predecessors, but their socioeconomic status should be more favorable. The next cohort of older adults will possess higher educational levels than today's aged and a larger and more secure income.

It is not yet clear whether the pattern of informal support networks that has been found to characterize inner-city neighborhoods will be found in other communities. Italian-American males in Columbia, Maryland, were not highly involved with their communities, and it remains to be seen whether the involvement of these middle-aged men will increase as they age (Gelfand & Fandetti, 1980). Gabriel (1973), examining ethnic communities in Rhode Island, also found a diminution of traditional values stressing interdependence among individuals who had migrated to suburban areas. With only limited literature available, we can assume that suburban communities will be characterized by relationships that stress weak ties, and that the lack of strong ties will make it difficult for older adults to fulfill their needs for intimates and a confidant within the local community. Given these difficulties it is important to look at other institutions in American society that may be able to provide an opportunity for the older individual to develop both strong and weak ties.

Voluntary Associations and Support Networks

One of the major social institutions that may be able to fill the gaps created by changes in the role of the family, community, and church in American society is the voluntary association. Studies of voluntary organizations have indicated a low degree of membership by the elderly. These low membership figures may, however, reflect the high proportion of low-income individuals among the present cohort of elderly, since higher-income individuals have always been more active in voluntary organizations. Older individuals who maintain membership in voluntary organizations are most likely to belong to church groups, fraternal associations, and veterans' organizations. The lessened membership in sport groups and professional or work-related organizations is related to loss of work roles after retirement and physical changes.

In an analysis of social class and voluntary association membership, Trela (1976) has noted that most older individuals belong to non-age-graded organizations. Higher-class individuals are more likely to join organizations in their later years than are their lower-class counterparts. These organizations are utilized to replace the loss of social relationships in work or professional groups. Because of the changes in their life, middle-income retirees tend to join new organizations that are age-graded. These new voluntary association memberships may serve as important links to the community, enabling the older person to maintain involvement in local activities. Trela hypothesized that these "voluntary associations can be a vehicle for delivering services, a hospitable social environment where new friendships are made, a means for pursuing common interests, and a context where older people can be socialized formally and informally about age related roles" (1976, p. 202).

Voluntary associations have the potential to foster incipient community support networks. In recent years as the network of organizations serving the aged has begun to expand, a number of service-delivery entities have become prominent. One of the most important is the multipurpose senior center, which has many of the characteristics of voluntary associations. These centers have not always been oriented toward being a major element in the community support network of older persons. In the remainder of this chapter the focus will be on the manner in which the multipurpose senior center can be developed and programs formulated to assist it in becoming a "focal point" for the support networks that are vital to the mental health of older adults.

Multipurpose Senior Centers

Although the Older Americans Act was passed by Congress in 1965, senior centers were first mentioned in the 1973 amendments to the act and major funding for the centers did not begin until 1976. In the 1978 amendments to the Older Americans Act, Title III mandated that local area plans for services in aging "designate, where feasible, a focal point for comprehensive service delivery in each community to encourage the maximum collocation and coordination of services for older individuals, and give special consideration to designating multipurpose senior centers as such focal points" (Older Americans Act of 1978, Sec. 306 (a) (3)).

The National Institute of Senior Centers (NISC) defines a senior center as "a community focal point on aging where older persons come together for services and activities which enhance their dignity, support their independence, and encourage their involvement in and with the community" (National Council on the Aging, 1975).

Senior centers offer a variety of services and activities in such areas as education, health, nutrition, social work, employment, recreation, and creative arts. Because of their holistic approach, senior centers can also provide individuals with a sense of belonging and security, improved self-image, and general integration into the community.

Facilities that are labeled senior centers vary in both their physical size and program components. Small senior centers often come close to approximating social clubs and may be located in churches or other existing community settings. Larger senior centers may be housed in a variety of "recycled" buildings that were formerly used as schools or firehouses. As their physical space increases, centers are able to offer more varied services, including both health and mental health programs. These centers thus begin to fall under the rubric of the multipurpose senior center. The model of the larger multipurpose center will be used throughout this chapter.

By participating in the activities of a senior center, older persons may be able to enhance their sense of belonging in the community. Besides the effects of its own programming, the senior center can help to foster informal support networks and what can be termed "quasiformal" networks. The senior center cannot expect, however, to meet all of the needs of the older person, but by paying attention to the needs of its members, senior center staff can ensure that the center serves as a linkage to existing informal and formal support systems. Before turning to all of these potential functions of a center, it is worthwhile briefly to consider the manner in which the physical design of a senior center can influence the development of informal support networks for older people.

In urban and suburban areas, ecological arrangements or transportation problems often make it difficult for older persons to meet and chat. The front entry lounge of a senior center can thus become an important meeting place. In this space older persons can meet new people and renew or extend their social network. For individuals who are not inclined to become actively involved with others, the front lounge offers them the opportunity to set their own pace for joining in center activities.

While the front entry lounge is of primary importance, it is also vital to provide small spaces where individuals can sit and converse. In these areas, discussions of personal matters can go on in an atmosphere devoid of any "fish bowl" feeling. The need for privacy is usually considered in formal counseling programs, but the need of individual center members for privacy and intimacy can often be overlooked.

Engaging in Center Activities

Joining and Belonging

Planning sophisticated approaches to activities that foster positive mental health among seniors will not be fruitful unless the center is first able to foster an interest among seniors in using its facilities. An older person entering a senior center for the first time may be brought by a center member who can act as host. An individual who enters with a member at least has a tie to one other person in the center. Individuals arriving alone may feel isolated in the middle of a large group of people. Some older persons coming to a center may be in the process of rebuilding a network to replace one that has been lost through deaths or moving. For this individual, the importance of the center "greeter" or receptionist cannot be overstressed. The "greeter" is part of the connection between the center and the larger community. If the greeter makes positive contact and helps the new individual feel welcome, the potential increases for the center to serve as a catalyst for the creation of new or expanded social networks.

Having formal membership helps the individual to feel that he or she belongs to a significant organization. A membership card in an organization can be of great importance to a person who has retired from a variety of work-related groups. The card can become an important part of the older person's identity even if he or she is not particularly involved in the activities at a senior center.

Confidant Relationships

Providing space for intimate conversation is important but does not guarantee that personal interactions will occur or that vital primary confidant relationships will develop. Eighty-four percent of the senior center members polled in a 1975 NISC report (National Council on the Aging, 1975) indicated that they had a confidant and that 49 percent of these confidants were also center members. It is impossible to determine whether these confidant relationships existed prior to these individuals' becoming center members, but we should not ignore the possibility of the center serving as a medium for the growth of confidant relationships.

Bley and colleagues (1973) argue that older persons come to a center to establish "secondary relationships" through general group affiliation, not to substitute for lost primary relationships. The need for secondary relationships can easily be met through centers that provide numerous opportunities for individuals to take part in group activities and make new acquaintances. Few centers offer many opportunities for the types of interaction that will develop into primary relationships. It is difficult to say at this point whether there is any specific programming that can be utilized to encourage the development of primary relationships, which often occur spontaneously. If staff are warm and sharing with feelings, this attitude may be communicated to members and adopted as a *modus operandi*.

Activities and Roles

Besides providing a sense of belonging, senior centers can help to foster meaningful roles for older persons feeling a loss of self-esteem. New roles can be developing through creative skills such as painting or through participating with volunteer programs in the center or in the community. Cuellar (1978) provides an exciting example of how older Mexican-Americans developed self-esteem through poetry workshops in a senior center. Apart from the activities themselves, these groups provide individuals with an opportunity to meet others with similar interests. Some of these contacts will develop into casual acquaintances, others into friendships, and possibly some into confidant relationships.

As these contacts increase and are combined with classes and discussion groups, the depression and poor self-image that characterize many people may begin to lessen.

Intergenerational Programming

Sharing with peers has obvious benefits in terms of the common life experiences of a particular age cohort. Age-segregated groups may maximize the potential for strong ties, but age-integrated activities may foster the development of important weak ties. As an age-segregated entity, the senior center must make special efforts to incorporate intergenerational programming into its activities. The key to successful intergenerational programs is allowing seniors to have some control over when and how they interact with younger age groups. In senior centers, specific opportunities can be developed for intergenerational activities.

These activities can flow in two directions. In one instance the senior is in the helping role and in the second instance the senior receives help. Seniors can provide a special program in a school setting or tutor students. In other instances a college student may volunteer to help seniors with shopping or letter writing. In both of these cases what starts out as a formal relationship frequently develops into an expansion of both individuals' informal support networks. The more opportunities for exchanges with other age groups a person has, the more opportunities there are to widen the social network. Neglecting intergenerational activities may result in the center increasing the gap between age groups. The gap isolates the older person from potential community supports as well as opportunities to engage in rewarding activities.

Ethnic Groups and Activities

Not all persons will be equally attracted by a senior center's program. When older persons have a strong identification with their community, individuals may decide whether or not to participate in activities depending on the ethnic background of individuals already enrolled in a program. Language barriers may make it impossible for an older ethnic to understand or take part in the center's programs. These language problems could limit the center to providing only food and shelter rather than activities that encourage the types of informal networks needed by older adults. Individuals with similar ethnic backgrounds can talk, share common histories, and assist each other in ways that are culturally accepted. The center staff must recognize the importance of ethnic culture and provide opportunities for older persons to reaffirm their cultural identity. Bilingual staff would help older ethnic individuals feel more comfortable and able to participate in the center.

Senior Centers and Support Networks

"Supporting" Informal Support Networks

Support networks within a center are primarily informal in nature. This does not mean, however, that there are no key individuals in these networks. Center staff should be able to identify individuals who are important in various support networks and reinforce their activity by providing verbal and concrete assistance. Reinforcing the ability of center participants to serve as important elements of support networks will enable older adults to better serve as effective links with their age peers. As part of the senior center's potential as a bridge between informal and formal support networks, members who are knowledgeable about community resources can provide outreach and referral for other older persons in the community. Outreach means contacting individuals and involving them in the center's activities in an effort to alleviate the depression, isolation, or other problems that may be bothering many of the local residents. Referral involves not only knowing what agencies can service particular problems but possessing an awareness of individuals who are part of the natural helping networks that exist in the community.

Quasi-formal Networks

Many of the informal networks that develop within senior centers can take on a quasi-formal nature because of the interest and energies of small groups of clients or a staff member. In this sense, *quasi-formal* means any activity that is not formally operated through paid staff and that functions primarily as a result of the interest of the individuals involved. Formal aspects derive from the fact that the functions were either initiated by staff or are acknowledged by staff to be an integral part of the senior center structure of activities. Space or other concrete assistance from staff also adds to the formal components of these networks.

One example of a quasi-formalized support network is a group of seniors who are friends and keep tabs on important events in each other's lives. When the group learns of a member who has suffered a loss of a spouse or relative, they send condolence cards, visit, and bring food. This group continues to maintain contact over a long period of time, and when they feel it is appropriate, they bring the individual back into the senior center to engage again in activities.

These preventive mental health activities become operative at the time of an individual's loss and at a later point when older individuals are most prone to becoming isolated and depressed. Despite their importance, there are a few potential problems with these arrangements.

Since word of mouth is the major source of information, members of the group may not know of all losses in a large senior center. If the group has no connections with the center staff, the possibility exists that as members of the group die, its functions will not be taken over by any other component of the center. To help alleviate these problems, a staff member can be designated as the link between the group and the formal service-delivery system. The staff member can refer individuals for additional help if there is a problem beyond the group's capability. Handled tactfully by staff, the suggestion that the group set up a mechanism for maintaining contact with the staff would be seen as supportive rather than an effort by the staff to take control of their activities.

The "buddy system" is another example of a quasi-formal service. The buddy system is operated by a group of seniors who take on the responsibility for calling each other on a daily or weekly basis to offer reassurance or check up on the health of the person being called. This system has the advantage that the members of the group also interact in the center. Some of the calling "buddies" often become close friends. The system can be coordinated by an older person who is paid to take the names of individuals needing to be called and those willing to do the calling.

Support for Family Networks

The above discussion has centered around older adults as individuals rather than as family members. Senior centers can also offer support to family networks. In New York a group of informal caregivers of different ages meet monthly at a local senior center. While this group is primarily educational in nature, it also affords participants the opportunity to share feelings and receive emotional support from others in similar situations. Such groups may be somewhat younger than the usual senior center patrons, but there are increasing numbers of individuals over age sixty who are providing care for an older relative and can utilize assistance. These older caregivers can benefit from a group organized through a senior center which provides concrete and emotional support.

Because of the increasing number of aged caregivers, a senior center is a natural place to offer assistance and to help prevent the older caregiver from becoming isolated and depressed with what he or she may view as an overwhelming burden. Along with attending the support group, the caregiver can also become involved in other activities. This will be more feasible if there is some form of adult day care attached to the senior center so that the elder needing supervised care can receive it while the caregiving older person enjoys the benefits of senior center membership. The senior center can facilitate linkages with other existing agencies if the development of an adult day-care center is not possible.

Links with Community Service Systems

As a facility that serves as a link to other service delivery systems, the senior center can establish working relationships with the local community mental health center. Having a mental health worker visit the center on a regular basis to conduct counseling and education groups helps to show support for the use of formal mental health services. The supportive atmosphere of the center is intrinsic to the success of a variety of activities including blood pressure checks and discussions of major life changes on the part of older persons.

Despite the positive environment it can provide, a senior center cannot and should not supplant other available community supports. These supports may include the pharmacist, grocer, and perhaps the newsboy or mailman. In many communities, a doctor, priest, neighbor, or friend may also serve as a vital element in the community support network. Aware of the potential for support offered by these individuals, the senior center staff can provide referrals and assistance if requested. The center staff can extend this information and referral function into the community by providing information or speaking to civic groups attended by older people. The key element in the center's role is its visibility as a part of the community and not simply as a building apart from the mainstream of community activities. Seen as an intrinsic element in the community, local helpers will view the center as a local resource.

To attain legitimacy in the eyes of formal, as well as informal, caregivers, a senior center needs to have continuing contact with community agencies. A center can be a source of referrals for mental health workers and physicians. These referrals may bring older individuals into the center who have been isolated in their home or a hospital for an extended period because of physical or emotional problems. Extended efforts may facilitate the provision of services to these clients by center staff. Additional staff may be required to work with older adults with special needs. Planned discussion groups and educational programs as well as individual support for all members may also be needed if individuals with mental health problems are going to find acceptance among established clients. With adequate staff support and open discussion, many seniors who have been recently discharged from intensive mental health services can be integrated into the center as well as into family and community networks. Unfortunately, despite all intensive efforts the behavior of some potential clients may be too disruptive for them to become involved in center activities.

Rather than viewing themselves as the only community resource, senior center staff should make efforts to assist the burgeoning self-help groups that exist in many communities. Self-help groups contribute to the integration of individuals with special needs into the community and provide either weak or strong ties for individuals whose mental health can best be served by being able to talk with someone with a similar problem. The senior center can support the development or at a minimum provide meeting space for ostomy patients, widowed persons, stroke victims, and other self-help groups.

Many of the physical and mental health services that senior centers now provide could be offered by other organizations including health clinics of community mental health centers. The negative attitudes of many professionals toward working with older people and the reluctance of older people to use many services has resulted in the older population being underrepresented in many community-based programs. In mental health, for example, the proportion of older people who are outpatients at mental health centers has remained at 4 percent for over a decade, a figure significantly below the representation of the older population in the United States. Ironically, the proportion of older adults in state mental health hospitals has always been significantly higher than the general population. Recently, nursing homes have become repositories for older individuals with mental health problems who might formerly have been relegated to state mental hospitals. As a community resource, the senior center does not carry the stigma that many older people attribute to mental health programs. The senior center thus has the opportunity to serve as a link to formal mental health services while also helping to strengthen the ability of the informal support networks that are indigenous to the community.

Limitations of Support Networks

Up to this point we have focused on the positive aspects of informal social networks rather than the potential limitations and negative aspects of some networks noted earlier. As already discussed, informal networks must be linked to formal support systems when specialized assistance is required (i.e., medical or legal aid). Assistance from formal caregivers may also be required as the older individual's support networks are reduced by illness, moves, and deaths.

Negative elements of support networks may exist both in the general community and in the senior center. In the community, a negative relationship with a family member may be the cause of a problem, which can be resolved only by moving the individual to a new living situation. An example is the recent discussions about the abuse of older persons by family members. While the prevalence of "elder abuse" is yet to be determined, it remains a possibility in many family situations. Abuse is particularly possible in situations where the older person is dependent on other family members for assistance and where this assistance can require a major shift in family routine and living patterns.

Within the senior center, as well as in the community, a social network can reinforce such negative behaviors as the overuse of alcohol. Less overtly negative groups may organize around opposition toward center programming or staff. Recognition of these negative groups is not always easy. If center staff become aware of their possible existence, then staff efforts must focus around finding more positive outlets for the group members, rather than dismissing complaints as bad feelings. Intervention with the group abusing alcohol may include the utilization of a counselor who can assist the senior staff in developing a program for older alcohol abusers. This new program can help staff avoid the necessity of ejecting alcohol abusers from the center.

Conclusion

The senior center has major potential as a reinforcer for positive support groups. A center's programs can reduce social and emotional isolation and alleviate accompanying depressive conditions. Accomplishing these mental health tasks depends in large part on staff abilities, attitudes, and training, clear delineation of center goals, and the ability of the center to attract new resources and utilize the existing resources of its members. While this chapter sets out a large agenda for senior centers, recent support for older Americans' programs would indicate that with flexibility and imagination these efforts can be successful. The senior center has the potential to act as a bridge between formal and informal support networks and to assist in the formation and strengthening of informal support networks. A concentration on support networks will help the senior center build upon important relationships the older person has in the community. Neglecting these support networks may mean that efforts by the senior center to have a positive impact on the older person's mental health will be only minimally effective.

12

The Chronically Mentally Ill: Sharing the Burden with the Community

Stanley R. Platman

Institutions were developed as an attempt to lessen the burden of the mentally ill upon the community. Today, the burden has been placed once again on the community, this time by "deinstitutionalization." Between these two extreme responses, there have been many efforts to create a balanced system.

The author of a paper published in 1847 urges that:

> Before a patient is returned to the environment that made him ill, he should be given specific instructions regarding his behavior outside the mental institution. Relatives should also be given appropriate advice. The patient has to be made aware of his weaknesses under certain conditions. The newly recovered patient needs help to regain "self and world-consciousness." He must learn to live among healthy people. It is necessary for him to develop new and constructive interests in nature, art, music and travel. The author suggests a "support fund" for the recovered insane, and a home for those with no family to return to [Harms, 1968].

Unfortunately, the polarization between adequate institutional and community care has not yet been resolved. It is even possible that both systems are not viable in tandem. Society may not be willing to provide a comprehensive community support system as long as it has also to support an expensive range of institutional services.

The purpose of this chapter is to document the critical issues facing the chronically mentally ill in the 1980s and to suggest that a neighborhood-oriented approach with special emphasis on self-help of former patients and support for the families of this population is superior to current "innovative" provider-dominated programs. In doing so we will describe the chronically mentally ill—who they are and what problems they face; reflect on society's attitudes toward these people; review examples of "innovative" programs; and discuss the role of the families of the chronically mentally ill, the movement toward self-help by former patients, and the need for a supportive neighborhood.

Who Are the Chronically Mentally Ill?

It is estimated that there are 400,000 chronic mental patients still in institutions today. Approximately 150,000 of this population are in the specialty mental health sector, and 250,000 are in nursing homes.

About 1.5 million chronic mental patients are currently living in communities throughout the United States. Of this total, there are about 400,000 chronic mental patients on SSI/SSDI, and another 350,000 on complete work disability. In addition, it is estimated that another 700,000 chronic mental patients with partial disabilities function in the community.

In general, mental disability may be viewed along two continua: duration of disability and severity of disability. The chronically mentally disabled are distinguishable as a subpopulation of the mentally ill according to both of these criteria: they represent extremes along both dimensions; they are severely and persistently disabled. These are the people who are, have been, or might have been in earlier times residents of large mental insitutions. They constitute the subgroup of the mentally ill for whom societal rejection has been and is most acute.

The Task Panel on Deinstitutionalization, Rehabilitation, and Long-Term Care of the President's Commission on Mental Health vividly described the serious problems of the chronically mentally ill as follows:

> The chronically mentally ill are a minority within minorities. They are the most stigmatized of the mentally ill. They are politically and economically powerless and rarely speak for themselves. Their stigma is multiplied, since disproportionate numbers among them are people who are also elderly, poor or members of racial or ethnic minority groups. They are totally disenfranchised among us.
>
> These individuals must be the concern not only of the mental health professions, but also of the total society. Although the problems, needs and fate of the chronically mentally disabled should occupy us all, this clearly has not been the case. Society has failed to ensure that those individuals are given opportunities to maximize their potential and autonomy. Deinstitu-

tionalization, ostensibly intended to assist the chronically mentally ill by taking or keeping them out of large, understaffed public mental hospitals and permitting them to be cared for in the community, has fallen short of its goal. Unfortunately, deinstitutionalization has too often occurred without adequate planning.

It is now widely acknowledged that deinstitutionalization has, in fact, often aggravated the problem of the chronically mentally disabled. All too commonly, no one reviews the requirements of disabled persons to assess whether hospitalization or community care is more appropriate to their level of functioning. Similarly, for these disabled persons who we hospitalize, there is often no one to assume the responsibility for assuring that their re-entry into the community is timely and desired by them. It is not uncommon for these patients to be released without adequate aftercare planning to community settings that are hostile and lack the flexibility to meet their needs. Stigma does not stop when they leave the hospital; it follows them wherever they go. The community rejection that may have contributed to their hospitalization is only increased when these patients are returned to the community without the supportive services they so desperately need [President's Commission on Mental Health, Vol. II, 1978b, p. 362].

Our Attitude toward the Chronically Mentally Ill

The word *stigma* is often used to describe the way in which society stamps those who have been mentally ill. Its literal meaning is "a stain on one's good name" or a "loss of reputation." Originally, the word referred to a mark placed on a slave or a prisoner as a sign of his status or lack of it. Whether it is a visible mark or an invisible stain, *stigma* acquires its meaning through the emotion it generates within the person bearing it and the feeling and behavior toward him of those affirming it (Cummings and Cummings, 1965). Cummings and Cummings, in a study in the 1960s of individuals discharged from a state mental hospital, noted the following comments: A patient's wife stated, "My children think he is just lazy. Of course, because of the kind of hospital he was in, the union probably doesn't think it was a proper thing to help him financially." His daughter interjects, "It was hard when he came home because there [were] all those stories in the paper about crimes, and they always turned out to be done by former mental patients" (p. 10).

The public backlash to community care becomes understandable when the research accumulated over the past twenty-five years on public attitudes is examined. This body of literature has almost consistently found that the mentally ill are feared, mistrusted, and rejected by the public. Cocozza and Steadman, in a recent study (1976), found that the public distinguishes the mentally ill from most people primarily in that they perceive the mentally ill to be dangerous and unpredictable and that over 25 percent of the respondents were not willing to interact with former mental patients in various social settings. Mike Gorman (1975) has noted that homeowners and businessmen in many urban communities complained that the existence of nearby halfway houses for the mentally ill constituted a threat to their lives and livelihoods. Aviran and Segal (1973) noted how communities in California created distance from discharged patients by use of the penal code to rehospitalize individuals, arrest and imprisonment of individuals for minor crimes, the creation of ghettos, the restrictive use of zoning laws, city ordinances and regulations, and a wide range of legal and bureaucratic maneuvers.

The Horizon House Institute for Research and Development was requested by the Pennsylvania Department of Public Welfare to undertake an assessment of the "quality of life" experienced by former patients of the State's mental hospitals. They found that, according to the patients, living in the community is far preferable to living in the hospital. In addition, despite the presence of problems and inadequacies in the community, a sizable number of the patients are capable of achieving satisfactory life patterns in society, and this capacity is highly related to the strength and cohesion of the community to which the patient returns (Horizon House Institute, 1975).

Many communities throughout the United States, however, have felt overburdened by the discharged patients, especially if the patient was disturbed and the community support systems were fragile. This led, all too frequently, to their rejection and recycling in and out of the state hospitals and, in some cases, the prison system. For some this "recycling" has been from one institutional setting to another—from the state mental hospital to the nursing home. Others simply disappeared and became part of an ever-enlarging group of homeless drifters that burden each major metropolis (Wing & Olsen, 1979).

As Ronald Peterson, a former patient at Pilgrim State Hospital in Long Island noted,

It's hard for me to express, but somehow the mentally ill in the community are looked at as a great and serious problem, and I don't think this is really the case. I know the needs of the mentally ill are great, but I only want to suggest that this is the case because so little is really being done. . . . One of the most important things you first have to think about is where you're going to live when you leave the hospital. In my case, I had no home to go back to. They got me on welfare and into a small hotel room on Times Square. I would get my check at the desk and sign it. They would take out the rent money, and I'd do this twice a month. You don't have much left over to live on when you're in a single room occupancy and don't get much space to live in for the money you pay. When you're all by yourself, you can really feel lonely even though there are lots of people you can see on the streets. But you're still isolated and by yourself. It was simply arranged for you [Peterson, 1978, p. 44].

He went on to express his and others' needs in the following manner:

We need, therefore, to be with others who believe that we are not at our best and that sufficient time will be given us to be at our best; maybe about as much time as the non-mentally ill have in order to achieve whatever their potential might be [Peterson, 1978, p. 42].

Ronald Peterson is saying that people like him need understanding, time, the right to make good and bad decisions, and a lot of tender loving care. Unfortunately, these essential elements as well as decent housing, sufficient money, responsive and quality mental health care, resocialization, and retraining are all too often nonexistent. The amazing thing is that so many Ron Petersons stick it out or, if they get recycled, go back and try again.

Provider-Managed Community Programs for the Chronically Mentally Ill

Service providers have created many programs to address the multiple needs of these individuals. Whereas it is recognized that quality and responsive mental health services are necessary and all too often lacking, it is also increasingly recognized by many programs that their availability is an insufficient singular resource for chronically mentally ill persons. These individuals have extensive needs beyond health and mental health care. They are poor and require the income maintenance and social support of impoverished individuals. If they have no supportive family, they need housing and food. They require advocacy, recreation, and rehabilitation. A number of programs have tried to develop a comprehensive approach to service delivery. However, all too few communities are equipped or willing to focus all these resources for the chronically mentally ill.

An example of "innovative" programs on the state and federal levels will help explain the operationalization of this new comprehensive approach. One program on the state level is the Mendotal Mental Health Institute in Madison, Wisconsin. This is a state hospital's program called

[Program of] Assertive Community Treatment (PACT), which, in the past seven years, has had remarkable success at maintaining an averge of sixty-five chronic patients in the community (*Today in Psychiatry, 1979*). In the PACT concept, it is required that needed mental health and social services be provided twenty-four hours a day and 365 days a year.

The program is expensive, and the philosophy is that many of the patients will need some form of care for life. Practical guidelines produced by this program for the care of the mentally ill include an assertive approach on the part of the staff, the use of social learning techniques rather than psychotherapy, and the holding of patients responsible for their actions, including taking the consequences for any law-breaking behavior.

On the federal level, the National Institute of Mental Health (NIMH) has launched a national pilot program entitled the Community Support Program (CSP). This program, in conjunction with state agencies, is attempting to overcome existing service fragmentation and defining one responsible agency in each geographical area. These programs perform the following functions: identification of the target population; assistance in making application for entitlements; crisis stabilization; attaining hospitalization, if necessary; psychosocial rehabilitation services; supportive services of indefinite duration; medical and mental health care; back-up support and involvement of families, friends, and community members; protection of client rights and case management; ensuring the continuous availability of assistance (Turner and TenHoor, 1978).

The Mendota and CSP models, frequently highly staffed and expensive to replicate, are motivated by doing things for the chronically mentally ill on a lifetime basis. There are a number of problems with these types programs that are thought to be innovative. They are highly dependent on significant leadership and enthusiastic staff. These attributes are difficult to obtain and maintain and are apt to be nontransferrable. Also, being staff dominated, they are apt to perpetuate the continued dependency of chronically disabled individuals and lead to a turf ownership by the designated agency caring for this target population. This competition for the patient is magnified by the fact that these programs are usually part of the mental health service-delivery system. Thus, clear boundaries with the state mental hospital and other mental health providers (CHMCs, private practitioners, etc.) are likely to be difficult to define around continuity of care. Each mental health agency is apt to claim ownership of the patient in their system and not be prepared to give up clinical and legal control to another mental health program. In addition, this new responsible agency is likely to claim "rights" to the patient in relationship to other non-mental service agencies in the community. This leads to continuing separation, stigma, and the avoidance of responsibility on the part of the disabled person, other individuals in the community, and other service providers in the geographical area.

These programs have tended to ignore the need to support families of the chronically mentally ill in the care that they provide and, by keeping patients dependent upon professionals, have not allowed for the development of self-help mechanisms by the chronically mentally ill and their families. Furthermore, sufficient attention has not been focused on the place to which deinstitutionalized mentally ill go—*the neighborhood*. It is to these concerns that we now turn our attention.

Family Support for the Chronically Mentally Ill

It is essential to recognize that most individuals discharged from a state hospital return to their family. In addition, many families maintain these individuals for many years. Some families, in fact, maintain a chronically mentally ill family member for years without the individual ever having been hospitalized.

Caplan and Killilea (1976) place high value on the family as a support system. They observed its value in providing a stable belief system, information and practical wisdom, a haven for rest and recuperation, and such practical assistance as transportation and child care. Relatives serve as active listeners, permitting grieving and offering support and love. Families have not been greatly assisted in these tasks. All too often, as the cause of chronic mental illness has not yet been discovered, professionals in theory and in practice blame the family environment. The difficulty with theories of this kind is that they are retrospective and depend upon studies of families now containing a chronically mentally ill member. All too often the caregiving system fails to recognize the burden on the family, the value of lightening this burden, and the importance of creating a helping partnership with the family.

Creer and Wing (1974) have studied this burden. Over 70 percent of the families who had chronically mentally ill members said that social withdrawal of the patient was the problem most frequently encountered, followed by underactivity and lack of conversation. Threats of violence were a problem for about one-quarter of the relatives. Sexually unusual or suicidal behavior was encountered quite rarely, although about one-third of the relatives said that depression was a problem. At present, it appears that the typical situation is of a man or woman aged about thirty, living with one or both parents aged sixty or more years. The individual has to cope with the aftereffects of illness, the possibility of relapse, continuous medication, and difficulties in picking up the threads of a normal life again. The parents have to cope with a grown-up son or daughter who is socially isolated and dependent on their care, but often demanding of time and energy and unpredictable from day to day regarding behavior or mood.

Such family members feel very isolated, feel they suffer from lack of information, and frequently complain of a lack of coordinated services and advice as to their best way of managing. These feelings are real and often due, at least in part, to a genuine failure on the part of professionals who, in turn, often feel at a loss in the face of long-term illness. One way around this is to help relatives who live with the mentally ill to help each other, since those who do manage well are potentially in an ideal position to share their solutions with others with the same problems. Such an organization of families of the mentally ill in Maryland is Threshold, which was organized in 1978 to provide mutual support, education, advocacy, and service. An older group with chapters throughout the country is the Schizophrenia Associations. These groups are primarily committed to a biochemical explanation of schizophrenia and inform their members through books and lectures of new developments. Through volunteer hot lines and small neighborhood groups, they give emotional support and advice on family management. Agnes Hatfield is a pioneer with these groups and has studied the family members of the Schizophrenia Association of Greater Washington (Hatfield, 1979). Members noted the need for information, someone to talk to, respite care, and responsive home visiting from providers. These needs are all too frequently unfulfilled.

The Movement toward Self-help

Unfortunately, a significant minority of the chronically mentally ill have no families or have rejected or been rejected by them. This is the group that is apt to be all too visible to the community, make up the homeless wanderers, and frequently recycle through the hospital and correction system. Many models have been developed throughout the country to bring such individuals together to help themselves. Many of these efforts followed the genesis of Fountain House, which was initiated thirty-five years ago by former patients on the wards of Rockland State Hospital in New York. These patients banded themselves together to help each other get out of the hospital and assist each other in getting jobs.

Once back in New York City, members continued to meet where they could—on the steps of the New York Public Library at Forty-second Street and Fifth Avenue, and later in coffee shops and the YMCA. In those days they called themselves "WANA," an acronym for "We are not alone." The little group had no backing and was under no sponsorship except for a few dedicated volunteers. As Fountain House grew, it symbolically accepted all patients as members of the extended family. They belong, and they are needed. They develop new attitudes and value systems; they learn to reach out and to help one another. They work together.

In the mid-1960s, George W. Fairweather further modified this model (Fairweather, Sanders, Cressler, & Maynard, 1969). It was based on the principle that a group, by working together, can succeed even when its individual members struggling alone would surely fail. He took a group of chronic patients with varying levels of ability and different strengths and weaknesses and molded them into a cohesive unit. He set up business for them, found them a house, and helped them grow into independent, productive members of the community. When the group matured, the professionals left them on their own. Many examples of such staff-initiated programs based on the Fairweather model leading to eventual independence for the patients have been created. There are now about seventy such lodges throughout the country.

More recently, this concept has progressed a step further. Groups have developed that completely reject professional input. This is not dissimilar to many other self-help groups—some as old as AA and Synanon, others relatively new in the human service area. For example, in November 1979, the Washington Network for Alternatives to Psychiatric Dependency had a meeting on building a separate support community for ex-patients. The meeting welcomed all those who had been institutionalized or were disenchanted with psychiatric solutions. They carefully noted that "professionals need not apply."

It probably makes little sense for these ex-patient–led groups to demand total independence from the caregiver system and even the creation of separate worlds from normal communities. However, it is understandable when one recognizes how poorly they have been treated by the caregiver system and how often they have been rejected by normal communities. I personally feel that, as with the history of the AA movement, this overreaction by all parties might be an initial healthy sign that will eventually lead to a better understanding of the problem and a meaningful compromise between the mentally disabled, other citizens, and various provider groups. The National Institute of Mental Health has recognized the importance of these mutual-help groups and has recently published a guide for mental health workers that attempts to strengthen the relationships rather than the differences (Silverman, 1978).

Thus, mechanisms are needed by which professionals can provide assistance, support, and encouragement to the deinstitutionalized chronically mentally ill that is consonant with the increasing self-help movement of this population and that does not foster dependency. The neighborhood is an important context in which such strategies can best be developed.

The Neighborhood and the Chronically Mentally Ill

It is evident that a neighborhood faces many important issues when it recognizes the presence of the chronically mentally ill in their community. A community examining this issue will discover that these individuals live in the following settings:

1. Most of the chronically mentally ill come from the neighborhood and live with their own families.
2. Some live in the homes of other neighbors and pay rent for their care and support to a caretaker.
3. Others live in special forms of lodgings such as halfway houses and group homes.
4. In addition, especially in transitional areas, some are visible only as homeless persons utilizing various temporary shelters.

On further examination, a community will discover that most of these individuals are linked to a caregiving system. The caregiving system may not, however, be within the community and may not be responsive to crisis situations. In general, the neighborhood is not aware of these people, except in an emergency and, when that happens, the normal response is to seek assistance for the individual. If help is not rapidly available, they seek the police and attempt to get the individual sent back to a state mental hospital.

It is essential to recognize that most successful deinstitutionalization programs have taken place in stable and supportive neighborhoods. In contrast, the use of transitional and disintegrating neighborhoods is frequently related to failures. This finding is not surprising, as decaying neighborhoods lack basic support systems and stable human relationships. Compounding the problems in discharging ex-hospital patients without family ties is that it is easier to place them in transitional areas due to their all-too-common rejection in stable neighborhoods. Thus, the simplest route is into neighborhoods in turmoil, lacking organized community resistance. In fact, because of the ease of placement in such decaying areas, the chronically mentally ill are frequently in competition with other deviant, unwanted groups: for example, former prisoners, juvenile delinquents, and the mentally retarded. The end result of this easy access for disabled individuals is to assure their failure, their potential destruction in a hazardous jungle, and continued stigmatization.

It is evident that deinstitutionalization of the chronically mentally ill can be destructive to the discharged person, to their family, and to their neighborhood. Success, as we have seen, cannot and should not be the total or even principal responsibility of government and private caregivers. In fact, success is probably more dependent upon the neighborhood, the chronically mentally ill person, and the family. Such success also requires, however, a responsive government and service providers.

The Neighborhood and Family Services Project Report notes that neighborhood residents want to take care of their own problems (Naparstek, Biegel, and colleagues, 1979). In this study of ethnic working-class neighborhoods, the researchers found that helpers in neighborhoods are clearly able to recognize psychiatric situations and feel that mental health professionals are important in dealing with them. The project's concept of a community mental health empowerment model is that there would be available local services and a neighborhood-based partnership among professionals and lay service providers that would help in overcoming stigma, increase utilization of services, reach people earlier, and create a constituency for mental health services. Essential to such partnerships is the "empowerment" of community residents.

The project has developed a neighborhood-run hot line as one mechanism to assist linkages between individuals with problems and community and professional service providers. In addition to such strategies, it is essential that a neighborhood organize a corps of volunteers to be "community friends" to the chronically mentally ill and also to offer respite relief to families and caretakers.

Although it is important for the neighborhood to integrate this population into the social and recreational network of the community, it is also important to recognize that the chronically mentally ill may require and want their own support system. This can often be achieved by helping the chronically mentally ill to develop a psychosocial clubhouse where they can expand their own network of contacts and friends.

It must be especially recognized that ex-patients may not be able to relate closely to their old friends. They may, in fact, be more comfortable with their new friends, other ex-patients, with whom they have shared certain intense common experiences. It may be good to encourage a group pride in their competence in dealing with this affliction. Members find each other jobs, room with each other, come to help one another in crises, and collectively apply skills that they learned together as a result of their special experience. It is the job of families and neighbors to support them in this effort, as in that way independence rather than dependence is created.

In addition, it is essential that neighborhood leadership ensure that the professional service system remain responsive to provide support needs, maintenance treatment, and crisis intervention. Adolph Meyer, writing in the early twentieth century, foresaw a concept of "neighborhood psychiatry." He proposed a mental health program in a single geographical area that would consist of an integrated program of prevention, treatment, and aftercare involving all caregiving agencies such as welfare, schools, and clergy. He suggested that the psychiatrists work together with the teachers, police, welfare workers, and family physicians in a given neighborhood (Meyer, 1952). To this statement we should now add an involvement with patient groups, families, community helpers, and community leaders in which the patients' capacities for self-help are maximized.

Part III
Professional Roles

A major and recurring theme throughout this book has been the need for partnerships between informal and formal support systems to enhance the provision of care to those in need. The articulation of such partnerships requires careful consideration to ensure that neither the informal nor the formal sector is undermined or weakened. The problem becomes more difficult when one considers that partnerships or coalitions require some form of parity to be successful. In other words, both the informal and the formal systems must respect each other's unique capacities, resources, and expertise.

Focusing upon this partnership theme, Jeger, Slotnik, and Schure's opening chapter presents a "perspective" of self-help/professional collaboration. They believe that such collaboration must have as an underpinning an integration of "experiential" and "professional" knowledge. Their perspective focuses on five specific areas—self-help group development, natural-helping-network enhancement, consultation and education, information and referral, and research—as providing opportunities for collaboration with documentation of successful "model" interventions by professionals in each of these arenas. The authors note the growing number of "resource exchange networks" among professional agencies, self-help groups and individual community residents that serve to both stretch limited resources and increase the sense of community as a positive indication that the self-help concept has many ramifications yet to be fully explored.

Building upon Jeger, Slotnik, and Schure's definition of natural network enhancement, Vallance and D'Augelli report the results of a NIMH-funded project aimed at expanding limited mental health resources through a prevention program that develops new services using natural helpers. A snowballing paradigm was instituted by which professionals provide training to natural helpers, who train other natural helpers, the process then continuing with little dependence on professional resources. Though the project's federal funding has ended, local activities are going on successfully. The authors argue that in working with natural helpers, professionals must not only be clinical practitioners but also consultants and advocates for social change.

Silverman's concluding chapter further develops the role of the mental health professional as consultant through the presentation of a model that enhances the ability of mental health professionals to work with mutual-help organizations. She notes that there has been considerable tension between self-help groups and professionals (a somewhat different perspective than Spiegel's in Part I) and that mental health professionals often have difficulty in consulting with mutual-help groups. Such difficulties arise because the knowledge and experience bases of professionals are more suitable to "clinical" interventions with clients and consultation with agency professionals and because professionals have nonempathetic attitudes toward mutual-help organizations. Silverman states that the mental health consultant should be a linking agent between mutual-help groups, helping the groups to share the expertise and knowledge that they each have. This recommendation is very similar to Jeger, Slotnik, and Schure's notion of resource-exchange networks.

13

Toward a "Self-help/Professional Collaborative Perspective" in Mental Health

Abraham M. Jeger,
Robert S. Slotnick, and
Matthew Schure

If I am not for myself, who will be?
If I am only for myself, what am I?

(Hillel, *Tractate of the Fathers*, 1:14)

Recent years have witnessed a dramatic surge in a grass-roots movement whereby people sharing a common need or problem band together to help one another. With origins in such established self-help groups as Alcoholics Anonymous and Recovery (for ex-mental patients), approxi-

The authors acknowledge the support of the New York Institute of Technology in establishing the Long Island Self-Help Clearinghouse. Our experiences at the Clearinghouse made possible the development of the perspective presented in this chapter. Special thanks are due to Dr. David Salten, Executive Vice President and Provost, and to Dr. Alexander Schure, President of the New York Institute of Technology, for their continued support and encouragement.

We thank Alfred Katz for his comments on an earlier version of this chapter and for granting us permission to quote from his unpublished paper. We also thank Leslie Borck, Thomasina Borkman, Leonard Borman, Bill Claflin, Alan Gartner, Dick Gordon, Ben Gottlieb, Leon Levy, Morton Lieberman, and Frank Riessman for sharing descriptions of their ongoing projects.

Portions of this chapter were presented by the authors as parts of symposia at the annual meetings of the American Psychological Association (September 1980) and the Environmental Design Research Association (March 1980), and as part of an Invited Address to the Association for Behavior Analysis, International (May 1980).

mately one-half million self-help groups exist for various problems and
populations (Gartner & Riessman, 1977). Groups exist for the overweight, compulsive gamblers, the physically handicapped, people undergoing surgery, schizophrenics, abusive parents, widows, to name
only a few. At the same time, mutual-aid groups have been formed for
purposes of "enhancement"—for instance, women's health collectives,
parent centers, skill exchanges and bartering networks, cooperative day-
care centers, and advocacy programs for the poor and ethnic minorities.
  Katz and Bender (1976b) defined self-help groups as:

> Voluntary, small group structures for mutual aid and the accomplishments
> of a special purpose. They are usually formed by peers who have come
> together for mutual assistance in satisfying a common need, overcoming a
> common handicap or life-disruption problem, and bringing about desired
> social and/or personal change. The initiators and members of such groups
> perceive that their needs are not, or cannot be, met by or through existing
> social institutions. Self-help groups emphasize face-to-face social interac-
> tions and the assumption of personal responsibility by members. They often
> provide material assistance, as well as emotional support; they are fre-
> quently "cause"-oriented, and promulgate an ideology or values through
> which members may attain an enhanced sense of personal identity [p. 9].

This definition captures the essential features of self-help groups that we
will be considering in this chapter.
  As the self-help movement has gained momentum, it has increasingly attracted the attention of mental health professionals. During the
1970s this interest was reflected in a host of developments—including
professional books on self-help, special journal issues devoted to self-
help, the establishment of national and regional self-help clearinghouses, and federal government initiatives (e.g., President's Commission on Mental Health, 1978b).
  In addition to the attention given to self-help groups, mental health
professionals are increasingly recognizing the roles of informal or natural
helping networks (Collins & Pancoast, 1976; Gottlieb, in press). These
networks consist of neighborhood helpers who offer support, advice, and
exchange of information without any group or organizational sanctions.
While they are less structured and less visible than self-help groups,
natural helping networks exist in every community in even greater numbers. We will use the term *self-help* in a more generic sense to include
mutual aid through informal or natural helping, rather than referring
exclusively to self-help groups.
  The increasing interface between self-helpers and professionals can
potentially result in new approaches to mental health service delivery.
One such approach is *self-help professional collaborative perspective*.

Our purpose in this chapter is to present a preliminary formulation of this approach. We will document the nature of existing collaborative relationships as reflected in major research/intervention programs and analyze the numerous roles of professionals and self-helpers vis-à-vis each other. The perspective will be operationalized by considering new knowledge bases necessary for effective collaboration between the professional and self-help communities. Our goal in this chapter is to systematize and discuss recent developments in the mental health field which we see as contributing to this evolving perspective. Thereby, we hope to provide a stimulus for its further conceptual development and refinement through analysis and application.

The theoretical perspective of human behavior that provides the framework for our conceptualization of a self-help/professional collaborative perspective is the ecological approach in the fields of community psychology and community mental health. To place our perspective in context, we present an overview of the ecological approach.

The Ecological Approach

According to Moos (1980), the ecological viewpoint is an alternative to the attribution of behavior to individual dispositions. The major features of social ecology, according to Moos, include a concern with the environment as a focus for mental health and an emphasis on person–environment transactions. The reciprocal influences between persons and environments, and the way that people cope with environmental stressors that they encounter and create, constitute the theoretical cornerstones of this perspective. Thus, emphasis lies in the capacities of individuals to design their environment, while at the same time considering the environmental influences on individual behavior.

The ecological orientation emphasizes practice in natural community settings, as opposed to institutional or clinic settings. Further, the approach emphasizes evaluation of all interventions, thereby merging research and service delivery in contrast to traditional mental health models, which separate research and clinical practice. The ecological orientation calls for broader roles for mental health professionals. Rather than the traditional focus on direct service roles, ecologically oriented mental health professionals are more likely to function as consultants, trainers, program designers, catalysts, participant/conceptualizers, resource persons, mediators, and evaluators.

A feature of the ecological perspective emphasized by Rappaport (1977) is that values are an integral part of the paradigm. The value guiding ecological interventions is that they should be aimed at enhancing the capacities of groups to strengthen their own communities in accordance with their goals. Ecological interventions should seek to strengthen the community's "mediating structures" (Berger & Neuhaus, 1977) such as family, church, neighborhood, and ethnic/racial subcultures. Along these lines, Rappaport (1977) suggests that programs should be federally financed but locally designed in keeping with the culturally diverse character of neighborhoods. Each community would then be able to develop new programs relative to its own unique needs and sensitive to the concerns that local conditions dictate.

In discussing the implications of the ecological perspective for community mental health programming, Holahan and colleagues (1979) called for environmentally oriented interventions to strengthen community support systems as well as individual-level interventions aimed at enhancing personal competencies. Examples of environmental interventions include the enhancement of natural caregivers (parents, teachers, neighbors) and the establishment of "artificial networks" when deemed necessary (e.g., self-help groups). Individual-level interventions include behavioral-skill training and personal-problem-solving training. Some of the projects discussed in later sections of this chapter exemplify such ecological interventions. (For additional programs that reflect the ecological perspective in community mental health, see Jeger and Slotnick, 1981.)

Toward a Self-help/Professional Collaborative Perspective of Mental Health Service Delivery

In this section we develop a perspective of self-help/professional collaboration, guided by the ecological approach in community mental health. We consider the knowledge bases for self-help/professional collaboration as well as action/research projects exemplifying such collaboration.

Knowledge Bases for Self-help/Professional Collaboration

Borkman (1976, p. 446), based upon her research with self-help groups, makes a distinction between "experiential" knowledge and "professional" knowledge. Experiential knowledge is acquired through personal experience and is said to be "concrete, specific, and common sensical." She introduces the notion of experiential *expertise*, which refers to the skills obtained through the application of experiential knowledge. Experiential expertise may serve as the basis for leadership in a self-help group.

Professional knowledge is "acquired by discursive reasoning, observation, or reflection on information provided by others" (Borkman, 1976, p. 446). Established by a formal profession and transmitted through socialization into that profession, objective knowledge is derived from systematic data collection and analysis. In the mental health field, professionalism is associated with degrees, credentials, and certification.

The knowledge base for a self-help/professional collaborative perspective is derived from an integration of experiential and professional knowledge. The assumption that the two knowledge bases are complementary follows from Borkman's view (1976) that experiential and professional knowledge can coexist and can be organized for sharing by self-help groups and professionals. As Borkman indicates, professional approaches vary in the extent to which they inherently share some of the attributes of experiential knowledge (e.g., client-centered therapy's emphasis on the subjective, behavior therapy's concern with overt behavior). In our view, an integrated mental health service-delivery system must acknowledge both knowledge bases and employ them separately or together as warranted.

While Borkman's analysis of experiential knowledge is limited to self-help groups, it can be extended to the informal or natural helping networks mentioned earlier. Informal helpers likewise develop their own experiential knowledge, which over time leads to the development of a notion that parallels Borkman's experiential expertise. Our integrated self-help/professional perspective draws upon the experiential knowledge acquired by self-help groups as well as natural helpers.

A collaboration that synthesizes the experiential and professional knowledge bases results in a new data base, one that we call "self-help/professional collaborative knowledge." Similarly, as experience with the self-help/professional collaboration expands, there will develop "self-help/professional collaborative expertise." This increased expertise will be reflected in new roles of professionals vis-à-vis self-helpers as well as new roles for self-helpers vis-à-vis professionals.

Self-help/Professional Collaborations in Action

Our perspective is derived from a review and synthesis of self-help/professional collaboration in five major areas: self-help group development; natural helping network enhancement; consultation and education; information and referral; and research. For each area we present specific projects or activities exemplifying self-help/professional collaboration and discuss some salient issues inherent in the collaborative relationship.

Self-help group development. A major activity exemplifying self-help/professional collaboration is the initiation of new self-help and mutual-support groups. A classic example is Silverman's widow-to-widow program (1970) at the Harvard Laboratory of Community Psychiatry. Since then numerous community mental health centers and human service agencies throughout the United States have sponsored support groups for widows. For example, groups for widows and widowers have constituted a priority activity at the Consultation and Education unit of the Rockland County Community Mental Health Center in Pomona, New York (Claflin, 1980, personal communication).

Groups for widowed persons constitute part of a network of eighteen self-help groups established at the Long Island Jewish Medical Center (New Hyde Park, New York). In addition, this hospital sponsors groups for people suffering from such chronic disabilities as diabetes, cancer, heart disease, and DES-related disorders. In the Long Island region, we (Schure, Leif, Slotnick, & Jeger, 1980) have identified thirty-two hospitals that sponsor groups or provide the setting for health-related mental health support groups to develop. What is significant about these hospital-sponsored groups is that they represent a trend toward establishing mental health supports for people with physical illnesses. The groups are necessary because of medical advances which, in turn, have led to the increasing chronicity of physical handicaps. As patients have to deal with chronic physical problems, they may require mental health support groups. These groups are stimulated by hospital-based professional staff in collaboration with their clients.

Our own activities at the college-based Long Island Self-Help Clearinghouse have included the development of a mutual-help group for drug-abuse clients in conjunction with a Methadone maintenance clinic, a support group for returning nursing students, several staff support groups for persons working in state-operated outpatient clinics, and a group for deinstitutionalized psychiatric clients residing in community-based adult homes.

A major issue surrounding the involvement of professionals in the initiation of self-help groups concerns the maintenance of the group's autonomy (Gartner & Riessman, 1977; Katz, 1979; Riessman, 1979). Consumers and citizens are all too often socialized to occupying passive or subservient positions when relating to professionals. This issue is especially critical in agency-based support groups. The delicate line between "collaboration" and "cooptation" is apparent in the conflicts surrounding CanCervive, a self-help program sponsored by the American Cancer Society which ended in failure (see Kleinman, Mantell, & Alexander, 1976). Related to the issue of autonomy is the need for both self-helpers and professionals to demonstrate mutual respect for each other's value systems and differential knowledge bases. Both parties need to keep in mind that neither knowledge base is superior and that an ideal collaborative relationship will successfully integrate the positive features of both knowledge bases. Professionals should not prematurely seek to impose their scientifically derived mental health technologies; rather, they should assist the self-helpers in determining when and how they wish to incorporate the professional knowledge.

It is our contention that most professionals presently engaged in initiation of self-help groups seek to shape "active" consumers. They are not likely to experience the fear of competition and the need to protect vested interests. Since the professionals are generally not in direct service roles, they are likely to prefer activated self-help groups. To accomplish this end, their roles as ecologically oriented mental health professionals are those of facilitator, resource person, and catalyst rather than expert and provider of direct service. We recognize that this is the case since most mental health professionals currently initiating groups are doing so voluntarily. As mental health budgets are reduced, traditional clinically oriented professionals may be mandated to initiate groups— thus possibly working with different motivations.

Natural helping network enhancement.   This area of collaboration refers to professionals forming an interface with informal or natural helping networks; such networks are less organized and less demarcated than self-help groups. The roles of professionals can range from initiating informal helping networks to enhancing existing networks. The following is a summary and discussion of projects that encompass the range of these activities.

At the Florida Mental Health Institute (Tampa), Gordon and his colleagues (Gordon, Edmunson, Bedell, & Goldstein, 1979; Edmunson, Bedell, Archer, & Gordon, 1981) have established the Community Network Development Project (CND) to improve the quality of community life for discharged patients and to prevent their future rehospitalization. Briefly, networks of twenty to fifty former patients living in proximity were developed and supervised by a lay Client Area Manager (CAM). The CAM's role was to lead weekly meetings of network members, provide peer counseling and referral information, and facilitate goal planning sessions among members. Network members often called each other, met socially, loaned each other money, helped with transportation, provided temporary housing, and manifested support for maintaining independent living. Professional staff roles included the development of modules and correlated training for CND members in such areas as pre-employment skills, peer counseling, group leadership, and community survival skills. Staff also serve as evaluators of the program. CND participants, relative to a control group, were less likely to be rehospitalized, spent fewer days in psychiatric hospitals, and were less likely to continue utilizing the services of mental health agencies.

Libertoff (1979) reported on a project of the Washington County Youth Service Bureau (Montpelier, Vermont) which sought to capitalize on the strengths of rural communities in providing help for runaway youths. In lieu of developing a central "runaway house" (typically an urban model), this agency identified and engaged natural helping families to offer temporary shelter and psychological support for runaway youth. The role of the professional agency was to coordinate service delivery for a network of over sixty families and to facilitate support (particularly through advocacy functions and provision of fiscal resources). Youth and adult peer counseling programs were an integral part of the project. Over 8,000 nights of temporary shelter were provided to hundreds of youths during the first three years of the program.

Norton, Morales, and Andrews (1980) reported on the Neighborhood Self-help Project, a joint effort of the Chicago Commons Association, the Taylor Institute for Policy Studies, and the University of Chicago's School of Social Service Administration. The purpose of this research/intervention project was to identify natural helpers in a low-income ethnic neighborhood, strengthen their informal helping capacities, and stimulate linkages with formal service agencies. Initial results of the project demonstrate that horizontal linkages (ties among individual natural helpers) were strengthened. Vertical linkages (ties between natural helpers and professionals) were also strengthened. Staff roles included serving as educators, advisors, resource persons, and "matchmakers." Similar goals were accomplished by the Neighborhood and Family Services Project in Baltimore and Milwaukee (Biegel & Naparstek, 1979). Additional programs that represent "professional partnerships" with natural helpers are described by Froland and Pancoast (1979).

Some of the issues concerning autonomy discussed in connection with self-help group development are likewise inherent in the type of collaboration considered here. For example, careful specifications of the roles of each party need to be made at the outset. Special sensitivity must be given to the impact of professional involvement on the natural helping process. Professionals must guard against disrupting the natural network and against "professsionalizing" the nature of their helping. Thus, when interacting with natural helpers, professionals should not model the traditional "psychotherapeutic role," lest natural helpers begin to "therapize" their peers. Rather, professionals should be guided by the ecological value that strengthening the natural helping networks involves promoting their capacity to mobilize and redistribute human and material resources, as well as increasing the resourcefulness of the individual natural helper.

On a community level, the goal of professionals working with natural helpers or informal community leaders would be to promote the "competent community." As defined by Iscoe (1974), the competent community is "one that utilizes, develops, or otherwise obtains resources, including of course the fuller development of the resources of the human beings in the community itself." As Iscoe noted, his notion of the competent community parallels Lehman's concept (1971) of positive mental health—namely, that the "utilization of resources," as opposed to the absence of symptoms, constitutes an index of mental health. In keeping with these values, the common goal of all the projects described in this section was to increase the self-helpers' resourcefulness, and thereby the self-sufficiency of their respective constituencies. While some of the projects mentioned reported increased utilization of professional caregiving agencies (which is congruent with the notion of utilizing resources), care must be taken not to encourage citizens to increase their dependencies on professional agencies. That is, while we view the interface between professionals and natural helpers as positive, there exists the potential danger that citizens may gravitate to and potentially over-rely on the professional caregiving system and that in fact professionals may implicitly or explicitly encourage natural helpers to make referrals to them instead of continuing to help people themselves. It is also important, however, that natural helpers learn to refer citizens to professional agencies when professional interventions seem warranted.

A final issue concerning collaboration with natural helping networks involves the unique significance of the "entry" process into the natural community. In his discussion on the role of process variables in community work, Kelly (1979) gives particular attention to managing entry into communities. He emphasizes that committing extra time and energy is especially crucial during the entry phase since this "makes it possible to take advantage of the unplanned and natural opportunities that occur as the new working relationship unfolds" (Kelly, 1979, p. 254). It is during entry that the setting is assessed in order to determine ways in which competencies can be expressed; entry also provides opportunities for learning new competencies. Further, Kelly states that ecologically oriented practitioners and researchers should begin by generating a support system for themselves, since the reward structure in mental health agencies all too often encourages "solitary activities." Extending one's relationship with other organizations is one way of creating a resource support system for the practitioner (see later section, "Future Directions"). According to Kelly, the basis for these guidelines rests on the notion of the "dignity of problem solving"—namely, the view that problem solving is an opportunity and that operating within a problem-solving perspective is energizing.

Consultation and education. While in the previous areas (self-help group development and natural network enhancement) consulting and service as educational resources clearly constitute significant professional roles, our focus in this section is on the roles of consultation and education in collaborating with *existing* groups and organizations. The activities engaged in by professionals in the projects described below include providing technical information and skill training, offering formal and informal workshops on specific areas identified by members of self-help organizations, developing technical resource materials to facilitate group functioning, and designing educational curricula to promote self-help awareness among students and the general public.

Mental health professionals working within a behavior-modification framework have increasingly been called upon by self-help organizations to focus their technical skills on facilitating behavior change. For example, in an early study, Miller and Miller (1970) successfully employed reinforcement techniques to increase the attendance rates of welfare recipients at self-help meetings. In the context of a "community consultation project," Miller (1978) offered eight weekly group sessions on applying behavioral techniques to staff of an Alcoholics Anonymous halfway house. The sessions included training in assertion skills, interpersonal skills, relaxation, and development of behavioral alternatives to abusing alcohol. As a result of the consultation, participants requested behavioral training to incorporate into the ongoing halfway house program.

Self-help groups for weight control have likewise interacted with professional behavior modifiers in order to enhance their programs. For example, Levitz and Stunkard (1974) added a behavior modification component to Take Off Pounds Sensibly (TOPS), the oldest weight-management program. It produced greater weight loss and significantly lower attrition rates than the alternative treatment methods. In a more ambitious project, Stuart (1977) developed eighteen behavioral modules (Personal Action Plans), trained group leaders working with Weight Watchers in their use, and actively involved program participants in module discussion. Following experimental evaluations that showed that the modules produced significantly greater weight loss, relative to control groups, these behavioral packages were integrated into the Weight

Watchers Program. Based on the success of this effort, Stuart suggested that a role for professionals vis-à-vis self-help groups is the development and evaluation of behavioral technologies, to be given to the self-help groups for dissemination to large numbers of people.

Over the course of several years, Fawcett and his colleagues (e.g., Fawcett, Fletcher, & Mathews, 1980; Fawcett, Fletcher, Mathews, Whang, Seekins, & Merola, in press) developed, evaluated, and disseminated behaviorally oriented "community education" materials as part of their Community Technology Project at the University of Kansas. These include materials in the areas of self-help technologies, living-skills education, employment preparation programs, and community support systems. Written modules were developed in collaboration with the low-income staff members of a local multipurpose neighborhood service center. Specific modules focused on developing community-based "open learning centers" to prepare nontraditional students for a high school equivalency degree; developing information and referral services for community service workers; operating emergency food and clothing centers; training in basic office skills; and training in problem-solving skills for use by nonprofessional counselors. The basic goal of the Community Technology Project is to enhance the capacities of local communities to help themselves and reduce their dependency on the formal help-giving systems.

Additional activities in the area of consultation and education have come from the National Self-Help Clearinghouse as well as the regional self-help clearinghouses in New York City, Long Island, and Westchester. For example, at the National Self-help Clearinghouse, resource materials on organizing self-help groups were prepared in the form of instructional guides (e.g., Bowles, 1978; Dory, 1979). Information contained in these comprehensive manuals ranges from finding a place to meet to group process skills. At the Long Island Self-help Clearinghouse, materials were developed for use by child-care workers in a community-run Mothers Center (Kohl & Marcus, 1979). They focused on developmental activities for enhancing cognitive, social, and motor functioning in children up to age four. Self-care modules were also developed for elderly community residents, focusing on their needs for medication (Marcus, 1979) and enhanced sensory functioning (Kohl, 1979). The Westchester Self-help Clearinghouse (Borck, 1980, personal communication) offered a series of six-session training seminars to leaders of self-help groups, focusing on enhancing their helping and group-leadership skills.

Self-help related course work has also been incorporated into the curricula designed for the preparation of professional and nonprofessional mental health workers. Influenced by our Long Island Self-help Clearinghouse, the New York Institute of Technology offered graduate and undergraduate seminars on "self-help in the human services." By featuring representatives of local self-help organizations, these seminars provided students with exposure to the experiential knowledge base of self-helpers as a complement to the academic material on self-help as perceived by professionals. As part of community mental health (and related) curricula, seminars of this nature constitute one vehicle for educating students in the practice of self-help/professional collaboration.

A major issue when consulting with self-help groups concerns the development of a truly collaborative relationship. Professionals and self-help group members alike need to be particularly sensitive to the processes inherent in sharing their respective technical skills. Self-help groups should have the final choice as to whether and how to apply the professional knowledge offered. Professionals should not attempt to mold self-help group members in the traditional style of delivering clinical service. At the same time, self-help groups need to be "ready" to receive professional consultation, acknowledge and respect the utility of professional knowledge, and contribute to the mutuality and reciprocity that make possible a collaborative working relationship. Finally, in the area of resource development, wherever possible, self-helpers should be involved in all phases of production and evaluation. This will not only facilitate widespread dissemination but will insure that the materials are suited for use by group members—in terms of readability, writing style, use of jargon, and contents.

Information and referral. Perhaps the most common way in which professionals and self-helpers have interfaced is their reliance upon each other as referral sources. For professionals to be able to refer community residents to self-help groups, knowledge of ongoing groups, their locations, contact persons, and so forth must exist. Toward this end, the special Task Force on Community Support Systems of The President's Commission on Mental Health (1978b) recommended that clearinghouses on self-help be developed throughout the country:

> [to]integrate information, to publish newsletters and other materials, to provide training and technical assistance, to sponsor periodic regional conferences on self-help, to enable professionals and members of self-help groups to learn from each other [p. 178].

The task force also recommended that directories of mutual-help groups be published and disseminated by community mental health centers.

In keeping with the above recommendations, national and regional self-help clearinghouses have been established. At the broadest level, clearinghouses serve to raise consciousness about self-help in a particular region. Typically, clearinghouses collect information on self-help and mutual-aid activities in a region and disseminate it to mental health and human service professionals, self-help networks, and community residents by maintaining a telephone information service, sponsoring conferences and self-help fairs, and publishing newsletters and directories. Directories generally contain basic descriptive information as to the purpose and activities of self-help groups, their address, telephone of contact person, time and location of meetings, and admission requirements. A unique feature of the directory published by the Long Island Self-help Clearinghouse (Schure et al., 1980) is the inclusion of human service agencies and community hospitals which sponsor groups—thereby giving particular attention to self-help/professional collaboration.

A critical issue relating to information and referral involves the organizational bases of clearinghouses and the influence of these bases on the nature of services offered. As Borman and Lieberman (1979) have indicated:

> There may be an important organizational basis for developing such clearinghouses independently of existing mental health agencies or clinics. One of the problems of tacking on an added function, such as a clearinghouse, to an existing large organization, such as a mental health center, is that the new task may be neglected or simply overwhelmed by other more important purposes of the organization. A clearinghouse is not a treatment facility. This fact alone suggests clear separation from clinical-treatment agencies [p. 425].

In keeping with this rationale, most of the existing clearinghouses are based in colleges and universities. An interesting feature of the Westchester County Self-help Clearinghouse is its co-sponsorship by a college (Pace University, which is its home), a state psychiatric facility (Harlem Valley Psychiatric Center), and the Westchester County Department of Community Mental Health. All three share the costs of operating the clearinghouse.

To improve the accuracy and success of referrals, Gottlieb (in press) suggested that collaborative evaluative research be conducted to ascertain the "fit" between potential client characteristics and the specific program of self-help groups. It should be emphasized that self-helpers require similar information on professional programs and consumers should therefore be involved in the evaluation process. While a great deal of research on professional treatment has been carried out, the tenor of the findings as to which type of intervention is best for which problems remains inconclusive, and, in any case, hardly available to the public.

Research.   As mental health practitioners have directed their attention to the self-help movement to develop collaborative interventions, social science researchers have likewise begun to carry out research on self-help groups and natural helping networks (Froland & Pancoast, 1979; Lieberman & Borman, 1979). Unfortunately, a great deal of this research evolved from a traditional research orientation, whereby self-helpers became subjects of professionally designed and executed research studies. The self-help/professional collaborative model calls for research that provides feedback to the self-help organization on its processes and outcomes.

We are calling for research guided by the values of the ecological paradigm—that the professional researcher consider him- or herself a partner with the self-help group, while striving to maintain scientific objectivity. Stated differently, the research should be conducted *for* the self-help group, rather than *on* it. The researcher's expertise and methodologies should be employed to the advantage of the group, not merely to contribute to the "professional literature." Borman's (1979) "action anthropology" approach, which is sensitive to working *with* a subject group, has guided the research conducted at his Self-help Institute (Northwestern University). This collaborative strategy merits attention by other researchers on self-help. Borman (1975) has stated that:

> Members of the [self-help] group should be involved in all phases of the research from the planning to the execution through the interpretation of findings. . . . Researchers should attempt to learn thoroughly the group's values and plan the total research process in a manner that respects and maintains the group's values. . . . Researchers should accept as a responsibility the training of group members in research in order to increase the capacity of self-helpers to solve their own problems. . . . All policy and operating decisions which might in any way be related to research being conducted should always be made by members of the group, not by the researchers [p. 274–75].

An exemplar of the action anthropology approach to research is the ongoing national collaborative program between researchers at the Self-help Institute and epilepsy self-help group participants (see Borman, Davies, & Droge, 1980). Through this effort the collaborators are developing materials to facilitate the growth and development of epilepsy self-help groups, while forming a national information network.

The work of Levy and his colleagues (e.g., Levy, 1979; Wollert,

Knight, & Levy, 1980) likewise reflects research compatible with a self-help/professional collaborative perspective. They studied the processes and activities of the following self-help groups, among others: Alcoholics Anonymous, Overeaters Anonymous, Make Today Count, Parents Anonymous, Take Off Pounds Sensibly, Emotions Anonymous, and Parents Without Partners. A twenty-eight-item instrument of help-giving activities to be rated by members of self-help groups was developed by the research team (see Levy, 1979). This constitutes a useful tool for monitoring group process over time by self-help group members. Also, in the course of their work, members of Levy's self-help research team served as organizational consultants to a chapter of Make Today Count, which resulted in improved group functioning (see Wollert et al., 1980). Thus, their research, carried out within a collaborative framework, was employed by the group for its own enhancement.

A "Conflict" Approach to Self-help/Professional Relations

Before considering future directions for our proposed "collaborative" perspective, we wish to call the reader's attention to a "conflict" approach of self-help/professional relations endorsed by Katz (1979), a student of the self-help movement for some thirty years. Katz's formulation is presented here for the sake of balance and to indicate some of the issues that need to be considered if a self-help/professional collaborative perspective will ever lead to an integrated mental health delivery system.

While acknowledging the usefulness of limited interface, Katz takes the position that self-help groups and professionals:

> seem to need each other not as complements, but in a sense as opposites. Each achieves vitality through opposition to the other. . . . The prospects for a future co-existence seem to lie not in the wishful belief that a greater degree of cooperation will take place, but rather in the maintenance of co-existing systems, with continuing tensions and conflicts [1979, p. 25].

This viewpoint is based on observations that relatively few professionals are "comfortable" with self-help groups to the point of accepting them as integral components of a professionally dominated mental health delivery system. He is not optimistic about most professionals separating themselves from their sources of power, status, and funding to join forces with the self-help movement.

In addition, Katz notes that professionals as a group tend to be uncomfortable with the style of helping in mutual-support groups—for example, the reciprocity, the personal involvement and self-disclosure, and the dependence indicated by continued group participation. Thus, due to the differences that exist in the kind and quality of help offered by the two systems, Katz maintains that both systems should be separately maintained, and that the values of each will be enhanced through remaining separate.

Whereas Katz's position clearly has a historical basis, we are optimistic about the prospects of developing collaborative relations for several reasons. First, since the early 1970s more and more professionals have begun to form interfaces with the self-help movement in ways that are not cooptive, but that respect the autonomy of the self-help organizations. Indeed, conflict-ridden interfaces may be the first step to collaboration in many instances. Second, there is support on the national level for such collaboration to take place. For example, the President's Commission on Mental Health (1978b) recognized self-help groups as integral components of natural helping networks and called upon professionals to enhance the group's roles. Finally, it may be that with increasing concerns about the prevention of mental health problems (relative to the almost exclusive concern with treatment to date), financial and professional incentives may be forthcoming for mental health workers who promote the self-help movement and develop collaborative working relationships.

Future Directions

In considering future directions for self-help/professional collaboration, we wish to draw upon Sarason's notion of the "resource exchange network" (REN) (Sarason, Carroll, Maton, Cohen, & Lorentz, 1977; Sarason & Lorentz, 1979). While support groups and informal networks among individuals have been discussed in various sections of this chapter, resource exchange networks constitute a specific type of support system among individuals while extending the notion of networks to settings or agencies.

Sarason and his colleagues began thinking in terms of "networks" on account of several observations. First, Sarason and co-workers (1977) pointed to the "unprecedented interrelatedness" in our society within and between various settings and institutions. They suggested that a failure of human service agencies to recognize the fact of "limited resources" and the fact that they are always "competing" for a share of limited funding for personnel and capital are critical factors contributing to the diminished "psychological sense of community" (Sarason, 1974). As a partial response to this situation, Sarason and a group of individuals from various educational and human service settings began to form linkages for purposes of exchanging resources in barter-style. As the number of participants increased, a greater diversity of institutions and resources became accessible and a resource exchange network (i.e., the Essex Network) evolved. As walls of agencies were permeated, the effect of the REN included an expansion of agency resources, satisfaction of the individual needs for support, and a sense of community. Thus, the rationale of the REN is based on the fact of limited resources coupled with the value of the psychological sense of community as in forming action. The opportunity for professional growth as well as self-growth for providers of mental health services is valued as much as the growth of the clients of those services (Sarason, 1972). Thus, the REN philosophy capitalizes on the interface between the individual and organization, thereby contributing to the enhancement of both.

According to Sarason and Lorentz (1979), the "ideal" type of REN is defined as:

> a voluntary, loose association of heterogeneous individuals willing to consider ways whereby each is willing to give and get needed resources from others, to seek to increase the number and diversity of participants, to place no restrictions on the substance or foci of exchanges, and to resist putting considerations of exchange and planning under the pressures of funding and the calendar [p. 178].

While recognizing that most RENs are not characteristic of this ideal, we wish to emphasize several salient features of RENs that are compatible with this definition. RENs redefine a resource need from "problem" to "opportunity." That is, RENs provide opportunities for redefining oneself and others as resources. Rather than dwell on deficits, the nature of REN transactions builds upon strengths, thereby serving capacity-building and empowerment functions in addition to improving service. The operating base of a REN is generally between agencies rather than within an agency. However, unlike federations, coalitions, and coordinating councils, which are comprised of member organizations and constitute major vehicles of interorganizational relations, RENs are composed of individuals who are also members of organizations but not necessarily representing their agencies in any official role. As such, RENs are loose, informal, and voluntary—with no formal decision-making structure or director; instead they use a "leader-coordinator," who functions more as a facilitator than as a conventional leader. His or her special abilities should include scanning the environment for resources, matchmaking, and being sensitive to interrelatedness. For example, the leader-coordinator should be able to see the possible connection between the needs of children, youth, and the elderly for its resource linkage potential—for instance, the utilization of teenagers and elderly in child care for the mutual benefit of all three groups.

What are the implications of the resource exchange network for a self-help/professional collaborative model? First, given the rationale of RENs—namely, their focus on strength building—we see RENs as providing vehicles for planning and implementing other mutual-support programs, such as self-help networks. That is, as RENs become more popular within professional mental health agencies, the kind of interventions likely to be supported would be compatible with the larger self-help, mutual-aid movement. Next, we point to developments with three types of RENs—among professional agencies, among self-help groups, and among individual community residents—that have implications for self-help/professional collaboration.

Among professional agencies, an interesting example of an interorganizational network in the Long Island region, one that is more "circumscribed" than the Sarason and associates (1977) Essex Network, was initiated by Rooney (1980, personal communication). She facilitated the development of a REN among directors of Long Island mental health and human service agencies funded by United Way. The aim of this network is to improve services to the constituency of each agency by having agencies develop a cooperative strategy of resource sharing—including the exchange of such concrete services and facilities as in-service supervision and printing. A similar project in the Long Island region is reflected in the Bayshore Resource Network developed by Topitzer and Green (1979, personal communication). The purpose of this network is to develop cooperative and reciprocal relationships among members of various human service groups, agencies, and institutions in order to exchange information, skills, space, material, and personnel.

Networks of self-help groups, while only a recent phenomenon, are already taking a variety of forms. These include a coalition of groups around a common problem or across problems, with or without professionals. Networks of mutual-help coalitions are also taking shape. Some examples follow.

In the context of consulting with self-help groups, Silverman (see Chapter 15 of this volume) developed a strategy for forming linkages among representatives of various self-help groups in order to share resources and information to their mutual benefit. For example, a self-help group that has become highly developed through establishing an appropriate organizational mechanism is now in a position to provide direct assistance to a new group that is just beginning to grapple with the issue of organizational structure. Such a network is perceived as preferable to professionals serving as "experts" when consulting with individual self-help groups. Silverman defined the role of the consultant as "resource linker" and encouraged its further development. While Silverman's project was not conducted within a REN framework, it can potentially provide a positive contribution in the further development of the self-help/professional collaborative perspective.

Borman's project (1980), whereby a monthly Self-help Epilepsy Workshop is held with representatives of epilepsy groups across the country, is likewise compatible with the REN approach. At the National Self-help Clearinghouse, Gartner and Riessman (1980, personal communication) are implementing an NIMH-funded Urban Brokerage Training Project. This project brings together representatives from the professional and self-help communities to exchange information, to discuss issues of mutual concern, and to provide a forum for the growth of linkages between self-helpers and professionals. A goal of this project is to develop a collaborative model that will be disseminated nationally. Clearly, national and regional self-help clearinghouses can provide the viable bases from which to facilitate the development of resource exchange networks among self-help groups, among professionals and self-helpers, as well as among individual community residents.

A most innovative direction in applying the network approach to self-help groups is apparent in the recently formed network of "self-help coalitions/councils" of six major cities. This network is made up of such "umbrella" coalitions as Toronto Self-help and Minnesota Mutual-help Council. Its purpose is to "initiate and strengthen self-help alliances by providing technical assistance, leadership training, help in writing funding proposals, and development of public relation skills" (Gartner, 1980, p. 1).

Conclusion

This chapter has presented an initial formulation of an emerging self-help/professional collaborative perspective of mental health service delivery which can contribute to an integrated and coordinated mental health delivery system. It is not offered as a "finished product" but rather as a guiding framework for self-help/professional collaboration. By presenting projects that exemplify collaboration in five major areas where professionals and self-helpers have formed interfaces and discussing major issues inherent in these collaborative efforts, we hope to stimulate more specific analyses to further the development of the self-help/professional collaborative perspective.

14

The Professional as Developer of Natural Helping Systems: Conceptual, Organizational, and Pragmatic Considerations

Theodore R. Vallance and Anthony R. D'Augelli

The rising costs and decreasing financial resources of mental health services require that less costly and equally effective means for providing direct services be discovered. This chapter addresses the problem of how the mental health professional can effectively assist in extending the manpower base of community mental health services through the involvement and training of natural helpers. The community mental health system cannot afford the luxury of having the mental health professional be the sole—or even the primary—provider of direct services to clients. The professional must be able to supervise paraprofessionals, consult with other diverse human service agencies, develop and administer mental health education efforts, and implement program evaluations. The view of the professional as an expert in indirect services, broadly conceived, is consistent with the ideology of community mental health. The appropriateness of this role is supported empirically by studies that find few outcome differences between professionals and less trained personnel in direct service delivery (see Durlak's review, 1979), clearly suggesting that the latter can perform many direct service functions under the training and supervision of the professional.

Recent interest in the use of natural support systems for mental health purposes provides yet another challenge to the mental health

Judith Frankel D'Augelli is thanked for her help on this chapter.

professional. Forging linkages to the informal system of caregiving in communities is an experience that is qualitatively different from the other role expansions noted above. The professional in this instance is contemplating working with a source of mental health personnel who often have no contact with mental health agencies, little ideological commitment to "mental health," and minimal interest in becoming extension agents of a mental health center. Problems of enlisting the interest and then ensuring the skill levels of members of this personnel pool make the task quite different from simply reorganizing existing agency personnel to provide quasi-professional services more efficiently and effectively.

The chapter will discuss issues important to professionals involved in developing new services using natural helpers—or other persons new to the mental health system—who perform a mental health function without labeling themselves "mental health agents." We will concentrate on the use of training as a skill-enrichment tool for such natural helpers.

The beginning focus of the chapter will be on general principles of personnel development in mental health and their applicability to natural support systems. We then present a way of thinking about the process of personnel development—admittedly a somewhat idealized and, for clarity, simplified model. The workings of the model will be illustrated in a specific field project directed toward enhancing the capabilities of natural helpers. The chapter closes with a discussion of the mental health professional's role in a community service delivery system in which natural helpers are effectively utilized.

Organizational Issues in Personnel Change in Mental Health Systems

Because the mental health system is so labor-intensive, the greatest opportunities for major improvements in system effectiveness and efficiency lie in personnel development. Improvement can result from increasing the quality of service from current personnel or through the creation of positions for new personnel who can provide similar, if not improved, benefits at lower cost. Among the improvements over the last decade in mental health systems, a number have occurred as a function of enhancing the skills of current professionals or by enlisting new sources of personnel such as paraprofessionals and nonprofessionals (President's Commission on Mental Health, Vol. II, 1978b).

Typically, human service systems are open systems that place heavier reliance on selection than on training of personnel. Usually, people enter the mental health system after completing a training program. Subsequent system improvement occurs by continuing education efforts. In addition to enhancing the competencies of staff, mental health systems can improve their processes of self-enhancement by refining training technology to reduce the time and cost of training. By both continually improving selection criteria and simultaneously evaluating and modifying training, considerable systemwide change can result.

The second major personnel enhancement strategy, the creation of new positions, is more challenging. A rational process can be pursued from the start. A cost and content analysis of currently performed duties and services can be undertaken using concrete service system goals as criteria. From these estimates of the efficiency of current positions, planning can begin for instituting new jobs that would facilitate the system's accomplishment of its service goals. After such jobs are identified, it is possible to consider issues of selection and training for these jobs: What aptitudes, skills, and competencies are required and how can acceptable levels of performance be maintained and improved over time? Thereupon job or task descriptions can be generated, selection procedures designed, and training models developed.

Such a rational process does not typically occur in mental health agencies. Normally, efforts to improve mental health personnel do not arise as intentional efforts to upgrade a system for which there are fairly clear-cut lines of responsibility and authority. In the human services, operating control and daily supervision tend to be rather loose and informal. In community mental health centers, heavy reliance on part-time independent professional practitioners is common practice, rather than having the full complement of such professionals on the payroll under the authority of the administrator and board. Likewise, it is common to have services of counseling, partial hospitalization, consultation and education, and others provided through contracts with external service organizations. Because of this, system improvement through personnel development frequently arises adventitiously as a result of studies of the potential for teaching new skills to non-mental health service providers and then trying to fit these resources into the mental health system. Examples are the numerous efforts to train people who are in frequent contact with the public—barbers, taxi drivers, hairdressers, firefighters—in skills that could be easily grafted onto the formal mental health service system. More typically, then, decisions to make improvements in utilization of personnel tend to be based on such external sources and on the hunches of wise observers more often than from formal program evaluations of the mental health service system.

The excellent review by Collins and Pancoast (1976) of over a dozen case studies of natural helpers working with agencies reinforces our feeling that such linkages are both feasible and practical. Further, it underlines our belief that a more orderly way of regarding natural helpers as a part of mental health services, when those services are conceived of as a system, would suggest improvements in how natural helpers can be recruited and trained and ways in which their usefulness in the community could be enhanced. We may also note that experience in our own work in developing natural helpers (see D'Augelli, Vallance, Danish, Young, & Gerdes, in press) led us to see the need for a more systematic conceptualization of how the natural helper can best be identified, trained, and supported.

Developing Personnel Systems

Given the discrepancy between the usual, haphazard process, and a rational, ordered model of personnel enhancement through training, we offer a generic framework for innovation through personnel development.

There are four stages, each identified with an actor or organizational "entity," in the process of which a labor-intensive human service system—such as a mental health system—attempts an improvement through personnel development. (We could use the idea of a "function" in place of "entity." We chose the "entity" concept because it lends itself to more explicit identification of roles and responsibilities.)

First, there must be an entity in which there exists a problem of operating efficiency that can be resolved through a personnel innovation. This *problem-posing entity* can be an outpatient clinic, a community mental health center, or a city or county office that has responsibility for and authority over agencies that provide services. Such a problem-posing agency should be able to recognize that a service is being performed inefficiently—or perhaps not at all. It should also be able to determine to its own satisfaction that the cost of having existing professional staff provide the service would be higher than trying to provide it through some alternative means. The poser of mental health service problems may be from any of a number of different kinds of agencies and at different levels of removal from contact with people being served. Mental health services, broadly considered, may properly be rendered by area agencies on aging, a visiting nurses association, a public health office, a freestanding counseling service, a social welfare office in almost any jurisdiction, or any of several other agencies whose general mission is to help people cope with problems of living. Formally constituted mental health services, either centers or county-based programs, since they are not targeted to a particular set or category of clients, generally have an excellent opportunity—and indeed are mandated if they are federally funded CMHCs—to work with other agencies in search of ways to improve the community's diverse mental health services. Prominent strategies could be the development of linkages with other helping services and with natural indigenous helpers in neighborhoods. The poser of problems of service effectiveness, whatever the agency might be, has the right and even the obligation to seek to develop such informal helping capabilities within the community as are believed useful to that service's objectives.

We propose that the community mental health center (or similar agency) be the primary sensor at the local level of problems in mental health service delivery and of opportunities for personnel improvement and linkages, mainly because of the breadth and noncategorical nature of its charter. (Other problem posers are state, regional, and federal levels of the mental health hierarchy, although people at these levels generally have relied heavily on ideas coming from the operating level.) At this stage an opportunity for potential improvement has been recognized.

The second entity involved, the *model-designing entity*, is an organization that is capable of designing, planning, implementing, and evaluating one or more alternative ways of improving service delivery. In this stage, the problems posed by the prior entity become clarified and various creative and innovative ways for testing and evaluating them are developed. Extensive familiarity with the problem-posing entity, its domain, and its associated services is vital, as is technical competence in design, implementation, and evaluation. In the past, the model-designing entity has been predominantly an academic institution committed to innovation in human service delivery systems. Such institutions, by dint of their personnel's conceptual skills and evaluation commitment, have been able to provide the technical underpinning for model design, development, and testing. In addition, many mental health centers can act in this role, and thus the problem-posing and model-designing entities may be one and the same. (It is interesting to note that federal agencies do not directly play the model-designing role. At NIMH, for example, intramural research is mainly basic research on clinical problems. This policy reflects the mandate of the 1963 Mental Health Act placing the responsibility for service delivery at the community level.) The model-designing and problem-posing entities in concert cannot as yet, however, produce a decision to proceed.

There is needed an entity that can provide several important ingredients to fuel the personnel innovation process—financial support, logistical-administrative support, and community credibility. This *support-generating entity* must be interested enough in the importance of the initiating problem and sufficiently convinced of the reasonableness of the proposed solution to initiate processes to promote financial, administrative, and community support. This entity could be the problem-posing entity first mentioned, or some other external entity. Beyond the practical matter of finances and logistics, this support entity must convince community people who will be affected by the effort that it is a worthwhile, credible, and nonthreatening endeavor.

Proposals for personnel innovation must include clear evidence of need, explicit information on feasibility, and detailed indications of payoff prospects. In addition, expected is such "entity-blurring" information as what formal agencies are involved, who would insure that new training of new personnel would be completed, and how commitments from personnel would be achieved. Thus, this "entity" is not a denotable organization, but rather a system of relationships and working agreements. Further, it is worth noting that this system becomes even more complex when the personnel involved are nonprofessionals such as natural helpers whose linkages to other formal and informal community systems may or may not be known.

This entity is by far the most complex for the mental health innovator since it represents a negotiation of interests of various groups: funding sources, agency administrators, local government officials, agency personnel, new personnel, and the "community-at-large," a heterogeneous and often ill-defined amalgam of interest groups, influential and informed citizens, and uninformed others. The complexity of this particular function makes specification of typical actors difficult. In the past, for example, the pursuit of financial support entailed the identification of a relevant state or federal agency or interested private foundations. The current sophistication in understanding the multifaceted nature of mental health problems and the increased competition for fewer (and inflated) dollars has resulted in the need for greater thoughtfulness in support-generation.

Even with the active cooperation of the foregoing three entities, there do not yet exist the necessary conditions for a decision to innovate. The fourth and critical entity, the *implementing entity*, is one that can reasonably ensure that an innovation in personnel use can indeed be successfully introduced into the system. In a highly controlled industrial or military system, this entity would typically be one with fiscal or command responsibility for the total operation in which the innovation would take place. This fourth entity would review data such as costs of implementation, potential savings or improvements in system efficiency, and estimates of unforeseen side-effects, and thereupon decide how to proceed.

In the mental health field this is the entity that will advocate an innovation and, given reasonable promise of success, make a commitment to adopt and nurture it. It is indeed likely that a mental health agency would be the Implementing Entity since this agency has ongoing and stable working relationships with professional mental health and often human service workers who would be affected by the innovation.

On the other hand, it is very unlikely that the model-designing entity and the implementing entity would, or even should, be the same. The model-designing entity, focusing on issues of research and development, takes an experimental stance: Others are assured that the innovation will be subject to considerable modification as a result of technical considerations (e.g., some training modules are inefficient) and community input. Contrary to the implementing entity, the designing entity is most often not part of the system undergoing innovation. The implementing entity has roots in the community, reputations to protect, alliances to maintain, and political support to sustain. Thus, while the model-designing entity is rewarded by the more abstract benefits of conceiving, creating, and teaching a new strategy, the implementing entity must deal with the very concrete contingencies of day-to-day mental health administration. Of course, the implementing entity must engineer the transition to the pragmatic context in which the innovation will in time become routine.

After all four entities have performed their respective functions, which eventuates in a decision to mount a personnel development effort, the final stage in the decision process is confronted. In this stage, a formal analysis of the costs and benefits of the innovation may be performed. This process in rough outline is essentially the following:

ESTIMATED VALUE
OF THE INNOVATION = ESTIMATED PAYOFF − ESTIMATED COST

where:

1. Payoff = value added to the system by each person affected × the number of persons affected
2. Payoff per person = performance unit gained × the estimated value of each unit + savings in actual costs of current short-term direct service + long-term savings through prevention
3. Cost = costs to entity providing administrative support + costs for entity financing the development project

The Community Helpers Project:
An Innovative Personnel Development Model

The following case example will demonstrate the usefulness of this four-entity model in the analysis of personnel innovation in mental health. The case will illustrate the decision-making processes discussed above and will lead to a consideration of how professionals are involved in the overall change process. (The Community Helpers Project was funded by NIMH Grant No. MH 14883 from July 1977 to June 1980.)

The Community Helpers Project was designed as a model prevention program for rural communities. Prevention programs are especially important for rural areas because of the prevalence of psychosocial distress and the difficulties, due to geographic distances, lack of trained personnel, and so on, in delivering mental health services in these areas. The Community Helpers Project has developed a system of community-based training for natural caregivers; natural helpers' helping skills are enhanced through a set of two skill-training programs of sixteen to twenty hours' duration and distributed over eight to ten weekly sessions. The project uses a pyramid scheme in which mental health professionals teach the helping skills to volunteers in the community who identify themselves as natural helpers to neighbors, relatives, or work associates in problems of everyday living. The helpers so trained are then given further training in how to impart these same skills to yet other community helpers, and they then conduct training sessions of their own. The project's long-run objective is to have in place a self-supporting system for training continuing groups of helpers that will endure independently of the professionals initiating it and that will provide a low-cost helping base within the community that will not be dependent in any way on continued funding from state or federal agencies.

The project was initiated by professionals (eventually project staff) who were based in a research and educational institution (Pennsylvania State University) and a community mental health service (The Mental Health/Mental Retardation Program of Columbia, Montour, Snyder, and Union Counties, Pennsylvania). Discussions by members of this initial group with other mental health service staff led to the conclusion that services to most parts of the four-county area were indeed thin and should be increased if resources to do this could be found. The financial means to extend services of the kind already being provided were clearly not available.

The prospect of developing a low-cost system focused upon primary prevention activities had considerable appeal to mental health service administrators and other local people actively interested in mental health matters. Consultation with providers of associated services and with the advisory board for the four-county mental health program led to a determination that a need did in fact exist for the kind of service that was contemplated. Thus the problem-posing entity was the local mental health system, which was provoked by both external and internal forces to contemplate an innovation.

The model-designing entity was Pennsylvania State University, more specifically, two cooperating human service graduate programs within the College of Human Development. Clearly, the University did not execute the project; but its name is important because the University is a legally responsible corporate entity that can assume and enforce responsibility in a contractual relationship. The actual project staff, working within the authority of this corporate entity, further elaborated the idea of a "helping skills" approach to personnel development and worked closely with the "problem-posing entity" to get the concept into a form that could be provisionally operationalized.

Soon thereafter, the third entity, the support-generating entity, was identified. This entity was in actuality a complex of organizations: the National Institute of Mental Health and a set of human service agencies in addition to the mental health program in the proposed project site. Consultation with NIMH staff led to the expectation that funds might be forthcoming; and consultation with the local service agencies supported a conclusion that assistance in recruiting natural helpers and local advisory boards and in disseminating information about the project could be anticipated. Both sets of consultations provided the basis for community credibility.

Finally, the fourth and critical entity—the implementing entity— appeared in the mental health program staff and the project's advisory boards; such a board was established for each of the two sites of the project. In addition, there was a commitment from the county commissioners to put up financial support to implement and sustain the program if the results of the developmental project were promising.

The four-entity model seems to have worked quite well. The major problems with it occurred in the early stages of the project when roles and distinctions between entities were being clarified. The project did not attempt to invoke the entity concept with all participants, fearing that this might introduce additional conceptual complexity in that already complex situation. However, were the project to be repeated in another setting it would undoubtedly be necessary to make explicit the use of the model and its concepts.

The project trained approximately 120 helpers. In the six months since the official termination of the project, evidence suggests that project activities are continuing in the two target sites. Twenty new helpers have been recruited and trained with no involvement from Pennsylvania State University. The boards in both areas remain active and are recruiting additional helpers to be trained; we are told that enthusiasm continues. The MH/MR Program Administrator has committed additional funds to help the boards publicize the program and print the necessary teaching manuals. The Community Helpers Project and its numerous outcomes and "how-to" lessons will be described in a monograph now being written.

We turn now to an in-depth examination of one topic especially relevant to our activities, that is, appropriate professional roles in working with natural helpers.

The Role of the Mental Health Professional

What is the role of the mental health professional in the process of developing linkages with natural helping networks, involving them in training, and in bringing them effectively "on line"? There are multiple roles that mental health professionals play in current service delivery systems. The mental health professional will likely be administrator, therapist, counselor, community consultant and educator, group worker, block organizer, psychometrist—to name some job-like titles. In addition to these roles, the mental health professional may be a competitor for professional turf, a seeker or defender of professional status, an adversary of the medical model of mental health service and proponent of some alternative model, an advocate of social reform and the dissemination of power to citizen interest groups. How does the professional mobilize "entities" to forge linkages with informal helping systems?

We see three roles for the mental health professional in this developmental process, each with some identifiable components: as a technologist-advisor in mental health, as a clinical practitioner, and as a humanitarian concerned with community development and change.

Technologist

As a technologist, the mental health professional can perform at least three functions in the development of linkages. First, the professional has an extensive competence in various techniques for helping, advising, counseling, teaching, and otherwise influencing the cognitive events and behavioral acts of people. The experienced mental health professional will be able to advise on the approaches to helping likely to be most appropriate for the kinds of natural helpers that would be the recipients of recruitment efforts and training. Likewise, he or she should be able to provide counsel concerning the target populations or helpees that will be most likely to respond to the new kind of helping service that might emerge. In sum, the qualified mental health professional should be able to help significantly in effecting the most workable match of a set of helper aptitudes and learned skills with a receptive consumer population for that set.

A second technological function is in the assessment of community needs for receptiveness to the kind of mental health assistance that could be provided through an innovation that highlights the use of non-professionals. Needs assessment is a procedure of considerable sophistication, and not every mental health professional will find comfort in its practice; nonetheless most will be able to provide useful guidance in the process and be able to locate more specifically trained assessors as may be necessary.

A cautionary note: Since a prophet is least loved in the prophet's own land, so would it be well to consider the use of a nonindigenous mental health professional in the needs assessment role. One could readily argue against this, noting that knowledge of the community gained from long residence would be indispensable. Such knowledge is very important, to be sure, and its facsimile would have to be acquired by anyone performing a systematic needs assessment. While it may seem expensive to invest the time and money in an outsider to develop the necessary community knowledge and trust by community members, the credibility of a properly executed needs assessment by an impartial outsider might well compensate for the corresponding disadvantages an insider might have.

A third technological function for the mental health professional is in the process of estimating and calculating benefits and costs. Here we are speaking of another sophisticated methodology, one in which economists are the prototypical and dominant practitioners. In any benefit–cost calculation, however, the skills of the economist are necessary but not sufficient for showing the potential—or later, the realized—value of an intervention. The nuts and bolts expertise of the mental health practitioner steeped in the technologies of the field and its traditions, folkways, successes, and failures is indispensable to a credible analysis. Research by Conley, Conwell, and Arril (1967) and by Holtmann (1965) estimating the costs of mental illness—and the value of its prevention—suggests approaches to the problem of estimating the scale of likely payoffs from investments in developing linkages with potentially helpful groups in the community. The costs of lowered human potential when matched with the probability of means to raise such potential could provide the basis for deciding on developmental innovations.

Perhaps the renewed thrust in NIMH toward assessing the efficacy of treatments will lead to increased credibility of this essential component of the decision formula. But again, caution is warranted. The expense of performing quality benefit–cost analyses can itself be rather high, and so its potential worth is partly a function of the likely cost of an intervention. Translation: Don't spend a lot of money to find out how valuable something that's cheap might be.

Clinical Practitioner

In clinical practice, the mental health professional can often become involved with both professional colleagues and nonprofessional helpers. Some mental health practitioners may perceive the natural helper as a threat to their interests. Even assuming such fears to be groundless, there remains the possibility of legitimate professional concern for the welfare of people seeking help from others who may not be competent.

We believe that it is a responsibility of the mental health professional who is called to participate in the development of an innovation based on the use of natural helpers to build into the process safeguards against incorrect use of the skills taught. Such safeguards would and should focus upon the potential recipients of the intended benefits. It would also have the additional effect of protecting the professional ethics of the established practitioner and his or her relations with professional colleagues and peers.

Humanitarian

Turning to the third major role of the mental health professional, that of humanitarian and concerned citizen, consider the Great Society programs in which the community mental health movement saw its most exciting years. Those were the days of "maximum feasible participation" by the citizenry in reshaping their communities. Model Cities, Youth Employment, Community Action Programs were but a few activities whose initial legislation made it possible for community groups to circumvent the formally elected and informally controlling power structure by going to state and federal agencies for money and authority to do good works. Such processes, intended as they were to bring a degree of self-determination to the theretofore powerless poor, had a distinctly humanitarian flavor. Mental health legislation has reflected this ethic in requiring that federally funded mental health centers have boards comprised of a majority of non-service providers, that is, community residents. The CMHC movement was able to attract a large number of professionals sensitive to the inequalities inherent in our society and inclined toward reform. The consultation and education requirement among the mandated services was often used as a means for initiating community improvement as part of primary prevention. (The Center for Metropolitan Mental Health reflected this thrust in NIMH and provided consultation and research support directed toward improving the quality of urban planning as a means for improving the quality of urban life and the mental health of citizens.)

The contemporary mental health professional still has the charter and thus the opportunity—and we should say the moral obligation—to maintain the tradition of improving the quality of community life through whatever means are available. The humanitarian impulses that still characterize much of the community mental health movement can be well expressed by the mental health professional in seeking the most economical and efficient ways to provide quality mental health services to the most needy and least served people in the community. By adopting a service ethic based on a social-contract philosophy of justice (we are each others' keepers and share in their benefits and griefs) as opposed to one based on utilitarianism (the greatest good for the greatest number), humanitarian values can be kept in the forefront of thought as the mental health professional surveys opportunities to engage the broadest linkages in the service of community mental health. (For further explication of this view, see Vallance and Sabre, 1981.) In this way, the mental health professional can provide the dissemination of this humanitarian ideal by inducing natural helpers to continue their good work.

Summary

We have argued that an important role for the community mental health professional lies in the development of means for identifying and training natural helpers within the community. To refine the process for making the decision to invest efforts to improve the functioning of a labor-intensive system such as mental health services, we have outlined and illustrated the working of a set of four related "entities" that are necessary to put personnel development innovations into effect. These are presented as entities that pose and validate problems, design potential solutions, provide logistical support and credibility to a development project, and implement successful outcomes. We propose three roles for the mental health professional in the process: as technologist-advisor on behavior change methods, needs assessment, and evaluation; as practitioner relating to colleagues and to professional standards of quality care; and as humanitarian seeking ways to improve the quality of community life through the development of human resources available in communities.

15

The Mental Health Consultant as a Linking Agent

Phyllis R. Silverman

Mental health professionals are constantly moving outside the borders of their own system to offer their services and thereby extend the influence of their expertise. Traditionally, this activity has been called *consultation* (Kadushin, 1977). Consultation as a helping method is poorly defined. Usually it describes a situation in which an outside expert provides advice to an individual or an organization about a problem that cannot be solved with the latter's current expertise. The recent beneficiaries of this outreach are neighborhood support systems as described elsewhere in this book and mutual-help organizations as defined below.

The offer of help by professionals to another system is often made without the prospective consultants considering the applicability of their knowledge base and related skills to the other system. A consultant cannot simply adapt clinical methods to this role. The work involves a new set of skills (Mendel, 1968) and often a new body of knowledge. Any provision of assistance has to be undertaken with an awareness of the differences between the recipient's system and that of the consultants (Rogawski, 1968). Without these considerations, a consultant may be at the least ineffectual or, in the extreme, disruptive. The problem is particularly serious with mutual-help organizations that have a value system and organizational structure different from other systems to which the professional may relate. The purpose of this chapter is to present a model of consultation that will facilitate the ability of mental health professionals to work effectively with mutual-help organizations. The model is based on the findings of a demonstration project designed to identify various organizational and substantive problems in mutual-help organizations and to determine ways in which mental health professionals could appropriately work with these groups to help solve some of their problems.* While the chapter focuses on the experience with mutual-help groups, the findings of this work and the model developed are applicable to other types of informal groups and networks as well.

The first section of the chapter defines mutual-help organizations and clarifies the ways in which they are different from the formal mental health service system. The next section continues by examining sources of tension and differences between these systems that represent barriers to their working together. The third section discusses aspects of the consultant's role that need to be considered in working with mutual-help organizations. Finally, in the last section, a model of the consultant as linking agent is presented. This model is proposed as one means of achieving successful collaboration between mutual-help organizations and the formal mental health service system.

Mutual-help Organizations

A mutual-help group is an aggregate of people sharing a common problem or predicament who come together for mutual support and constructive action to solve their shared problem. The help offered is based on the participants' experiences in coping with their problems and is not a result of any professional training or education group members may have. Most of the time this type of help takes place in informal exchanges in one's family or among friends and neighbors. Often, however, these informal exchanges evolve into a formal organization with its own governing structure to which people with the same problem are recruited to join as members. Mental health professionals are most aware of these formal organizations and it is with such organizations that they are most likely to consult.

Every mutual-help organization can be identified by (1) its helping

*This was a two-year project funded by the National Institute of Mental Health under a contract # 278-77-0038 (SM) awarded to the American Institutes for Research in the Behavioral Sciences, Cambridge, Massachusetts. The official title of the project was Development of Special Mental Health Technical Assistance Materials for Self-Help Groups in Particular Populations. The contract required that the focus be on groups that were concerned with family violence, minorities, families and children, the elderly, displaced homemakers, and ex-offenders. Based on their experience, the staff of this project prepared six pamphlets to be used by mutual-help groups in general. These unpublished pamphlets deal with organizational and substantive issues. A seventh pamphlet, for professional audiences, describes the professional role and serves as the basis of this paper. The project was called the Mutual Help Project. This designation is used when it is referred to in this chapter.

program and (2) its organizational structure that distinguishes it from other types of helping programs. In a mutual-help group, people are helped by receiving information on how to cope; obtaining material help if necessary; and by feeling cared about and supported. These types of help are uniquely effective because people find others "just like me"; learn from the group experience that other people have similar feelings and that these feelings are "normal"; have the option of becoming a helper, in turn, and are thus not bound to the role of recipient in order to remain in the organization. Thus, in a mutual-help group helpers are approached by others because of their own personal experiences with the problems facing group members.

Help in a professional mental health organization is offered only by someone who is trained and has the appropriate credentials. Professionals develop a work ideology that stresses the technical superiority of their work and their capability. This ideology justifies and legitimates the exercise of professional authority with clients. Mutual-help groups, on the other hand, value experiential knowledge and do not require credentials for participation as a helper in the group. These two sources of knowledge, "experiential" and "professional," are often sources of conflict at the interface between the two systems (Borkman, 1976).

The organizational setting in which the work is carried out and the helpers' relationship to that organization affect the nature of the help offered. In contrast to the formal organizational structure of bureaucratic or professional organizations, mutual-help groups are fluid organizations. In mental health organizations, people typically relate in a hierarchical order, with each position regulated by specific rights and duties.

Unlike the professional organization, mutual-help organizations have a structure which allows for mobility in the system—from recipient to helper—and which enables the consumers or members to control resources and policy. Many groups, such as Parents Without Partners, take the form of a club or voluntary association depending on their members' prior experiences. Some, such as the Gray Panthers and the Mental Patient Liberation Movement, develop a consensus, anti-hierarchical way of governing themselves. The latter groups often come into being as alternate systems with a strong anti-establishment bias because they feel they have been poorly served by establishment agencies. They spend a good deal of energy maintaining their differences and therefore avoid any type of hierarchical organizational structure, sacrificing efficiency to ensure maximum participation of all their members in the life of the organization.

Some groups, such as the La Leche League, are organized as service delivery systems with authority coming from the national office down. Leadership is appointed through an elaborate state–national ascending hierarchy. However, leadership is always recruited from among people who come to meetings and have been helped by the group. Other groups follow parliamentary procedures with established committees and regular election of officers. However, even when a hierarchy exists, leaders lack a reward and sanction system to enforce their power. Members leave when a group stops meeting their needs. Most often an informal consensus determines group policy and often organizational viability is maintained through the application of new rules, which can be invented as needed.

Most groups are small with limited memberships, from ten to twenty people, are constantly struggling to maintain themselves, and seem to have similar problems. They need help in developing and maintaining leadership and in developing procedures for involving more members in the work of the organization; they have difficulty in defining their goals, in developing helping programs that meet all their members' needs, and in implementing their goals and program ideas. In order to get things done they tend to let one or two people carry the burden of the organization. Some groups are only partly aware of the value of the help that group members provide to each other. Such groups feel self-conscious when interacting with professionals, feeling that what the group is doing is not adequate. Sometimes they place a greater value on professional assistance than upon self-help. These groups need approbation and support about the appropriateness of their own activities. One way in which they can find stability and enhance their organizational effectiveness is to turn to community agencies and ask for help from their staff. Some groups have formed alliances with established and prestigious national organizations such as the American Cancer Society, but the price of this affiliation often involves some loss of autonomy (Tracy and Gussow, 1976). In such cases members feel constrained by controls imposed by boards of directors of the parent organization, which are often dominated by medical and organizational professionals.

Groups have also found ways of sustaining themselves by joining with each other. They form local federations or coalitions of organizations with similar agendas. Such coalitions exist, for example, for battered women's groups and for parent groups for children with various special needs.

The most effective way for groups to sustain themselves in the long run is to be affiliated with a national organization from which they can receive direction and advice on programmatic and organizational issues. There are several types of national organizations. The simplest form is a loose network of autonomous groups. However, the most common form

is a formally organized national association that authorizes the establishment of local branches or chapters that use its name. Dues from these
affiliated chapters often support a national office and its paid staff, who
develop program materials for the local groups. Some groups also provide consultants from regional offices to help promote strong chapters.

Interface between Mutual-help Organizations and Mental Health Services

While mutual-help groups have a specific ideology, value system, and
structure that differentiate them from more formal mental health helping systems in a community, they nonetheless share a common goal with
professionals of promoting the well-being of their constituents. Occasionally, both groups have the same people as members and as clients,
respectively. Various theories exist about how these two systems ought
to and do relate to each other. Baker (1977) believes that the two systems should engage in free communication and collaboration with each
other and should supplement each other's services. Other professionals
urge the promotion of a psychological sense of community that would
strengthen the relationship between informal and formal organizations
(Sarason, 1974). Gartner and Riessman (1977) want mutual-help groups
to be change agents and believe that they can help humanize the human
services. Caplan (1976a), Dumont (1976), and Silverman (1978) caution
that the distinct qualities of each system be maintained. Gottlieb (1976)
suggests that each part must recognize the presence and legitimate functions of the other.

Baker (1977), while recognizing the separateness of the two systems, observes that they nevertheless interface with each other in important ways and that this interaction is often characterized by tension
and competition. Sources of competition relate to such issues as clients,
political sanctions, financing, volunteers, and information. Huey (1977b)
identified feelings of power resulting from the professional's need to
maintain a superordinate position as "expert" as a major determinant
affecting the ability of the professional to cooperate with mutual-help
groups.

Another area of tension between the two systems often results
from a difference in perspective about the helping value of each system. The nature of the help given in mutual-help groups is sometimes
judged by professionals to be superficial (Silverman, 1978). The implication is that "real" help must involve restructuring and rebuilding the
personality. In addition, the professional often sees continual participa-

tion in the mutual-help group as an indication of dependency rather than as a demonstration of newfound strength to help others (Silverman, 1978). Further, professionals traditionally value objectivity and detachment and are uncomfortable with the level of personal involvement exhibited by members of mutual-help groups. Finally, professionals feel that credentials are required to work with people who are experiencing serious personal difficulties.

Members of mutual-help organizations for their part have often had poor experiences with the formal helping system. At times they denigrate the services offered, encouraging members to rely on each other for any and all assistance they require. Because, historically, professionals have often attempted to co-opt mutual-help organizations or to impose professional knowledge only, mutual-help organizations have considered professionals to be intruders (Katz, 1961; Collins and Pancoast, 1976). Collaboration and cooperation between the two systems may be more an ideal than a reality. Borman (1975) writes that:

> successful consultants have had to behave in nontraditional ways, not typically associated with their role as a professional and as a mental health consultant. Many of them [self-help groups] have been initiated and supported by professionals. Many of these have had to "bootleg" their efforts since they were never sanctioned by the agencies for which they worked. In order to enhance the experience of people who are trying to help themselves and each other, these professionals have had to abandon many customary approaches to helping troubled individuals. They had to learn to play a subsidiary role and to have their opinions rejected as often as accepted.

These qualities that Borman describes are in fact attributes of a successful consulting relationship. The mental health system is only now beginning to legitimate the role of consultant to mutual-help organizations and to analyze what qualities would facilitate a successful relationship. What are the attributes of a good consultant who does not intrude and who does not need to "bootleg" his or her activity?

The Professional as Consultant

As we have stated, consultation is a professional activity which, in its simplest sense, refers to a process by which an expert attempts to help a less knowledgeable consultee solve a problem (Rapoport, 1971). However, there is little agreement, beyond this definition, among mental health consultants as to what they do as consultants.

Despite the general assumption among mental health professionals doing consultation that they are operating within a set of principles which distinguish their consultation efforts from traditional treatment modalities, there is an absence of consistency in the way consultation is conducted [McClung & Stunden, 1970].

Students of the consultation process stress the importance of establishing and maintaining an effective relationship between consultant and consultee; assisting in diagnoses of the problem and the development of alternative solutions; and achieving a satisfactory terminal relationship. Implicit in these activities are the essential elements of gaining the sanction of the key staff of the consultee agency and of developing a contract that specifies the consultant–consultee relationship and the goals and expectations of the consultation (Rapoport, 1963). The consultant has no responsibility in the consultee system for carrying out any recommendations made, nor does he or she have any administrative responsibility in the host system, so that his or her recommendations can be ignored as easily as implemented.

In many types of consultation, the consultant never has contact with the consultee's client, who nonetheless is often the main subject of the consultation. Typically, consultation is often an ongoing process in which consultee and consultant meet on a regular basis to discuss problems as they arise, approximating for mental health consultants the long-term relationship they may have with clients in their own system (Caplan, 1970). The role clearly has similar elements to those found in the role of therapist. Levenson (1972) describes consultation more in terms of a task-oriented approach in which the consultant role is defined as coming in and studying a problem, making a diagnosis, and recommending a solution with suggestions for implementing the recommendations.

Havelock and Havelock (1973) point out that the role of mental health consultant is expanded to include dimensions other than the traditional roles presented by Caplan and by Levenson. He notes that since the consultant is there to effect some change in the system, he or she can be identified as a change agent. Another function Havelock identifies is that of "interpersonal linking agent." The function of the interpersonal linking agent is to serve as a channel between resources and the consultee system. One kind of linker is the conveyor, who takes knowledge from expert sources and passes it on to nonexpert users—someone who takes a fully packaged and fully usable product and places it in the hands of the user. In the role of linker the consultant is a facilitator, helper, objective observer, and the specialist in how to diagnose needs, how to identify resources, and how to retrieve expert sources. He tells "how" in contrast to the conveyor, who tells "what."

There are special behaviors or considerations that result in more successful consultation. Most researchers agree that whether the consultant acts in the traditional roles of a study/diagnosis and treatment consultant, or as a change agent or linking agent, the relationship between the consultant and the consultee must be coordinated and nonhierarchical for mutual trust and respect to develop. Kadushin (1977) focuses on the need of the consultant to have expert knowledge. Sometimes, he notes, "egalitarian peer" relationships are confusing and run counter to the consultee's expectations that the consultant is an authoritative expert, which is why he or she was called in. Rogers and Shoemaker (1971) found that the degree to which the consultant and client are alike is an important factor leading to effective diffusion of new knowledge within the client system. Larson, Norris, and Kroll (1976) drew the following conclusions about the behavior of a good consultant:

he or she listened
he or she did not step in or out of a role, rather he or she interacted with the staff in all situations
he or she was a storehouse of information
he or she made use of past experiences
he or she functioned as a pipeline and information conveyor
he or she suggested action alternatives
he or she saw the consultation as a personal learning experience
he or she suggested clients work on problems they would realistically be expected to solve
he or she acted as a catalyst

All of this research on consultation has dealt with situations in which the consultant and consultee have come from similar organizations, with similar structures and ideologies about the work they do, and have had similar or parallel positions in the hierarchy. Typically, these are professional and bureaucratic organizations providing consultation to other similar organizations.

Sheldon (1971) points out the difficulty in using this personal interactive approach when dealing with fluid and changing organizations—that is, when the organizational structure changes and the client population is not stable. Mutual-help groups are examples of fluid organizations. A consultation approach applicable to the mental health system may not be appropriate to a mutual-help system. Warren (1963) wrote of the difficulties in consultation which resulted from the differences between the subculture of the practitioner and the subculture of the consultant. The failure of the mental health system to successfully consult with mutual-help groups may be a result of the former's inability to adapt the consultation model to the needs of the mutual-help system. In this latter system, the client is often difficult to identify, and meetings of the organization may be informal *ad hoc* groupings. It may not be possible to establish regular formal meetings, and the consultant's position may not be valued any more than that of any other group member. Consultants need a different model for relating to this system than the one they customarily follow.

Still another reason for failure emerges from the deficiencies in the mental health professionals' knowledge base. Clinically trained mental health professionals are not typically schooled in organizational theory and development, or in understanding voluntary organizations. Their expertise lies in identifying psychopathological processes and in applying personality theories and therapies. As mental health professionals, with some few exceptions, are not trained in consultation skills, neither are they educated to deal with these organizational issues.

Finally, the consultation fails when the professional needs to, but does not, have an empathic attitude toward the group and an interest in working with it as a separate system (Silverman, 1978). Professionals who are concerned with issues of power and control and who have doubts about the viability of "untrained" people helping others with very personal problems should eliminate themselves from consulting with mutual-help groups.

As observers have become aware of the problems potential consultants face, many have suggested that professionals should not work with mutual-help groups or should do so only with additional training. Another approach, which does not necessarily require retraining, is proposed in this chapter. It utilizes other aspects of the professional role such as the ability to facilitate group process and to mobilize resources while capitalizing on the existing knowledge and experience generated by mutual-help organizations themselves. This model, reported on below, evolved from the experience of the Mutual Help Project staff while providing technical assistance to the mutual-help groups cooperating in the project.

A Model for Consulting with Mutual-help Organizations

Initially, the Mutual Help Project staff recruited, from among the mutual-help groups in the greater Boston area, those groups who had identified problems or issues within their group and who were interested in cooperating with the project in trying to solve these problems. Problems included questions on how to increase the involvement of members in the organizational life of the group; how to expand their helping program; and what organizational structure would be most effective in achieving their goals. The project staff was concerned that in providing assistance they do nothing to weaken the integrity and independence of the groups. The following guidelines that would be respectful of the group while permitting a good working relationship to develop were established for the consultant:

- The relationship between consultant and consultee is that of colleagues.
- Consultants must appreciate that groups have value systems of their own by which they judge their own work and whether or not they have achieved their goals.
- The consultant cannot tell the consultee how to integrate into the group's functioning the additional information provided.
- The consultant is a visitor, not a group member, and can take no responsibility to see that suggested ideas are implemented.
- The consultant can be dismissed at any time.

In trying to identify who the consultees would be in each organization, it became very apparent how fluid these organizations are. While in most situations the primary relationship was with the president, chairperson, or designated leader (where groups rotated leadership), with some groups the entire steering committee that governed the organization wanted to meet with the consultant. At some meetings the consultant could be asked to react to events that were taking place at that moment, or about his or her own personal situation as it related to what the group was discussing; or the consultant was asked to meet with an *ad hoc* committee to work on a particular problem. The informality of most settings made it impossible to have a clear delineation of roles. The consultant could be asked to help serve coffee or share in a pot luck supper to which he or she would be coming. In addition, membership in these groups changed frequently as people's needs were met or other pressures took precedence. The consultant needed to be flexible and to match his or her activity with the uneven rhythm of the organization.

It became necessary to establish a body of relevant knowledge and experience from which to draw for solutions to these problems. A review of the literature developed by mutual-help groups themselves revealed a good deal of excellent and appropriate material. The consultant began to report on relevant literature to the groups. None of the groups had any knowledge of other mutual-help organizations' experiences. They tended to idealize those that seemed to be functioning well and presumed themselves to be unique in that they were having difficulties. The groups became interested in what was happening in other groups the consultants were seeing. The main thrust of the consultation became the sharing of material and observations about what other groups were doing.

The same process was being repeated within each group. It seemed appropriate to bring them together since, in spite of the disparity among the groups in terms of the problems to which they addressed themselves and their organizational styles, they had a good deal in common. When the groups came together they discovered that the differences between them were less important than their shared interest in strengthening their organization.

They formed themselves into a working group and decided to plan a meeting inviting leaders of exemplary mutual-help groups, such as La Leche League, Parents Without Partners, and Movement for a New Society, to discuss with them how their groups solved the problems of leadership, expanding the involvement of members, and enhancing their helping programs. La Leche League and Parents Without Partners are hierarchical organizations, while the Movement for a New Society follows a consensus model. This workshop was very successful. The working group discovered in the course of planning this day and evaluating it afterwards that they had within themselves hidden resources to help solve each other's problems. They convened several subsequent meetings to provide a forum for sharing their own expertise with each other.

The consultation process involved several phases that applied to activities both with individual consultee groups and with several mutual-help groups together:

- There was a need to develop mutual trust, understanding, and respect.
- The group was able to identify its problems to reveal difficulties it could not deal with alone.
- The consultant was able to point out that other groups had the same problems—the group was not unique—thus legitimating the group and its concerns.
- Ideas, experiences, and written materials from other groups were presented to indicate how they approached similar problems.
- There was a review on how to use the new data.

By the end of the project, it became clear that the primary function of the consultant was that of linking agent—that is, "middle man" between groups in need and available resources (people, ideas, and materials) which would help solve their problems.

The concept of consultant as linking agent described by Havelock most accurately described this activity. Generally, linkers, defined earlier, stand between two parties, and the way they are seen may have considerable effect on their ability to introduce users to information or services (Havelock, Guskin, Frohman, Havelock, Hill, & Huber, 1971). A linking agent has the task of building awareness and understanding of a body of information in the consultee. The consultant's primary task was to link groups directly with each other or to provide them with relevant information gathered from other groups when they could not meet directly.

From the consultee's point of view, three stages can be identified in the process:

1. Discovering that the group's problems are not unique; there are commonalities across divergent organizations.

2. Sharing respective experiences of successful and unsuccessful solutions, members engage in a mutual learning exchange, identify with each other, and provide models for how to implement new knowledge.

3. Searching for additional answers, solutions, and techniques together, mutual helpers help each other.

The reader will recognize that this is a replica of the mutual-help experience that takes place for individual members in their organizations. In an atmosphere in which people can identify with each other, they find their dilemma typical rather than unusual and learning is enhanced. People seem to be able to integrate and use new knowledge when it is presented by peers with whom they can identify and who have had similar experience (Bandura, 1977). In duplicating the mutual-help experience, some of the institutional barriers that exist between the two systems are minimized. The role of the professional is (1) to legitimate the groups' learning from each other using experiential rather than professional knowledge, (2) to facilitate groups meeting each other, (3) to help mobilize resources, and (4) to share skills in group process. Above all, the professional has to know when to step back as groups take over this process for themselves and each other without additional help.

In conclusion, the successful consultant develops a mutual-help experience with his consultee that parallels that of the system to which he or she is relating, thereby mobilizing the most relevant help available. This process will most likely maximize the utilization of this help by the consultee.

Part IV
Policy Perspectives

The final section of the book is concerned with the relationship between community support systems and public policy. There is no universal agreement among community support system scholars as to the appropriate role of the government vis-à-vis community support systems. While many scholars have called for a "partnership," there is little agreement on the operationalization of this concept. For example, some, including the Editors, have advocated direct government funding of neighborhood organizations and self-help groups for support system building efforts. Others fear that government involvement with support systems will weaken them and lead to their demise, and therefore urge more of a "hands off" approach. Still others argue that we do not know enough about support systems as yet to make any policy recommendations.

Frol and reveals the complexity of these issues by raising a number of important but as yet unanswered questions. He reports that three approaches to community support systems have been suggested: *in* the community, which stresses decentralization and locus of delivery; *by* the community, which stresses community control; and *with* the community, which stresses shared responsibility or partnerships among professionals, families, and community members. Froland believes that the *with* community approach is the valid perspective and states that while there is general agreement on what values such an approach should stress—responsiveness, involvement, equity, efficiency, and accountability—we do not as yet have a handle on how to implement these values through true partnerships.

Naparstek and Biegel, building on issues raised in the Froland chapter, discuss the operationalization of partnerships. They state that for partnerships to be successful from their perspective, there must be two prerequisites. First, the interaction must be on a peer or colleague level; and second, partnerships should be locality-based, suggesting the neighborhood as the locus and focus of the partnership. In order to promote partnerships, capacity building for both community representatives and professionals is needed, consisting of both skill building and a focus on interpersonal relationships. They urge policymakers to make sure existing policies do not have negative, unintended consequences for local capacity building; to develop flexible programs; and to create incentives for the development of partnerships.

The need for neighborhood-oriented policy proposed by Naparstek and

Biegel is cited by Owan as especially applicable for members of racial and ethnic minority groups. Owan notes that the present mental health system is inadequate to meet the needs of these population groups, citing problems of differential treatment, negative outcomes of therapy, underutilization of services, and noncompliance by services with civil rights mandates. He proposes a neighborhood-based mental health approach that utilizes cultural and organizational networks in minority communities and that provides financial resources directly through contracts with minority groups for the delivery of culturally acceptable mental health services.

In the final chapter, Lewis presents an ethical perspective of support systems, arguing that a guiding goal of the welfare state should be to promote distributive justice. He notes that professional services, by focusing on the rights of individuals, have tended to isolate people from one another. He compares this with informal systems in which the fraternal concern for the common good is paramount. Lewis urges the professional sector to work toward promoting the fraternal spirit by developing linkages with informal networks.

16

Community Support Systems: All Things to All People?

Charles Froland

Discussions of the concept of a "community support system" have almost reached the point where what was once something may become nothing by virtue of being seen as everything. If anything serves to spark a rally, it would seem to be the belief that individual needs for care and support are most appropriately handled within the milieu of everyday social life (Abrams, 1978). Of course, the arrangements needed to operationalize this belief into some sort of "system" vary considerably in scope and emphasis according to the predilections of various constituencies. Even so, there does seem to surface a consistent argument for including a fairly long list of potential providers of community support traditionally unrecognized: clients, families, friends, neighbors, workmates, pastors, shopkeepers, hotel managers, and so on. Invitations are issued with an implicit request to put aside usual lines of allegiance, whether this be a matter of professional discipline or agency affiliation or more broadly a call for joint action by public, private, and voluntary sectors. A further point of emphasis is the knitting together of the contributions to care made by such actors into an explicit system; this "knitting together" is seen to be accomplished by various means from establishing communication linkages, carrying out systematic planning processes, and providing forums for community involvement, to a more ambitious structuring of community-wide networks among professional providers, clients, lay helpers, and the public at large.

The philosophical underpinnings of the concept are perhaps attrac-

This research was supported by Grant #18-P-00088, Office of Human Development Services, DHHS, Natural Helping Networks and Service Delivery.

tive, but they must face up to a number of basic realities that are certain to impede easy success. Some of these realities have to do with the way services are presently constituted among the helping professions and the settings in which care is formally provided. Other realities center around the ambiguities of how life in communities is either organized or disorganized in respect to a diversity of social divisions, the distribution of individual motivations to provide support to people in need or to participate in broader social affairs, and the nature of social need which one may be concerned to take on. (Finally, there are the realities of trying to sort out what professional service providers should do, what people should do for themselves, and where the two should meet.) In short, the concept faces the realities of finding bridges between two worlds: one formally organized and seeking the comfort of reliable and routine care and one with an informal organization relying on a more spontaneous order for its sustenance (Robinson, 1978; Froland, 1980).

Before we get to the point of attempting to fashion society into some form of a community support system, a prudent detour is warranted to question some of our assumptions about professionals, clients, and communities and the demands for performance that we may expect to make of them. In particular, what do our assumptions say about the involvement of lay helpers and citizens in providing for community support and the roles played by professionals in facilitating this involvement? What do these assumptions say about the respective rights and responsibilities of those in need and those who might make a contribution to caring for that need? What distribution of coverage and reliability in meeting needs is possible among people within different communities, and what sorts of strategies might usefully sustain, reinforce, or expand a community's capacity for dealing with different individual and social problems? These questions ask us to take a more sober look at the promise of a community support system in understanding its viability as a contribution to policy in social care. They are also the sort of "wicked" questions (Rittel & Webber, 1973) that are not perhaps even answerable but in any event need discussion. In this chapter, I would like to take a closer look at what these questions ask us to consider when we think about the prospects of policies advocating the development of a community support system.

Raising Questions of Involvement, Responsibility, and Control

The idea of a community support system runs into several enduring issues that have been consuming a fair amount of printed space for some time. These have to do with how much involvement in the provision of mental health care we want and can expect from clients, family members, neighbors, self-help groups, and others outside the fold of public auspice. It is not long after we begin to consider the type and level of involvement desirable (not to mention what involvement means) that we also have to come to grips with questions of where professional, agency, or governmental responsibility for care begins and ends. How we consider the issues of involvement and responsibility will also bring us a long way toward addressing the question of who controls the provision of care and support.

These rather broad-ranging issues are not readily handled at a global level of abstraction, but we can get a better view of how they get worked out by looking at three alternative orientations that seem implicit in the way advocates discuss the development of a community support system. These orientations suggest views of the system in which the provision of care is alternatively carried out *in* the community, *by* the community, or *with* the community (Bayley, 1978). The simple substitution of prepositions implies markedly different visions of how a community support system will deal with questions of community involvement, social responsibility, and public control.

The model of care *in* the community generally starts with the articulation of a plethora of explicitly structured, publicly supported, professional services that are seen to be provided locally in communities and neighborhoods (cf. Joint Commission for Accreditation of Hospitals, 1976; Turner & TenHoor, 1978). Support systems *in* the community become a matter of the appropriate location, arrangement, and dispensing of formal caring resources. Considerable attention is given to the administrative arrangements necessary to orchestrate the system in the development of mechanisms for ensuring efficiency and accountability in operations, case management, and client tracking systems to guarantee continuity in care and ways to establish local, state, and federal intergovernmental cooperation. The responsibility for providing support essentially comes to rest in the public domain, with client needs factored into a continuum of way stations from hospital to home where professionals wait ready to administer their remedies. To the extent that the community becomes involved in a model of care in the community, it seems to be by formal invitation or induction either as advisors on boards, volunteers under supervision, or recipients of support or advocacy services.

A contrasting orientation to developing a community support system is held by advocates of the model of care *by* the community. Here, the development of community support systems starts from the social milieu of the community through "the cultivation of effective informal caring activities within neighborhoods *by* local residents themselves— discovering, unleashing, supporting and relying upon indigenous caring agents and locally-rooted helping networks" (Abrams, 1980, p. 12). Aside from the suggestion that most people would rather be helped by informal means anyway (cf. Gourash, 1978) and are woefully dissatisfied or distrustful of public services (cf. Katz, Gutek, Kahn, & Barton, 1975), the new "populism" evidenced by the growth of grassroots neighbor-hood involvement (Perlman, 1978) and self-help initiatives (Katz & Bender, 1976b) has served to further buttress arguments for the model of care by the community. Community involvement and control is seen to eclipse the public and professional role, although there is still ground left open for professional responsibility. The focus of this responsibility centers on legitimizing and developing linkages among community or-ganizations, religious support systems, and support found in the work-place, in medical care settings, in criminal justice settings, and in schools as well as within other specialized self-help groups and mutual-aid networks.

While I have sketched these two orientations toward community support systems in somewhat exaggerated terms that perhaps few are dogmatic enough to adopt, I do think they represent two polarities that characterize the conflicting positions one sees among proposed policies addressed to various populations in need. To some extent, these orienta-tions imply different conceptions of what needs and resources are, with one seeing an expanded public role in the wake of a perceived break-down in traditional family functions and social institutions and the other viewing such expansion as undermining and misappropriating the com-munity's capacity for care (Moroney, 1976). They also reflect different responses to questions of responsibility for care and how this responsi-bility is best carried out. Care *in* the community promises equity and reliability with public responsibility for meeting needs, while care *by* the community argues for responsiveness and self-determination; in many ways each sacrifices what the other argues for.

Because neither position is tenable in the extreme, many have sought a policy choice "in between the aimless wandering of communal life and the authoritarian direction of the community which is not a compromise between the two extremes, but an entirely new approach" (Sennett, 1970, p. 103). Imagination runs rampant in attempts to envis-age what such a new approach to care *with* the community might look like, and the search seems to move beyond earlier notions of "ladders of citizen participation" (Arnstein, 1969) or the volunteer roles that have often been fashioned for "the other helpers" (Gershon & Biller, 1976; Levine, Tulkin, Intagliata, Perry, & Whitson, 1978). What is starting to surface is the notion that a balance between more localized formal ser-vices and stronger informal systems might be struck within arrangements that foster shared responsibility for care among professionals, families, and community members (Moroney, 1976; President's Commission on Mental Health, Vol. II, 1978b; Parker, 1980). The idea of shared care with the community would pursue a direction in which the informal help provided by families, friends, and neighbors is recognized by public service agencies and supported within a collaborative partnership whereby responsibility for meeting needs is vested equally among all parties to care—formal and informal. A further direction pursues ways to share care among a variety of informal caregiving sources within a community to reduce the burden of need on any particular source (Bayley, 1978; Froland, Parker, & Bayley, 1980). Whether shared care is possible or practical or holds any value to the concept of a community support system will be a matter for testing.

Further work is required to know whether the test is of the "true–false" or "multiple choice" variety, but for now we can expect two major sets of issues to determine the prospects for a policy of shared responsibility for care. The first of these has to do with issues of the capacity of a community to provide support: What is the distribution of informal caring resources, what is the potential for mobilizing support, and who is not likely to be helped? The second set of issues involves the capacity of formal services to engage in care with the community: What is the impact on organized agencies? What demands are made on professionals and how likely are they to respond to those demands? As we begin to inquire into this rather large list of issues, we will also be presented with choices that, once made, will tell the difference between policies that disadvantage the community, provide for an unwieldy public sector, or have a chance to promote improvements. Fortunately, we have some evidence to suggest what these choices may entail.

Community Support

The idea of arranging for some sort of shared responsibility with the community in the provision of direct support demands that we also have a better understanding of the distribution of informal help bearing on the question: "Who cares for whom?" Our appreciation of the phenomenon of informal helping networks is still moving through fairly rudimentary stages as it has taken us some time to realize first that they exist and later that they make a difference in whether people seek professional help, how well they adjust to different problems, and, indeed, what sorts of problems they experience (cf. Pilisuk & Froland, 1978). At this point it would seem useful to move a little closer to the phenomenon of supporters and supported and ask who the informal caregivers are, what is required of them, and how willing or able they are to meet these requirements.

These questions take on further significance when we think about the special needs of populations who are most often the focus of building community support systems: the old, the young, and the dependent, who are the major consumers of institutional resources. At the very least these individuals' problems are much more severe than the range of stresses and strains faced by a general population. That needs for support are great among those populations requires that we begin to appreciate who now provides informal care for these needs and how these caregivers respond to the demands placed on them.

What evidence there is on the identity of informal caregivers can easily lead to the conclusion that the phrase, "networks of informal helping" is really a euphemism for wives, mothers, and daughters (Abrams, 1980). The vast bulk of care received by the chronically impaired is provided principally by family members (National Center for Health Statistics, 1972), and women are the primary "kin-keepers" (Lieberman, 1978, p. 496). Two recent British studies focusing in particular on the informal caregivers of dependent individuals give insight into the experience of providing support. One study identified 120 caregivers within a general population that cut across both urban and rural areas (Equal Opportunities Commission, 1980). More than 60 percent of those identified were caring for an elderly relative, and roughly one-quarter were caring for a disabled adult, with the remainder caring for a handicapped child. Female caregivers (usually mother, wife, or daughter) outnumbered male caregivers (usually husband) three to one. Most caregivers were providing extensive help with activities of daily living (e.g., shopping, cleaning, transportation) as well as companionship and emotional support. The effect of providing care on the caregivers' lives was telling. More than one-quarter experienced profound economic limitation, having either to give up a job altogether, cut back in hours worked, or forgo job advancement. Most experienced a financial burden in meeting the extra costs associated with transportation needs, special foods, clothing, and various aids. Needless to say, the social life of the informal caregiver was severely curtailed and family stress more pronounced. Another study looking at informal caregivers of 100 long-term psychiatric patients generally confirms these findings (Lonsdale, Flower, & Saunders, 1980). Two-thirds of the patient sample were men, one-third were under forty, and one-third over sixty; 40 percent were unemployed; thirty-six out of the sample of 100 had no one they could name as a caregiver. Of the sixty-four caregivers identified, women outnumbered men two to one and almost two-thirds were married to the patient; parents, siblings, children, and friends comprised the remaining one-third. Less than one-third did not live with the patient, although most of these lived in the same building or neighborhood. The majority of caregivers (two-thirds) reported being the primary source of support, receiving no help from other relatives; only a minority felt that formal services could be relied on if they were not able to provide care. The impact of providing care was significant: one-third reported financial hardship, one-half reported diminished health and well-being from being tired, anxious, depressed, or nervous. These effects were more pronounced for those caregivers of patients with more severe problems. Most caregivers saw their role as being both "companion and watchdog." There was also at times some divergence between what the caregivers perceived as needed and what the patients' own perceptions of their needs were. A common finding of both studies was that caregivers helped out of a sense of moral responsibility, that their understanding of the problems they were attempting to care for diverged from that of professionals, and that they were often unaware or mistrustful of available services.

Whether or not the experience of the informal caregivers revealed by these studies applies more generally, there seems ample evidence to suggest that family isolation, breakdown, and ultimate rejection of a dependent member is not altogether a rare occurrence (cf. Kreissman & Joy, 1974). The studies also point up the potential pitfalls of basing care on the assumption of moral responsibility, not only because of the likelihood that this may become a burden to the caregiver (with implications for the resulting experiences of the cared for), but also because this responsibility seems to be disproportionately taken on by women. This is not to suggest that we raise a suspicious eyebrow about those who act on moral obligation but rather to ask whether this is by choice, particularly since the obligation seems to severely limit one's social and economic opportunities. If we are serious about developing a partnership with informal caregivers in a community support system, we need to begin to consider the disadvantages that seem to attend the experience of providing informal support for the dependent and to find a more equitable distribution of the tasks of being supportive. Part of this issue will entail developing a better understanding of the demands made on informal caregivers (Parker, 1980): for example, for how long will it be necessary to provide care, what will be the appropriate intensity and complexity of caring tasks, will the situation get better or worse? We also need to understand the conditions that foster a fairer allocation: "Once we bring ourselves to see care as an essentially calculative involvement, we can go on to ask a large number of questions about the specific sorts of calculation that will make specific sorts of caring worthwhile to specific sorts of people" (Abrams, 1978, p. 86).

In the final analysis, we must also come to terms with the limits of informal caregivers and with the realization that for some needs, formal resources must be brought to bear. However, we should not be too quick to assume the benefits of our formal facsimiles of informal support. If the experience of providing formal home-based care for the elderly is any indication, formal substitution for informal care may not be particularly effective, may not relieve stress on informal caregivers, and may not be equally sensitive to different populations at risk (Dunlop, 1980). On balance, the overriding issue here is how standards of effective care can be assured among informal caregivers. Recognizing that informal caregiving activities may be attractive only under conditions of limited reliability (Leat, 1979), will an attempt to promote community support be one of strengthening the effectiveness of informal caregivers on their terms or, rather, a reconstruction of informal support to fit a conception of effective care quite incompatible with the terms of informal caring relationships?

Enlisting the Community

The necessity of seeking out ways to broaden the range of persons providing support also means we must bring ourselves to look more closely at the community to find the relevant points of contact to establish a basis for informal support. When we do, we run into the almost classic argument over the relevance of "place versus nonplace" attachments in community life (Webber, 1964). Are the relevant social bonds of an individual those bounded by geographical location or are people linked together into networks of interest determined by kinship, religion, occupation, or ethnicity which may only coincidentally fall into geographical areas? The evidence from some general population surveys of helping patterns (cf. Sussman, 1965; Litwak & Szelenyi, 1969; Lieberman & Mullan, 1978) suggests that neighborhood ties may have only a small part to play in providing support, particularly if we think about the needs of dependent populations at risk of institutionalization. Because of these limitations, some argue that the relevant social bonds of communities are more effectively serviced by systems of self-help groups and mutual-aid networks based on shared race or ethnicity, religious affiliation, occupation, and so on—shared care through shared concern (Gladstone, 1979). On balance, the choice between community of interest or community of propinquity is not an either/or proposition but rather a matter of understanding how much of both makes sense in developing support systems (Wellman & Crump, 1978).

Another line of inquiry takes us beyond what presently exists for building a community support system and into an examination of what we think should exist. If neighborhoods are not now supportive, should they be? Is the type of support provided by self-help groups what we want to promote? If kinship ties are breaking down, should we put our energies into strengthening families or establishing alternatives? I have no special vision to offer on these matters, but I do think we should pause to consider whether our well-meaning policies (once granted effectiveness) may add to a sort of "social gentrification" of the kind witnessed in neighborhood reinvestment strategies (Levy, 1978). Before we get too far into establishing a system of support in which almost everyone is engaged in helping almost everyone else—listening, emoting, providing well-informed and reasoned advice—we might wonder whether we may be really asking one social class to accept another's prescriptions for the good life. One need not take the position of a "slum romantic" (Sennett, 1970, p. 81) to appreciate that support means different things to different people and that even among marginal populations living in adverse circumstances one can find "supportive" patterns of exchange (Jacobs, 1961; Cohen & Sokolovsky, 1980). This issue stresses the importance (and difficulty) of maintaining a sensitivity to and tolerance of diversity among different populations while also maintaining an equitable allocation of rights and resources among those whose needs require different responses.

The Demands on Professionals and Organized Services

If issues of equity and reliability seem to dominate the community side of the shared care question, issues of responsiveness and credibility seem ubiquitous in discussions of the professionalism and bureaucracy that have become hallmarks of formal services (Wolfenden Report, 1978; Sosin, 1979). While many have raised the hydra-headed specters of the encapsulated professional walled-off from the realities of clients' needs (Lightfoot, 1978; Robinson, 1978), bureaucratic malaise and insensitivity (Hugman, 1977), the colonization of a community's caring resources by the welfare state (Abrams, 1980), and, indeed, the professionalization of everyday life (Illich, 1975), launching into a polemic on the evils of public services will not get us very far with our task. What seems more germane in understanding the prospects for policies of care *with* the community is to know more about the demands made on professional providers and formal service organizations in developing partnerships with the community and to explore ways that these demands can be met.

Probably the primary source of these demands stems from the discontinuities that result from attempts to bridge two systems that have very real differences in their assumptions about what help is and how it should be provided. When formal service providers attempt to develop partnerships with informal caregivers in the community, I have suggested, they face a number of fairly basic dilemmas in trying to reconcile their different expectations about care (Froland, 1980). These dilemmas are illustrated in the following sorts of tradeoffs:

Responsibility. Professionals and agencies deal with "clients" and must operate under certain ethical or legal standards for assuming responsibility while informal sources of help "care for those they care for" (Abrams, 1979) within relationships that range in emphasis from encouraging dependency to encouraging autonomy. Where is the line drawn between "standing back" in respecting self-determination and self reliance at the risk of violating formal standards and "stepping in" to take responsibility for client needs at the risk of disenfranchising informal supports?

Knowledge and identity. Because of the responsibilities they must often assume, agency workers may tend to give greater credence to a technical knowledge base and a professional frame of reference while informal caregivers may emphasize practical and subjective understandings within the terms of an indigenous group. From an informal perspective, an individual may be "well-meaning, easily misunderstood, temperamental" while the professional view may refer to the person as "paranoid, rejecting, and abusive to her children" (Goldberg, 1965). Where is the line drawn between accepting informal conceptions of needs and solutions that may meet suspicion in professional circles and adopting the stance of an "expert" that may conflict or lack credibility with informal caregivers?

Authority. The responsibility accorded formal service providers and the training or credentials that seem necessary to justify it often translate into an assumption of authority and status in deciding "what's best." Informal sources of help draw their authority from those they serve through implicit votes of confidence for help received in the past or perhaps even through charisma. Conflicts in purpose and ideology can exacerbate the differences between these two sources of authority and status, but there is ample room for tension in deciding when to bargain with those who have legitimate claims and when to construct barricades to keep out those with an "axe to grind" (Darvill, 1975; Steckler & Herzog, 1979).

Accountability. The assumption of responsibility and authority for the needs of dependent populations by unelected agents of public service creates the need to assure accountability to elected officials and the public at large. This typically devolves into a system of reporting requirements built around explicitly defined target populations, eligibility rules, and categories of service for documenting that money spent carries out the terms of legislative authorization. Because problems presented by informal caregivers may often not fit the form specified, cut across several target population definitions, or require activities not defined by usual taxonomies of service, a substantial number of tensions can arise in trying to conform to a formally prescribed agenda for excellence while responding to the often naturalistic and spontaneous demands of the informal system of helping. The comment, "we do a lot of work in coffee shops but the State doesn't see this as counseling," suggests one way these tensions can present themselves.

There are other dilemmas that could be discussed (cf. Riessman, 1970; Lenrow, 1976) but, for starters, these four areas provide some indication of the demands that will be made on professionals and service organizations in pursuing a policy of shared responsibility for providing support. Of course, there are also more specific demands that come in the form of training, skills, staff assignments, organizational arrangements, and resource investments, but it seems to me that these matters follow from first considering how the basic structural differences between formal and informal support systems get worked out. Because these differences reflect a continuing dialectic among alternative value positions about how care should be provided (cf. Alford, 1975), they are not likely to be put to rest and, indeed, may even provide a useful disorder in our pursuit of simple solutions (Sennett, 1970).

Rather than assuming that these dilemmas should be left to political negotiations altogether, we might look for avenues that provide the conditions for adapting to the demands of working out what shared responsibility can mean, perhaps to find some sort of "mutual coercion, mutually agreed upon" (Hardin, 1968). What such conditions might be in the abstract and how they are likely to fare in practice seems open to speculation at the moment and some of the proposals are not entirely unfamiliar to us. For example, some views suggest that the way to deal with the uncertainty and tension that will likely be involved in adapting to conditions of shared responsibility is through the promotion of strategies of gradual decentralization, de-standardization and de-professionalization (Gladstone, 1979). Rather than a policy of dismantling formal services, this position argues that formal services are still vital but better provided within organizational conditions that are more likely to respond to the demands of working closely with local communities. Locally based services, greater staff autonomy, integrated packages of services, and more decentralized and flexible systems of authority are some of the elements of organization that may facilitate a more sensitive response (cf. Froland et al., 1980; Hadley & McGrath, 1980). Finding the proper form of organizational and management arrangements may provide the suitable conditions for a policy of shared care with the community, but this approach offers no guarantees. Review of earlier experiences in promoting locally based services (O'Donnell & Sullivan, 1974), service integration (Gans & Horton, 1975), flexibility and autonomy in staff roles (Leighninger, 1980), and decentralization policies (Aldrich, 1978) suggest that these strategies are not without their hazards to matters of coordination and accountability, among other things.

That organization and management will not provide all the answers demands that we jointly pursue other alternative strategies. One possibility is to look for various incentives that might promote more shared responsibility, for example, providing staff with a budget constraint for each client and allowing them to provide financial incentives to informal helpers (Challis & Davies, 1980) or providing tax incentives to promote self-help (Gollub & Waldhorn, 1979). Obviously, incentives must be found that are effective without commercializing informal relationships or otherwise proving disruptive in their implementation. As another alternative, some are attracted to the idea that the promotion of greater shared responsibility may come from the creation of expanded opportunities for local governance, arguing that "good clients make bad citizens" and what we really need are good citizens (Dewar, 1978). Local solutions to local problems might come from fostering the development of groups and associations within the community that are sufficiently empowered to participate or otherwise make an impact on formal service delivery (Berger & Neuhaus, 1977). Whether the conditions for working out the demands of shared responsibility are found among various strategies of organization and management, incentives, or governance is waiting to be discovered from something now in the making, but the complexity of negotiating trade-offs among different expectations about care suggests a commensurate need for pluralism of means and ends if the systems of community support we try to develop are to be viable.

Prospects for Community Support Systems

A community support system has come to mean many things to many people. Whether or not the concept has a future is basically a matter of having a clearer idea of what it is we seek to implement. In the first instance, we should be more explicit on the subject of purpose: Should the system reflect the principles of care *in*, *by* or *with* community? I have explored the notion of care *with* the community as a possible avenue to pursue because, at least in the abstract, it seems to offer a more tenable solution to questions of community involvement, public versus private responsibility, and local control in the provision of support for dependent populations.

Care *with* the community reflects a philosophy of shared responsibility between professionals (*qua* public resources for providing support) and informal caregivers (*qua* community resources for providing support). This philosophy emphasizes a balance of roles and responsibilities such that professional support is neither intrusive nor neglectful while opportunities and incentives for informal support provide for involvement without resulting in burden (cf. Froland et al., 1980). This statement of purpose will become rather meaningless, however, unless it can be articulated into a set of principles and procedures for practice in which the reliability of means can be tested. My intent here has been to suggest a number of points of reference that must be accommodated in articulating the means for care with the community.

Viable policies will need to be concerned with the demands made on informal caregivers and the community as well as on professionals and the public sector and in some ways will need to be advocates for both sides. If too much emphasis is given to the virtues of informal support with the result that people are left to "get on with it," informal caregivers will be burdened and community needs unmet; likewise, emphasis on professional responsibility and control as a way to assure reliability and equity may undermine the contributions made willingly by informal caregivers and may prove insensitive to individual needs and situations. Because of the list of issues that goes into creating such a balance, some may conclude that the principle of shared responsibility is really "fool's gold"—glittering and causing much interest but worthless as a currency.

Such a conclusion can easily lead one to throw one's weight behind other orientations to what a community support system might mean, for example, more localized professional services or stronger informal support systems. Arguments will be further clouded by future uncertainties. For example, the changing role of women and the increase in working mothers has led to a call for greater public involvement in child care (Bane, Lein, O'Donnell, Steuve, & Wells, 1979; Waldman, Grossman, Hayghe, & Johnson, 1979). If, as evidence reviewed earlier suggests, women are also the primary informal caregivers of other dependent populations (particularly the elderly, whose proportions will be swelling for the rest of the century), will this trend not also call into question the reliability of informal support and increase the need for more formal services? Alternatively, some point to the decline in GNP, citizen tax revolts, and the increasing ability of the public sector to finance professional support for meeting social needs (Janowitz & Suttles, 1978; Central Policy Review Staff, 1978). Observers of this trend will find grounds to argue for the development of self-help initiatives to enhance the community's capacity to care for its own. One does not have to spend a great deal of time on the subject of futurism before realizing that philosophical adherents of either care *in* the community or care *by* the community will both find ammunition in future uncertainties to support their respective positions.

Reconciliation (if that is the desired end) would seem to hinge on how we come to terms with the conflicting policy criteria reflected among these alternative positions. Equity, efficiency, accountability, responsiveness, and involvement are benefits few would not want reflected in a community support system. The trouble is that these criteria must be translated into strategies for action wherein we are likely to find that not all may be achieved at once (cf. Rein, 1972). The competing expectations about care and the dilemmas they raise are not just matters confronted by policies of shared responsibility and escaped by pursuing alternative policy orientations. Trade-offs among competing values are implicit in any policy proposal; very simply, something cannot be everything. In this respect, the prospects for a community support system depend on a better recognition of where and how the process of compromise may be approached. Experimentation with a view toward tolerating a pluralistic diversity in matching needs and resources and mutual respect for the different contributions professionals, clients, and informal caregivers can make to a community support system may provide a useful foundation to begin this process. Complexity and conflict are also likely to be abiding characteristics of the process and we might usefully adopt a perspective that accepts the legitimacy of untidiness. On this point, Schiller's comments on the French Revolution may provide a timely guide: "The political or educational artist must learn to approach his medium with genuine respect for its individuality and potential for dignity . . . and beware of damaging its natural variety" (Schiller, 1797, quoted in Gladstone, 1979, p. 123).

17

A Policy Framework for Community Support Systems

Arthur J. Naparstek and
David E. Biegel

In recent years mental health and human service professionals in the United States have earnestly sought to bring services back into the community arena. However, in spite of significant developments, such as the community mental health movement and many important research efforts, providers and consumers have not been satisfied during the past two decades. There are those who still claim that services are delivered in a fragmented manner, that services are often offered in an inefficient, duplicative, and bureaucratically confusing fashion to those in need, that services are lacking in accountability, and that service delivery systems do not provide for attention to prolonged needs or for comprehensive analysis of clients' problems (Agranoff, 1977; National Conference on Social Welfare, 1977; Biegel & Spence, 1978; Naparstek, Biegel, Sherman, Andreozzi, & Coffey, 1978; President's Commission on Mental Health, 1978b; National Commission on Neighborhoods, 1979).

After reviewing the genesis and scope of these problems, this chapter will propose a neighborhood-based partnerships approach linking informal and formal service-providers as a means of addressing them. Partnerships are not easy to develop or maintain; specific atten-

The authors wish to thank Chester Haskell and Wendy Sherman for assistance in developing the themes of this chapter.

tion will be paid, therefore, to necessary prerequisites for partnerships and capacity-building efforts needed to ensure success. Finally, policy implications of this approach will be presented.

Service Delivery Problems and Issues

The New Federalism and Great Society initiatives in mental health and human services have led to a proliferation of federal programs since the early 1960s—each with its own target populations, regulations, and funding channels. This has resulted in considerable fragmentation of services. Several years ago, the National Conference on Social Welfare (1977) reported its findings and recommendations of a major study funded by DHEW of problems in the delivery of social services. Of interest is their documentation of the extraordinary number of social service agencies and programs. Their research shows that over 300 social programs were made available by DHEW alone, with the average state having 80 to 100 service programs. There are over 79,000 state and local governments, each administering a variety of service programs to their constituents. The average large city has some 400 to 500 private and government programs and/or agencies.

A single community mental health center may receive money from federal, state, and local governments, from the United Way, from national and local foundations, from fees for services, and through grants, contracts, purchase of service, insurance reimbursement, and so forth. These different levels of funding sources and different funding mechanisms make the development of a coordinated service-delivery network extremely difficult, as they entail conflicts in regulations, eligibility criteria, funding levels, funding periods, and the like.

Obstacles to accessibility can also prevent people from seeking and receiving help. Among such obstacles are services that are provided at inconvenient hours and locations, that are narrowly defined, that cost too much, that are delivered in an inappropriate or insensitive manner, and that are poorly designed in that they do not account for class and ethnic differences among clients. Accessibility issues often arise from legal obstacles present in the conflicting eligibility criteria for given services due to the multiplicity of funding sources and their requisite spending regulations. Legal obstacles at present also prevent mediating institutions such as churches, ethnic clubs, or community organizations from receiving, for example, federal mental health monies despite the advantages of access they offer for the development of community-based preventive and rehabilitative programs.

Lack of awareness of helping resources by service providers also hinders accessibility since helpers are limited in their ability to martial a range of resources for multiproblem clients or to make adequate referrals. In fact, Naparstek, Biegel, and Spence (1979) found that professional and lay helpers are not aware of resources outside of their own sphere of interest and those resources which they name most frequently present few choices for people in need.

Accountability is an important element of service delivery because interactive relationships are necessary between the individuals being served and the service decision makers in order to insure that clients can influence decisions that affect them and to assure sensitivity to their needs and interests (Gilbert, 1973). Agranoff (1977) points out that services often lack such interactive relationships and that this causes severe accountability problems. For example, we know that considerable and significant helping services are provided by community helpers who have firsthand knowledge of problems and concerns of people on the neighborhood level. Yet professional agencies often do not understand or respect the roles that these helpers perform and thus allow them little input into agency planning, service delivery, and evaluation.

Finally, it is increasingly clear that no one sector of the mental health or human service system has the resources—fiscal, political, administrative, legal, or personal—to deal singlehandedly with these issues. To further complicate matters, although categorical programming is often cited as a major cause of these problems, categorical programs were developed in response to the legitimate needs of interest groups representing high-risk population groups.

In summary, fragmentation, lack of accountability, and lack of accessibility are major problems in mental health and human service delivery. Cutting across each of these problems is the fact that we have attempted to develop only large-scale or macro solutions. In doing so, we have bypassed an important small-scale or micro resource- community support systems. These systems—family, friends, neighbors, coworkers, natural helpers, clergy, neighborhood organizations, mutual-help groups, and so on—are an unrecognized, underutilized, and unintegrated service resource. Despite the knowledge that currently exists about these support systems, they have been ignored, in large part, by professional service providers.

Community mental health centers may be located *in* communities, but, in the sad majority of cases, they are not truly part *of* communities. In fact, mental health programs have too often been "parachuted" into a community and are operated with few, if any, ties to neighborhood-based organizational and cultural networks. A full understanding of the intercultural dimensions of neighborhood life, particularly in relation to service delivery, has not yet evolved. A consequence is that the inherent strengths of neighborhood residents have not been utilized in prevention, treatment, or rehabilitation programs. The problem is made more complex because of our insufficient understanding of the interdependencies among race, ethnicity, social class, and well-being.

These themes were stressed by the report of the President's Commission on Mental Health (Vol. II, 1978b), which revealed that even those support systems that work well are often ignored by mental health professionals. Furthermore, the Commission stated, many professionals are not aware of, or do not recognize, the significant roles of these community support systems. The Commission feels that professional services should be built upon these informal networks. The report states that,

> Mental health services should be offered to individuals which would build first on their own assets and strengths, maintaining and cultivating their membership in social networks and natural communities in the least restrictive environment. This would mean developing methods which could identify and assess the functioning of an individual's natural support systems, and establishing, where appropriate, linkages between the natural support systems and the professional caregiving systems based on a respect for privacy and on genuine cooperation and collaboration, not cooptation and control. . . . Helping people where they are and assisting them to help themselves allows entry into the help giving and receiving system without requiring that a person be labeled patient or deemed "sick" [Vol. II, 1978b, p. 154].

We believe that effective mental health programs need to be operated on a genuinely human scale. This requires the empowerment of people in their neighborhoods so that they themselves may develop and direct appropriate service systems relevant to their own needs. Working partnerships need to be created between empowered neighborhoods and mental health institutions.

In fact, the notion of partnerships is being discussed a great deal in government these days. It was a theme of the final reports of the President's Commission on Mental Health (1978a) and the National Commission on Neighborhoods (1979). President Carter's Urban Policy message of 1979 called for the development of partnerships among all sectors—local, state, and federal government; business and the private sector; the voluntary sector; and the neighborhood—as a necessary process for solving complex problems faced by urban and rural communities alike.

While such partnerships already exist in some cases, their development and maintenance are neither automatic nor obvious. It is to these issues that we now turn our attention.

Developing and Maintaining Partnerships

A Neighborhood-Based Approach

Rather than search for new program and administrative models for mental health services, a whole new approach seems to be required for us to avoid the pitfalls of the past. During the past two decades, most human problems have been defined in the context of macro social and economic forces. The persistent failure of programs developed by governments to be directly relevant to the needs of people can be traced to policymakers' insistence on diagnosing and prescribing for all ills on the grand scale almost exclusively. The assumptions and beliefs underlying the service initiatives and theoretical systems of the 1960s and 1970s were not directed toward the micro-aspects of problem solving in a neighborhood context. Virtually all efforts to halt the decline of our cities have been marked by a failure to define national policy on a human scale.

Therefore, policymakers have not developed policy initiatives that serve the varied needs of differing neighborhoods. If we are to speak realistically of preconditions required for effective changes, it must be recognized that the neighborhood—not the sprawling, anonymous megalopolis—is the key. In real terms, people live in neighborhoods, not cities. In real terms, their investments—emotional as well as economic—are in neighborhoods, not cities. The city cannot survive if its neighborhoods continue to decline.

We propose a new analysis of the potential of a neighborhood approach in policy and programs terms. We recognize that any model for a neighborhood approach ought to fulfill four general prerequisites. First and foremost, involvement of all concerned sectors in a city—public and private human service providers, community residents, and government representatives—is required. Second, the approach must be pluralistic to be successful, cognizant of the diverse needs of different groups of people. Third, the need for "approachable scale" is crucial. This is not a question of absolute size, but rather of determining the appropriate scale for what we are trying to do. Some activities are best undertaken on a large scale. In Schumacher's words, "For his purposes, man needs many different structures, both small ones and large ones, some exclusive and some comprehensive" (Schumacher, 1973). Fourth, the effort must build on the strengths and resources of neighborhood-based community support systems.

As we have stated, community support systems have been largely ignored by professionals. Before discussing prerequisites for the development of partnerships, we will discuss these support systems in further detail in order to provide additional evidence of the advantages of a neighborhood-based approach.

Building on Strengths: Community Support
Systems and Neighborhood Networks

Mental health and human service providers focus upon people's weaknesses and problems. Too often providers overlook the strengths and resources of people and the systems of support in their communities. There is a rapidly increasing body of research about community support systems (Litwak, 1961; Breton, 1964; Slater, 1970; Glazer, 1971; Caplan, 1974; Collins & Pancoast, 1976; Warren, 1977; Naparstek et al., 1978; President's Commission on Mental Health, 1978b). Community support systems serve preventive functions by contributing to individuals' sense of well-being and of competent functioning. They can assist in reducing the negative consequences of stressful life events (Cobb, 1976; Dean & Lin, 1977). They can reinforce or hinder the effectiveness of professional treatment rendered to persons in need.

Community support systems serve all of us in some degree, and in different ways. More specifically, however, community support systems serve many population groups that are unable or unwilling to seek professional help or for whom professional services are currently lacking: specifically, ethnic and racial minorities, women, and the aged. Community support systems offer help in a culturally acceptable manner without stigma or loss of pride. The individual seeking help does not need to identify himself as having a problem, being weak, sick, a client or patient as he would when seeking professional help.

Many community support system elements have a neighborhood locus. There is much evidence that neighborhood-based cultural and organizational networks can play important roles in assisting professionals in the delivery of mental health services (Collins & Pancoast, 1976; Berger & Neuhaus, 1977; Biegel & Naparstek, 1979; Warren, 1981) and evidence that the effectiveness of professional treatment rendered often depends on the social supports or lack of support in an individual's neighborhood (Myers & Bean, 1968; Caplan, 1974).

Naparstek (1976), Doughton (1976), and Berger and Neuhaus (1977), among others, argue that people need to feel that daily life is on a manageable scale and for most people that means the neighborhood. These authors speak of the importance of locally relevant institutions—family, church, neighborhood associations, civic and voluntary associations—which mediate between the private world of the individual and the public world of the system. They argue that people working in small groups around concerns of the neighborhood strengthen their internal networks and make it possible to link with other systems for mutual problem solving.

It should be noted that people determine their resource needs quite subjectively guided by interrelated principles of equity, security, and sufficiency. Citizens must feel that their investment is equal to their return; that they are economically, physically, and socially secure; and that they have the sufficiency to participate in government, to deal successfully with the problems of their community, and to exercise some control over institutions that have direct impact on their lives.

The degree to which people feel sufficient is often determined by how a neighborhood defines itself and how others define it. People in neighborhoods, then, with a sense of who they are and a feeling of capacity and competence, have the greatest ability to deal with their problems. When people have a sense of their own efficacy, their investment in their community creates both psychological, social, and physical supports leading to healthier individuals, families, and neighborhoods. We believe that partnerships between neighborhood organizations and mental health and human service professionals can enhance the sense of sufficiency and reduce alienation of urban residents.

Prerequisites for Partnerships

There are a number of prerequisites to the establishment of partnership between the neighborhood, that is, community-based organizations, self-help groups, clergy groups, and the like, and professional mental health and human service providers.* First, all relevant actors, be they mental health professionals, human service administrators, or community representatives, must be able to interact with each other as peers. Appropriate and effective partnerships assume some type of rough equality among all partners. Such equality is often difficult to achieve, since professionals usually control important resources—money, staff, and expertise—and may be unwilling or unable to interact as peers with lay persons felt to be less than their equals (Biegel, 1979). Andy Mott, Director of the Center for Community Change, has commented, "It is difficult to conceive of a true partnership in which one partner has a stranglehold on the resources which are crucial to the other partner's

---

*The neighborhood sector partner will vary in different communities. In some areas, it may be a funded, coalition-type, community-based organization. In others, it may be a ministerium, self-help group, ethnic club, or church organization. The aim over time should be to broaden the base of the neighborhood partner to include a representative sample of the lay leaders and helpers in the community.

ability to function." Too often partnerships are not roughly equal in terms of either power or resources. Under these circumstances, such partnerships are doomed to failure. A critical ingredient of any approach to building partnerships, therefore, must be the development of means that enable and encourage peer relationships among diverse, and often competing, parties.

Another crucial prerequisite is that such partnerships, by our definition, are locality-based, that is, they relate to a specific neighborhood or subsection of a city. This does not mean that the locality is the only perspective but that the neighborhood is both the locus and the focus of the partnership. All neighborhoods are not alike. Neighborhoods, like people, have distinct personalities. Middle-class Italian neighborhoods in Baltimore deal with problems differently from Jewish neighborhoods in Chicago, whose residents in turn face crises and seek help differently from Hispanic, black, Polish, or Irish neighborhoods elsewhere. The above may seem like a truism, yet planners of government programs have often acted as if American urban communities were uniform building blocks, waiting to be fit into some enormous superstructure with the "made in Washington" or "made in the State House" label—a label that many people with emotional and economic investments in city neighborhoods have learned to distrust. The tendency has been to diagnose and prescribe for mental health problems exclusively on the grand scale, not the human scale.

Finally, each partnership must have its own financial resources so as to allow for independence from the other partners. Thus, neighborhood organizations may require small amounts of seed money for staff to assist their capacity-building processes.

Building Capacity

The building of capacity for partnerships includes the following key elements:

1. Helping all actors to recognize that each sector brings strengths, as well as weaknesses, to any partnership.

2. Helping all actors to recognize that empowerment of citizens enhances the ability of neighborhood residents to interact with the professional sector without threatening or diminishing professional roles.

3. Moving people away from zero-sum, confrontative (the us vs. them syndrome) views of power to emphasizing interrelationships and mutual gains.

4. Enabling all actors to understand the service delivery systems, formal and informal, within which they operate.

5. Enabling all actors to recognize the existence of fiscal, legal, and administrative obstacles or disincentives to partnerships, and assisting partners to develop strategies to address these issues.

6. Enabling citizens and public officials to build on the existing network of organizations and institutions that are the infrastructure of any neighborhood [of special interest here is the concept of "mediating institutions" discussed by Berger and Neuhaus (1977) and the locality-relevant support systems discussed by Naparstek and Biegel (1979)].

7. Helping citizens and neighborhood organizations develop the technical and administrative skills required to operate in a decentralized system; this includes resolving questions of funding.

Every potential partnership is faced with meeting a range of needs in order for it to develop into an active, problem-solving process. First, each partner, independent of the others, must be able to mobilize its own resources and knowledge. To make sure each sector is "up to speed," capacity building—technical assistance, funding, and consultation—is required. The key is making certain that each actor has the wherewithal (however appropriate or defined) to fill his or her partnership roles effectively.

Given the fact that different neighborhoods have differing needs, there are numerous ways of fostering these abilities. We have already indicated that technical assistance in the form of seed money to community organizations may be a prerequisite. Other types of technical assistance may include help in needs assessment and planning, program development and evaluation, leadership training, communication skills or basic organizational skills—planning and chairing meetings, setting agendas, and so forth. Through this technical assistance, neighborhood organizations become aware of their own strengths and resources and develop the capacity to interact with professionals.

Equally important, we must not assume that only the neighborhood sector needs capacity building. Professionals are also often quite lacking in the skills needed for successful partnerships (Silverman, 1981). Thus, capacity building must occur in both the neighborhood and the professional sector. This does not mean that the same types of assistance are required for each actor. Indeed, a primary concept must be the necessity of targeting development assistance to meet the particular requirements of each partner at a specific point in time.

Second, each partner must develop the ability to perform cooperatively with regard to both specific problems and the ongoing process. In other words, suppose a partnership between a community organization and agency professionals in a neighborhood coalesced around the need to enhance social support for the unemployed. The task goal is to develop a program or service to meet the needs of the unemployed. Even more important, the process goal is to develop the program or service in such a way as to enhance the interest and ability of the partners to work collaboratively around future needs—in other words, to lay the groundwork for an ongoing partnership. In this way, specific programs or projects are both ends in themselves and also means toward a larger goal insuring a continuing partnership.

Such ability requires the development of a range of skills, both substantive and interpersonal. All too often programs designed to provide support for various partnership efforts end up dealing only with certain types of needs, usually technical skills or expertise. What is commonly forgotten is that working with people requires more than just substantive knowledge. Indeed, probably more important over the long run is the human ability to work together; to be able to utilize interpersonal, process-oriented talents. The core of a partnership is not expertise or objective data. Those can always be acquired. What is absolutely necessary is a capacity to interact mutually in moving toward common goals.

Third, the composition and needs of the partnership will change over time, thus requiring a constant process of capacity building and support. This is especially true in terms of the need to target partnership efforts in particular areas, since neighborhoods and their problems are hardly static.

Ideally, the objectives of neighborhood capacity-building efforts should include a focus on the following issues:

1. *Equity*. All individuals and groups needing services should have access to them. With limited resources, however, choices must be made in allocating these resources. Equity requires that priority in resource allocation go to those most in need and least able to afford services.

2. *Accountability*. Accountability is not a one-way street; that is, not only the public sector should determine what services are delivered to a neighborhood, and whether they are delivered appropriately and effectively. Procedures for insuring mutual accountability are necessary in which consumers are accountable to providers, and providers are accountable to consumers. In this way we can help ensure that the system remains relevant. Without procedures for mutual accountability, providers are often unable to identify the strengths and needs of individuals and their families. A delivery system cannot be effective if whole individuals are viewed only in relation to separate programs. By building mutual accountability procedures into the system, consumers will be assured an opportunity to make their views

known and to make those views count. This implies, for example, citizen involvement in the development of a mental health service from planning to evaluation stages.

3. *Accessibility*. Accessibility issues are multidimensional, with objective and subjective elements. Objective elements include convenient location within the neighborhood, transportation to and from services, and services offered at convenient times, such as evenings and weekends. Subjective characteristics include flexibility, identity, and empathy. Flexibility of the delivery system suggests a pluralistic approach in which economic, social, and cultural differences of clients are taken into account. The notion that different groups of people deal with crises and problems differently is given a high priority. Identity means that the program should be designed to reinforce people's positive view of themselves. Through the neighborhood approach, the delivery system will preserve a sense of human scale rather than having consumers feel like cogs in an impersonal machine. Building on the natural helping networks in a neighborhood also assures empathy among professional mental health practitioners. By linking helping networks to service agencies it is likely that personnel will be able to identify with the aspirations and problems of the consumer.

The joining together of different people with various backgrounds to work on a problem of general concern can engender a spirit of cooperation. As the team grows and people's experiences with each other increase, the advantages of bringing to bear different perspectives and skills may be realized in ways that were not previously obvious. Partners can see that by working together they can change things in a way they could not do on their own. They see they are capable of solving problems as a group and positively affecting the neighborhood, its people, and its institutions. At the same time, they learn and grow personally, coming to understand the value of cooperation and communication with others (Biegel & Naparstek, in press).

Over time, success breeds success. Every time a partnership successfully deals with a problem in this fashion, the opportunities for personal growth, confidence, and satisfaction are increased.

Finally, the partnership approach forces the tailoring of any capacity-building or technical-assistance effort to deal with particular, specific situations. Therefore, any partnership-building effort must account for at least six major variables:

1. *People*. Who are the people involved? What are their backgrounds, positions, goals, and values? What constraints do they operate under?

2. *Needs*. What are their various training and technical-assistance needs from their own perspective, as well as those of others?

3. *Policy*. What are the formal and informal policies, rules, and ways of getting things done?

4. *Problems*. What are the major problems facing each of the actors? Which of these are seen as common and which are peculiar to each actor?

5. *Skills*. What competencies does each actor bring to the partnership? What weaknesses? Where are there deficiencies that must be overcome before the partnership can operate?

6. *History*. What has happened in the past that colors each actor's outlook on the problems and upon the other actors?

Thus, any attempt to build a partnership in a particular setting must take into account a host of variables relevant to the situation. Partnerships do not just occur. They require a great deal of hard work by everyone involved.

As we see it, there are three levels of capacity building. The first, as noted above, is development of the individual partner's capability to be able to perform partnership functions. Such development is primarily unilateral and is directed at any of the partners.

Second, there is the development of interactive, ongoing, local problem-solving partnerships. As noted above, this multilateral effort is the central point of any partnership strategy, focusing as it does on cooperation, teamwork, and mutual assistance in the quest for the resolution of common local problems. Again, there is a broad range of potential approaches, including the provisions of external, group process facilitators, the funding of partnership staff or technical support, and the building of common data bases. While most current programs that support local partnership are limited to one or two areas such as counseling services or health care, the crucial factor is that the emphasis in partnership building is the development of tactics, mechanisms, patterns of behavior, or political processes that are internal in nature. The focus is intergroup.

The third level is the development of interpartnership networks. Once the local partnership is formed and has begun an ongoing process of problem solving, it can begin to interact beyond its boundaries. However, it is important to note that the other steps of partner development and partnership building must come first. Locality-based partnerships can deal with larger, more comprehensive partnerships only when they "have their own act together." In other words, the local partnerships precede the expanded network. Another implication of this approach is that local partners will build a sense of community and shared goals among themselves, thus facilitating their interaction as a unit with other local partnerships, city-wide organizations, and county, state, and federal government. This approach explicitly recognizes that many neighborhood problems cannot be resolved with a strictly local focus.

Using the Partnership Approach: Field Experiences

The neighborhood-based partnership approach we have described has been developed and utilized in several projects sponsored by the University of Southern California, Washington Public Affairs Center. The first of these, the Neighborhood and Family Services Project, funded by NIMH, was a four-year, two-city (Baltimore, Maryland, and Milwaukee, Wisconsin) research and demonstration program designed to (1) mobilize ethnic neighborhoods around mental health issues; (2) develop program models to overcome identified obstacles to service delivery; and (3) develop policy initiatives on the national, state, and local levels to institutionalize project findings. This project has been extensively reported in detail elsewhere, and therefore will be discussed only very briefly here (Naparstek et al., 1977; Biegel & Naparstek, 1979; Biegel & Sherman, 1979; Naparstek & Biegel, 1979; Biegel & Naparstek, in press; Naparstek & Biegel, in press).

The project succeeded in developing a number of preventive interventions aimed at serving hard-to-reach populations (i.e., self-help groups for divorced, widowed, and agoraphobic persons; family communication, parenting, and stress workshops; clergy/agency/community seminars and case study luncheons; referral directories and a community hot line, among others). Even more important than the creation of programs to meet unmet needs, the project created a process approach, the Community Mental Health Empowerment Model, for strengthening lay and professional helping networks and then linking them together. Policy recommendations stemming from the project have been included in the final reports of the President's Commission on Mental Health (1978b) and the National Commission on Neighborhoods (1979).

Building on the Neighborhood and Family Services Project, the Washington Public Affairs Center, through a HUD/IPA (Inter-governmental Personnel Act)-funded fourteen-month grant in two small (less than 30,000 population) suburban communities (Hyattsville, Maryland, and Pittsburg, California) expanded upon the partnership notion. This time instead of mental health and human service, the focus was commercial redevelopment, housing, and transportation revitalization. The aim was to assist citizens, government officials, and business people in using local resources to tackle revitalization issues. The project involved intergovernmental partnerships at state, county, and city levels together with partnerships of the local business and citizen sectors. The project led to the establishment of significant broad-based cooperation between local government, citizens, and the business community in both cities. Specific accomplishments have included the following: formation of a local community development corporation by citizens and business persons; adoption of citizen-initiated land use plan for the central business district; downtown revitalization of the central business district through a UDAG (Urban Development Action Grant); development of a neighborhood revitalization needs survey leading to the formation of neighborhood associations; development of a Directory of Community Services; formation of a Citizen/City Anti-Crime Program, among others. Further details about this project can be found in the Final Report to HUD/IPA (Sherman & Haskell, 1980).

Policy Implications of Neighborhood-Based Partnerships

The experiences of the 1960s and 1970s suggest that policymakers and politicians still have a tendency to respond to complex human problems with dramatic, but simplistic cure alls. More often than not the more grandiose the scheme, the messier the unintended consequences.

Thus, we can assume that the decentralization of services and a straight resource approach to neighborhoods, by themselves, will not support a viable neighborhood climate. Although the community mental health movement was predicated on the notion that its programs could improve the overall quality of community life, little attention has been given by mental health professionals to the complex set of legal, administrative, and fiscal policies that independently and/or collectively make it difficult or impossible to bring about change. These obstacles to change are structured into the urban system and act to create a set of disincentives for neighborhood viability. For example, neighborhoods cannot maintain a viable infrastructure (network) if local and state policies, ordinances, regulations, and judicial decisions have negative impact on a community. Further, such public actions often serve as legal obstacles inhibiting participation and fostering a sense of insufficiency among residents. Another example is the relationship between general municipal services and neighborhood approaches to the human services. The interdependencies among the delivery systems of various types of services is essential to a healthy community environment. The inequitable distribution of city services stimulates conditions in which people will not stay in a given neighborhood. Such disincentives serve to break down neighborhood-based networks and thus permit and engender conditions of inequity and insufficiency. Thus, a primary precondition for change must be the identification of such disincentives, their removal, and the concomitant creation of incentives for the maintenance and enhancement of neighborhood-based networks.

The decisions facing local mental health professionals on neighborhood-related issues are complex and politically hazardous. Often practitioners are confronted with a dwindling tax base, aging housing stock, increased numbers of aged and dependent people, underemployment, and a breakdown in social service delivery systems. All these elements lead to varied conditions of alienation and make it difficult to decentralize services in any meaningful way.

Mental health and human service legislation needs to be enacted which will facilitate a comprehensive approach toward restructuring the processes of governance through a mixture of centralization and decentralization of public and private service delivery systems. Legislation aimed at eliminating systemic origins of neighborhood decline also needs to be developed. Perhaps the greatest challenge confronting mental health and human services is to meld federal funds and programs with local conditions in ways that increase utilization, build upon neighborhood strengths, and allow for the uniqueness among communities.

18

Neighborhood-Based Mental Health: An Approach to Overcome Inequities in Mental Health Services Delivery to Racial and Ethnic Minorities

Tom Choken Owan

Despite significant contributions made by the Community Mental Health Center movement in increasing the range and quantity of community-based care, there are still major gaps, particularly those services targeted to racial and ethnic minorities, who represent large segments of the high-risk, underserved, and unserved population groups. To a large extent, the CMHCs, federal, state, and local governments have not adequately responded to the special needs of pluralistic and culturally diverse communities, especially within our major metropolitan areas. We have not taken seriously that race and ethnicity are very important variables affecting utilization, treatment modality, and treatment outcome. Indeed, the present caregiving mental health services to racial and ethnic minorities, by and large, have been inappropriate and ineffective (President's Commission on Mental Health, Vol. III, 1978b).

In *Beyond the Melting Pot,* Glazer and Moynihan state: "The notion that the intense and unprecedented mixture of ethnic and religious groups in America was soon to blend into a homogeneous end product

Views expressed herein are those of the author and do not necessarily reflect the opinions, official policies, or positions of the National Institute of Mental Health.

has outlived its usefulness, and also its credibility" (1963, p. 47). The point about the melting pot, they continue, is that "it did not happen." Ethnic groups today embrace the concept of cultural pluralism—the right to share fully in the benefits of American society while retaining pride in their cultural heritage, distinctive religion, and language. Professional literature is replete with data indicating that new immigrants, refugees, foreign-born residents, and senior citizens of Hispanic, Asian/ Pacific, and Native American origin do not—more likely cannot—adapt to the current methods of service delivery. The continuing major reliance on the Western European tradition and practices, the "Anglo" approach to serve "people of color," has lost its credibility; it is in direct conflict with Hispanic culture, Asian/Pacific culture, American Indian culture, and Afro-American culture. In addition, ethnic minorities simply do not fit into the well-known picture of the YAVIS patient (Young, Attractive, Verbal, Intelligent, Successful) who is considered by the psychotherapist as best for treatment (Schofield, 1964). Further, they neither fit nor share the contemporary values of the majority, in relation to, for example, independence (versus interdependence), individualism (versus familism or groupism), and nuclear family (versus extended families) (Yamamoto, 1978). There is a commonality of harsh experiences that "people of color" encounter as service users, and there is much evidence that they continue to be subjected to inferior treatment in mental health services delivery (Finan, 1975; Hogan & Hartson, 1978).

Since the inception of the community mental health movement in the early 1960s, the providers have forced racial and ethnic minorities into an unnatural amalgamation in their quest for mental health services. Crowded into generally contiguous areas, sharing severe social and economic problems, yet needing widely varying approaches, a conventional model of mental health services delivery was superimposed on the entire group. This has led to a growing sense of conviction among racial and ethnic minorities that existing governmental entities have ceased to adequately respond to the major problems caused by an environment that these very entities have in fact created.

What we need now is not more of the same sterile platitudes of the past—namely, the reiteration of major barriers to services delivery replete in the literature and monotonously mentioned at conferences— but instead a bold new strategy that takes a quantum leap. We need, as T. S. Kuhn describes in his book, *The Structure of Scientific Revolutions,* a new paradigm—a tradition-shattering achievement or model that attracts an enduring group of adherents away from the tradition-bound or accepted modes of activity. This paper will present such a new paradigm, namely, The Neighborhood-Based Mental Health (NBMH) services. This approach is being increasingly advanced by proponents based on preliminary evidence that it is more successful in meeting needs of minority groups than other approaches. Indeed, from the users' perspective, it has been found to be vastly more Accessible, Available, Appropriate, Acceptable, and Accountable for minorities (Five As) than are the existing models. The following sections address in a systematic fashion the justification for this new paradigm so that providers will become more keenly aware of its viability. Research to strengthen the scientific underpinnings for NBMH will be supported, and, more important, a realistic and responsive NBMH policy declaration can be enunciated for the 1980s.

Inequities in Mental Health Services Delivery

Differential Treatment

Numerous investigators provide continuous and widespread evidence of differential mental health treatment based on race and ethnicity. Gross (1969) found that diagnosis becomes less accurate and disposition more nonspecific as the social-cultural difference between the therapist and client increases. Lowenger and Dobie (1966) found that therapists' attitudes and recommendations for treatment are related to the race of the client. Blacks, compared to whites, are seen more often only for diagnosis (Jackson, Berkowitz, & Farley, 1974). Whites are likely seen by psychiatrists, while blacks are more likely to be seen by paraprofessionals (Sue, Allen, McKinney, & Hall, 1974). Participants for insight-oriented therapy are more likely to be white than black (Rosenthal & Frank, 1958) despite indications that lower-income blacks and Mexican Americans can also profit from such therapy (Acosta, Yamamoto, & Evans, in press).

Minority groups frequently receive "qualitatively inferior" or "less preferred" forms of treatment (Yamamoto, James, & Palley, 1968). For example, of the 143 chronically mentally ill Chinese American cases carried by an "Aftercare Program" (N.E. Health Center, San Francisco), forty cases (28 percent) were randomly selected to determine their state hospital experience: average stay in the state hospital was seventeen years and the nature of treatment most received was chemotherapy (83 percent) (Wang & Louie, 1979). Length of stay and percentage receiving chemotherapy were significantly less for white patients.

A combination of factors, including the lack of insurance coverage, have perpetuated a two-class system of mental health care (Goldman, Sharfstein, & Frank, 1980). The authors based their findings on data reported to the Division of Biometry and Epidemiology, National Institute of Mental Health (1975), which indicate that the uninsured, non-white patients with chronic and more severe diagnoses (organic brain syndromes, schizophrenia, alcoholism) predominate in public institutions (state and county mental hospitals, VA hospitals, and CMHCs) when compared to private institutions serving a better insured, white population with less severe, acute disorders. Thus, we have a dual system of care that often relegates non-whites to custody instead of treatment.

These kinds of issues have prevailed for a long time and have never been resolved. Minority groups have continuously raised serious legal questions based on Title VI of the Civil Rights Act, 1964, on issues of discrimination in services delivery (*Association Mixta Progresista et al.*, v. *HEW et al.*, Civ. No. C-72-882-SAE, N.D. California, May 16, 1972; *Lau* v. *Nichols*, 414 U.S. 563, 1974; Hogan & Hartson, 1978; American Indian and Alaskan Natives Subpanel, President's Commission on Mental Health, 1978b).

Negative Outcomes

Premature termination of psychotherapeutic treatment by patients is a commonly recurring problem. This problem occurs even more if these patients are poor, working-class, and minority individuals (Yamamoto, James, Bloombaum, & Hatten, 1967; Sue, 1977). Unilateral termination of therapy among minorities reflected the expressed dissatisfaction with the therapists and therapy that clients received as reported in follow-up contacts (Kline, Adrian, & Spevak, 1975). Sue (1975) found that 52.1 percent of blacks dropped out after the first session as compared to only 29.8 percent of whites. Various researchers have attributed this behavior to unmet patient expectations about their potential improvement, about their role as patient, and about the role of the therapist in the psychotherapy process (Overall & Aaronson, 1963; Acosta, 1979).

In citing the conflict in expectations of the lower socioeconomic groups toward psychotherapy, Lorion (1973) indicated that such persons typically prefer advice for the resolution of "social" rather than intrapsychic problems. This point is supported by Abad (1974), Yamamoto (1978), Murase (1977), and Sue, Wagner, Ja, Margullis, and Lew (1976). They concluded that unlike the passive "Anglo" approach, which relies on the patient to talk about his problems introspectively with the therapist taking the neutral, nonjudgmental, and noncritical role, the Puerto Rican and Asian/Pacific patients' expectations are for the therapist to be actively involved in their relationship, giving them advice and prescribing medication or some tangible treatment. As Goldstein (1980) emphasized, social workers need to rely less on abstractions and to become more active in pursuing knowledge of real-life problems that clients face and in utilizing specific interventions that are effective. Thus the goal for therapists in these situations should be less often insight and more often better coping with the problems by their patients.

Sue and McKinney (1975) found in their study of seventeen community health centers in the greater Seattle area over a three-year period, the dropout rate after the initial intake session for Asian patients was 52 percent, or almost twice the dropout rate for white patients. Karno (1966) has also documented high dropout rates among Mexican Americans and Puerto Ricans.

These studies strongly reveal that "people of color" are usually found to have less positive treatment outcome than others in the general population. A recent NIMH report concludes that when patients come from minority groups or low socio-economic classes, the difficulty of determining the appropriateness and efficacy of treatment is particularly great (Segal, 1974).

Underutilization

A comprehensive review of mental health literature documents widespread underutilization of mental health services by Hispanics, Asian/Pacific Americans, and Native Americans. For example, patterns of underutilization by Hispanics have been reported for California state mental health facilities (Karno & Edgerton, 1969), San Jose California Mental Health Center (Torrey, 1973), Denver Facilities (Kline, 1969), and Texas State Mental Hospitals (Pokorney & Overall, 1970) among others. Burruel and Chavez (1974) and Ramirez (1980) indicate that the patterns of underutilization are primarily the result of culturally irrelevant services which are being provided to the Mexican Americans. Conversely, when specific mental health programs are culturally relevant, services tend to show an increase in the rate of utilization (Morales, 1978; Chavez, 1979).

In Los Angeles County, which has the largest concentration of Asian/Pacific Americans in the United States, their admission rate for inpatient and outpatient mental health services in 1971 was 0.9 percent of the patient population, although their representation in the county was close to 4 percent (Hatanaka, Watanabe, & Ono, 1975). Despite the Synder Act, which authorizes services for all Indians no matter where they live, the lack of funding has caused the Indian Health Service (IHS) to limit mental health services only to Indians who reside on reserva-

tions, thereby excluding the urban Indians and students who are entitled to such services. Comprehensive community mental health centers
have described grossly inadequate services to tribal communities (President's Commission on Mental Health, 1978b). Thus, for the Native
American who is worse off in any comparative analyses measuring the
quality of life, underutilization is far from being only academic in nature;
it has now reached epidemic proportions.

   It is clear that to the extent that providers of services remain unresponsive to the basic needs of racial and ethnic minorities, minority
users will, very likely, drop out of treatment and discourage their
family, friends, and associates from seeking help.

Noncompliance

In the following, noncompliance issues will be discussed that demonstrate the manner in which "people of color" are subjected to differential
treatment, raising serious questions of legal accountability and indicating
the urgent need for affirmative action to remedy inequities. Title VI of
the Civil Rights Act of 1964, 42 U.S.C. S 2000 et seq., mandates that:
"No person in the United States, shall, on the grounds of race, color, or
national origin, be excluded from participation in, be denied the benefits of, or be subjected to discrimination under any program or activity
receiving Federal financial assistance" (42 U.S.C. S 2000 d).

   HHS, in compliance with the foregoing Congressional mandate, has
issued the implementing regulations aimed at assuring equal treatment of
all qualified persons under programs receiving Federal financial assistance (45 C.F.R. S 80 et seq.). Despite the existence of the implementing
regulations, however, a consortium of national minority organizations
(League of United Latin American Citizens, IMAGE, ASPIRA of America, Inc., Japanese American Citizens League, Chinese for Affirmative
Action, Mexican American Women's National Association, Association of
Mexican Educators of California, El Concilio de Fresno, Inc., Mexican
American Political Association, National Council of La Raza, and Leadership Conference on Civil Rights) found that the very acts of discrimination
that are prohibited by these regulations are persistently and extensively
practiced in HHS-funded social service, health, and mental health programs against non-English (NE) and limited English-speaking (LES) individuals (Hogan & Hartson, 1978). The group found further from their
experience that this situation is the result of HHS's failure to mandate by
regulation that compliance with Title VI and its implementing regulations
requires recipient agencies to provide bilingual staff and printed matter.
As a result of these findings, Hogan and Hartson, in a letter to Secretary

Califano in November 1978, requested that "rule-making proceedings" be instituted for the purpose of requiring bilingual staff and printed matter in any program receiving financial assistance from DHHS and whose service area population is at least 5 percent NE or LES persons.

The Office for Civil Rights, DHHS, has determined that in DHHS financially assisted health and social service programs an absence or insufficient number of bilingual staff in "public contact positions" to serve NE or LES persons erodes the quality of services, increases differential treatment, and greatly discourages participation on the part of some potential program beneficiaries. The Office of Civil Rights, DHHS, Title VI Compliance Review of California Welfare Agencies provided the following relevant findings:

> Spanish surnamed and Asian persons have been subjected to unequal treatment in the delivery of public assistance benefits and social services not because of a lack of eligibility or legal entitlement to benefits and services but because of their national origin. Because of these clients' language and culture, their limited knowledge of the English language, and the failure of both State and County Welfare Departments to adequately take account of these characteristics, such clients frequently received inferior treatment and services. County departments failed to utilize staff with an understanding of the culture of, and with language skills necessary to communicate effectively to non-English speaking persons [DHEW, 1973].

The effective exclusion of NE and LES persons from programs that do not employ bilingual staff and do not use bilingual printed matter is dramatically demonstrated by programs in which bilingual staff and notices are made available to such persons. The "Chinatown Project" involved the establishment in June 1975 of a branch office of the Social Security Administration in Chinatown, New York City. The office was staffed entirely by Japanese, Chinese, and Filipino workers and used bilingual literature and signs. A study of that office was designed to examine the extent to which bilingual/bicultural service delivery could improve the productivity of the staff and equality of services to NE and LES persons. The project clearly demonstrated that the utilization of indigenous bilingual/bicultural staff can significantly improve productivity, quality of services, and the overall effectiveness and efficiency of services delivery (Owan, 1978).

Clearly, these findings indicate that NE and LES persons suffer greater difficulties in program participation than do English speaking persons in terms of waiting delays, expense, misdiagnosis, breaches of confidentiality, improper findings of ineligibility, and unwarranted termination of benefits. As the Office of Civil Rights has explicitly noted,

NE and LES persons are denied equal services on the basis of race or national origin in violation of Title VI and its implementing regulations (Hogan & Hartson, 1978).

In the implementation of the CMHC program, there are adequate provisions to ensure racial and ethnic minorities equal benefits and opportunity to participate in the CMHCs comprehensive mental health program. For example, the CMHCs program is governed by legislation first passed in 1963 (The Community Mental Health Centers Act, P.L. 88-164) and later amended in 1975 (P.L. 94-63) and in 1978 (P.L. 95-622). Two references to ethnic minorities appear in the legislation:

> The [community mental health] center's services . . . (b) shall be available and accessible to the residents of the area promptly, as appropriate, and in a manner which preserves human dignity and assures continuity and high quality care and which overcomes geographic, cultural, linguistic, and economic barriers to the receipt of services. . . .
>
> An application for a grant under this part [Part A, Planning and Operations Assistance] . . . shall contain or be supported by assurances . . . that . . . (d) in the case of a community mental health center serving a population including a substantial proportion of individuals of limited English-speaking ability, the center has (i) developed a plan and made arrangements responsive to the needs of such population for providing services to the extent practicable in the language and cultural context most appropriate to such individuals, and (ii) identified an individual on its staff who is fluent in both that language and English and whose responsibilities shall include providing guidance to such individuals and to appropriate staff members with respect to cultural sensitivities and bridging linguistic and cultural differences . . . [Sec. 206, (c) CMHC Act].

The standards referred to clearly mandate the CMHCs to bring about equitable mental health services delivery to racial and ethnic minorities. A recent NIMH study, however, reveals that unless strategies are developed to remedy service inequities, the scenario for the 1980s will remain undistinguishable from that of the 1970s:

> In 1974, out of a total of 98 CMHCs in HEW Region IV, 42 CMHCs were serving non-whites at lower rates than whites. The 42 CMHCs were provided technical assistance to improve their utilization to non-whites for a period of three years (1974–77) through ADAMH regional staff. Despite these efforts, the 42 CMHCs showed little or no improvements. It seems apparent that even with special efforts, non-compliance remains a critical issue [Windle & Wu, 1979].

The aforementioned identification of differential treatment, negative outcomes, underutilization and noncompliance issues merit profound reassessment of policies, and detailed evaluation as to how we can reshape the delivery of mental health services to substantially improve access and utilization by racial and ethnic minorities.

Since the existing models serving minority groups have, in large measure, failed to fulfill the need of these patients and especially the NE and LES persons, it is obvious that some alternate method of service delivery is necessary. It is doubtful that, with current models of delivery, a mere redirection of philosophical emphasis will accomplish anything more than a cosmetic improvement. An obviously effective and thoroughly accepted procedure must be provided. The Neighborhood Based Mental Health (NBMH), the new paradigm, offers a promising alternative choice to overcome the long-standing inequities in mental health services delivery directed to racial and ethnic minorities.

Neighborhood-Based Mental Health: "Front-line Caregivers"

There have been a number of major trends within the field of mental health since the beginning of the nineteenth century: moral treatment, custodialism, psychoanalysis, use of psychotropic drugs, CMHCs and a relatively new frontier—Neighborhood-Based Mental Health (NBMH). NBMH represents a progressive modification of the CMHC movement of the 1960s, focusing orientation from large, amorphous catchment areas into smaller and more realistically sized ethnic or destiny-related geographic areas (Klerman & Borus, 1977). Sharfstein (1974) cites the advantages of "Neighborhood Psychiatry" (akin to NBMH) as a new community approach—early intervention in crisis with individuals and agencies, increased accessibility to the entire family, integration with general health services, easy follow-up and aftercare of recently discharged psychiatric patients.

From the minority groups' perspective, NBMH is a concept in which services are organized and staffed along ethnocentric lines, giving primary attention to needs of specific minority groups in a manner that ensures acceptance and participation. Its mission is to fit professional resources to the specific needs of the client instead of fitting the client to the resources and framework of professionals. Such a strategy enhances positive outcomes within the context of the neighborhood.

Neighborhood-Based Mental Health as an approach to the delivery of mental health services has a number of important and distinguishing characteristics:

1. Provides services where people live and work.

2. Seeks greater involvement from neighborhood residents than "paper" compliance with consumer involvement guidelines of the 1975 amendments to the CMHC act. This neighborhood involvement is sought in order to help achieve the Five As (Accessibility, Acceptability, Availability, Appropriateness, and Accountability).

3. Builds upon and is linked to strengths of informal networks— blood kin, non-kin, self-help, and mutual-help.

4. Provides treatment as well as preventive services to previously unserved/underserved people.

5. Considers services to the chronically mentally ill as one of its most important challenges.

NBMH provides an important link in mental health services delivery to minority groups. It complements the services of the CMHCs particularly in filling major gaps and deficiencies in the delivery of services to such diverse groups as the Asians/Pacific Islanders (Vietnamese, Laotians, Cambodians, Koreans, Chinese, Filipinos, Japanese, Hawaiians, Samoans, Guamanians), Hispanics (Mexican Americans, Cubans, Puerto Ricans), American Indians/Alaskan Natives, and blacks.

The thrust for NBMH has been fostered by enthusiasm among the users of NBMH and by reports of promising beginnings. In general, the providers report that when visible culturally relevant programs are provided, there is a significant increase in the number of racial and ethnic minorities seeking their services.

Sue and McKinney (1975) report that in Seattle the number of Asians utilizing an Asian American Counseling and Referral Service in one year was approximately equal to the total number of Asians utilizing a total of eighteen other community mental health centers over a three-year period. In San Francisco, after the establishment of a mental health facility specifically designed to serve Asian Pacific Islanders (Maxi-Center, Richmond, California), more Asian/Pacific patients were seen in the first three months of operation than were seen in the previous five years (Wong, 1977). In addition, Maxi-Center had the lowest no-show rate for first appointments of comparable outpatient centers in District V, San Francisco—over 90 percent of all clients who called for services showed for their first appointment. There is no waiting list for its services (Wong, 1979). True (1975) reports that an Asian community-based mental health program in Oakland saw 131 Chinese Americans in the first year of operation, in contrast to three Chinese out of a total of 500 utilizing a central outpatient facility. Hatanaka and co-workers (1975) also report that their data for Los Angeles suggests that the presence of comprehensive, accessible, and ethnically appropriate services increased by approximately 200 percent the rate of utilization of Asian/Pacific Americans over a three-year period. The South Cove Community Health Center, "Chinatown," Boston, Massachusetts, reported decreased stigma attached to mental health when mental health services are part of a general health care program rather than separate and that psychosomatic illness is more effectively treated in an integrated setting (Lee, 1980).

La Frontera Center, Tucson, Arizona, serves a catchment that has the highest concentration of minorities (51 percent) with 41 percent Mexican American. Prior to 1971, client visits to the outpatient clinic were less than fifty a month. Today, the average visits are over 2,000 a month. Forty-five percent of the clients are Mexican Americans. The "cultural responsiveness" program was responsible not only for the substantial improvement in the utilization rates but also in the completion of treatment (Chavez, 1979).

While these findings must be regarded as preliminary and tentative, they are nevertheless immensely suggestive of a new paradigm in which mental health services for racial and ethnic minorities should be considered as alternative approaches to existing service delivery needs in order to achieve optimal utilization and effectiveness. As Glaser and Marks (1966) stated:

> It is destructive and wasteful that people should be frustrated and often defeated by difficulties for which somebody else has found a remedy. The gap between what we know and what we put to effective use bedevils many fields of human activity—teaching, business, management and organizations which provide health and welfare services [p. 6].

An important issue for consideration is the relationship between NBMH and CMHCs. Today, two critical issues confront the future of CMHCs: (1) Because the 1975 amendments to the CMHC Act imposed seven additional services onto the original five mandated services without correspondingly increasing financial support to centers, these extra service requirements have placed a tremendous burden on the CMHCs. (2) CMHCs are "graduating" from federal support and often have not been very successful at replacing an equal amount of lost federal dollars from other sources. Thus serious concerns have been expressed as to whether CMHCs are headed for extinction or whether there will be new vitality for this national program into the 1980s (Sharfstein, 1978). Under these critical circumstances, there is increasing skepticism among minority groups concerning the capabilities of the CMHCs to meet the massive unmet needs of the non-English, limited English-speaking, unserved and underserved, racial and ethnic minorities.

Given these circumstances, NBMH services can be initiated in several ways. First, a CMHC recognizing the inability of its current services to meet the needs of racial ethnic minorities might set up a special service, program, or neighborhood satellite with minority staff and active consumer participation to deliver specialized services. Second, an independent minority community group or agency may receive a subcontract of funds from a CMHC to develop and deliver services to residents in their community. Third, and probably most often, a minority community group or agency will seek funding through a variety of public and private sources to develop and deliver services to community residents without going through a CMHC. An important fact to consider is that there are currently only 675 federally-funded CMHCs covering half the country in operation. In those areas without a CMHC there are great differences among state and local programs in the degree to which they are meeting the needs of minority residents. Thus, minority groups may need to develop their own programs for lack of a suitable mental health agency to be linked to.

It must be clearly understood that different groups of people solve problems and meet needs in differing ways, so no mental health program that is prepackaged in Washington with identical programs and services will work. Services have to be tailored to meet the needs of specific groups. It is not enough for a CMHC to hire a bilingual staff person if the design of the services does not take into account racial and ethnic differences. Since many catchment areas are multiracial and multi-ethnic, it makes sense for service providers to contract with minority organizations for consultation in program planning, development, and evaluation and/or for the actual delivery of services.

In order to facilitate and enhance the development of the NBMH for racial and ethnic groups, four essential components will need to be integrated into its program focus and mission: (1) alternative service delivery models, (2) neighborhood support systems, (3) research, and (4) evaluation.

Alternative Service Delivery Models

The development of alternative service delivery models is crucial if we are to increase utilization substantially among racial minorities at the neighborhood level. For heuristic purposes and to develop eclectic approaches, consideration should be given to the social support model elucidated by Sotomayer (1980) and Dean and Lin (1977). In addition, Margolis and Favazza (1977) have identified seven current mental health models: sociocultural development model, community psychiatry–community mental health model, medical model, behavioral model, psychodynamic model, humanistic model, and general system model. Of these eight models, those meriting special attention for NBMH are the social support model, the sociocultural development model, and the community psychiatry–community mental health model.

The *social support model* may be defined as support (mutual-reciprocal) accessible to an individual based on informal networks of family members, kin, friends, acquaintances, and neighborhood organizations. These networks are utilized by individuals on an ongoing basis for social and emotional support and vary by group norms and/or expectations. In the *sociocultural model*, the dynamic interface between culture and mental health is brought into focus, that is, mental illness is strongly influenced by culture: it is culturally constructed involving social issues rather than a discrete disease process. Thus, from the bilingual/bicultural population's perspective, the exclusion of culturally syntonic treatment modalities would be tantamount to the practice of veterinary medicine on humans. The *community psychiatry–community health model* implies that the community is the unit to be worked with and analyzed. For example, a specific group is served, the service is accessible to the client, community resources are extensively utilized, mental health rather than mental illness is strongly emphasized, mental health services are integrated or linked with general health care programs, and the community shares the responsibility for solving the problems. Thus, these three approaches should form the basis for the development of alternative services delivery models to minority groups. It is interesting to note that especially the last two models were the theoretical underpinnings of the CMHC movement. It is clear that practice has not followed promise.

Neighborhood Support Systems

NBMH should build on the strengths of the neighborhood. In all neighborhoods, in varying degrees, there is a web of helping networks that link the individual to the indigenous formal and informal social fabric—the extended families, church, social clubs, credit associations, mutual-help/self-help, pharmacist, doctors, barbers, and so on. The importance of these neighborhood-based natural, cultural, and organizational networks has been noted by Naparstek, Biegel, et al. (1977), Biegel (1979), Murase (1977), Sanchez (1977), Kitano (1969), Sotomayer (1980), Warren

(1977), and American Indians and Alaskan Natives Subpanel, President's Commission on Mental Health (1978b), among others.

In the Leighton et al.'s Sterling Study (1963), ten indices were developed against which to determine the degree of "integrated" or "disintegrated" state of community. The ten were: (1) poverty—instability of income as well as low level; (2) cultural confusion, that is, confused and conflicting values; (3) secularization, that is, absence of religious values; (4) frequency of broken homes; (5) few and weak associations in the group, both formal and informal; (6) few and weak leaders; (7) few patterns of recreation; (8) high frequency of hostile acts and expressions; (9) high frequency of crime and delinquency; and (10) fragmented network communications. NBMH has strong potential to become an integral part of neighborhood efforts to act as a counterforce against the disruptive effects and influence which tend to rapidly erode the neighborhood, keeping in mind the limits of any one program, especially mental health, to be able to successfully address the complex issues of neighborhood decline and decay. Neighborhoods with strong ethnic identities have a sense of pride and coping styles that may serve far more effectively to lessen the deleterious effects of stress and hence the risk of mental illness. The research by Lin et al. (1979) strongly supports this empirical method. Their preliminary findings suggest that social support contributes significantly toward reducing the severity of illness symptoms. In contrast, stressful life events (SLE) are positively related to illness. More specifically, the stronger the social support an individual can amass, the less likely the individual would experience episodes of illness; also, social support performs a valuable mediating role between SLE and psychiatric symptoms.

Undeniably, we are poor in tapping the rich resources of the neighborhoods, and it would seem far more productive to redirect our energies to developing culturally syntonic neighborhood support systems than to continue the counterproductive practices that have contributed to the severe underutilization of mental health services.

Research

In David Hapgood's inelegantly titled book, *The Screwing of the Average Man* (1978), he provides harsh criticism of how big government and big business victimize the average man through questionable practices. Among racial and ethnic groups there is growing disillusionment that despite the annual billions of dollars poured into research and development, its purported benefits to improve the quality of life are simply not "hitting the streets." We have despaired at repeated waves of "wheel reinvention." A greater effort must be made to make researchers and program managers aware of the ways research findings can be effectively transferred to the community. Davis (1978) discusses eight key factors for increasing the probability of successful adoption of innovation and change: ability, values, information, circumstances, timing, obligation, resistance, and yield.

A critical area of research needed in this field is the obvious one—to determine whether the NBMH system will work. In order to determine the effectiveness of NBMH, Klerman and Borus (1977) suggest two prominent hypotheses to be tested: (1) can the neighborhood delivery system decrease the incidence of mental illness by providing more effective direct and indirect mental health services, and (2) can a neighborhood delivery system itself help to better Gemeinschaft communities (those organized around face-to-face contact, common values, and informal modes of control). An examination of these two hypotheses provides some meaningful research questions. For example: What services are most appropriately delivered at the neighborhood level? How does delivery of mental health services at the neighborhood level compare in terms of accessibility, acceptability, and utilization with alternative delivery systems, such as private practice and free-standing community mental health centers? Can neighborhood delivery of health and mental health services increase neighborhood organization and cohesion? Does such a delivery system increase community acceptance and readiness to deal actively with the chronically ill in the neighborhood setting? Will these new service delivery systems help define a more functional consumer constituency in the neighborhood to work cooperatively with professionals? Can such a system be cost-effective and self-supporting and prevent costly hospitalization? How do the costs and benefits compare with other systems of care?

Evaluation

Evaluation is the measurement of program performance (efficiency, effectiveness, responsiveness), the making of comparisons based on those measurements, and the use of the resulting information in policymaking and program management. A number of program managers and policymakers are aware of the need to provide effective services to the underserved and unserved minority populations. Several exemplary and innovative projects have been implemented at the neighborhood level. Little, however, has been done to document or measure specific cultural and language-based program achievements and outcomes. The appropriate language/cultural-based program objectives, evaluation criteria, and techniques for assessing performance have not been recognized or used in the mental health evaluation repertoire. Lacking these, policymakers, program managers, and civil rights enforcement staff are severely hampered in their efforts to bring about desired and necessary program changes needed to make mental health services delivery more effective and responsive to the needs of linguistically and culturally diverse groups.

Consumers and citizens are conspicuously absent in evaluation. There is increasingly frequent discussion about how evaluations are designed and conducted from the providers' viewpoint and how different the results might appear if more could be learned about the view from the clients' perspective. The key to better decisions and better government programs is the establishment of realistic measurable objectives and measures of program performance information to bring about management of change in program activities (Wholey, 1979). In order to facilitate evaluation processes and the development of program performance standards, an approach suggested is the utilization of the Five As. While the following Five A's are by no means applicable in all situations, they provide an effective framework to ensure quality of services and valuable data on understanding the causes of achieving or failing to achieve priority program objectives.

Accessibility connotes the ability and opportunity to approach, enter, and communicate. Is the facility located in relation to specific population groups targeted? Is there convenient access to public and private transportation, within reasonable travel time? Are services available during evening hours and on weekends? Is the waiting time before appointment and at appointment reasonable?

Availability considers the adequacy of the range of services provided. Are a variety of inpatient and outpatient treatment modalities offered? Are services tailored to needs of varying at-risk population groups? Are preventive services offered?

Acceptability reflects the consumers' assessment. Are the patterns of utilization consistent with nonethnic groups? What is the no-show rate for first appointments; the dropout rate? How do the outcome and length of treatment compare with the clients' expectations?

Appropriateness considers the delivery of mental health services that are culture-specific, to overcome major barriers of language, cross-cultural misdiagnosis, and clashes between Western European thoughts and traditions in the Hispanic, Asian/Pacific American, and Afro-American cultures. Are there bilingual/cultural staff at both the professional and paraprofessional level? Are linkages made to folk healers and the subculturally preferred patterns of seeking, giving, and receiving help? Does the ambience induce warmth, informality, and receptivity by use of familiar decorations, furniture, photo displays, and the like? Are the social support systems an essential component of services delivery? Is use made of bilingual literatures, ethnic newspapers, radio, and T.V. programs?

Accountability deals with the mandate of Title VI, Civil Rights Act (1964), Department of Health and Human Services implementing regulations, and P.L. 94-63 in which CMHCs are required to evaluate their impact of services to the unserved and underserved populations. Is the size and balance of the minority staff adequate to reflect the catchment area served? Is there sufficient representation on the Advisory-Governing Board to reflect the neighborhood served? Have patients' rights and advocacy programs been implemented to protect particularly the non-English and limited English-speaking persons?

The Five As are intended to determine the strengths and weaknesses of mental health services targeted to racial and ethnic minorities and to provide technical assistance to correct major deficiencies. They are to facilitate decisions on whether support for culturally relevant programs is warranted and/or whether these efforts are wasteful or duplicative. Furthermore, the use of the Five As will provide necessary data to reward effective and efficient program performers and deny the funding of programs that consistently fail to achieve acceptable standards of performance.

The Need for a NBMH Policy Declaration

If federal policies and programs targeted to ethnic minorities had been successful, the general public and elected officials would now be our strongest allies and would enthusiastically support these efforts. However, not only have few programs been demonstrably successful but many others have been viewed by the users as ineffective, wasteful, and even harmful in mental health services delivery to racial minorities. Given this negative assessment, it should become increasingly evident that our policymakers are out of step, that is, federal policies are no longer congruent with or responsive to the changing demographic texture of our inner-city populations. For example, in the State of California 35 percent of the population is already made up of minorities; it is estimated that by 1990, over 19 million of California's total population of over 31 million will be members of minority groups—a staggering 60 percent (Francisco, 1977). California will thus become the first "Third World" state in the Nation. On a nationwide basis, Hispanics will number well over 20 million by 1990, placing them ahead of the blacks as the largest minority group in the country (Russell & Satterwhite, 1978) and the Asian/Pacific Americans should exceed three million by 1980 (Owan, 1975).

We urgently need for the 1980s a NBMH policy declaration that strongly supports the development of alternative services delivery relevant to the true needs of racial minorities, other ethnic groups, and the neighborhoods. Such a policy should provide for contracting, especially with minority organizations in the areas of rendering specific outreach services, training, research, and evaluation. Indeed, a NBMH policy will have significant implications for effective intervention in the improvement of general health care, especially for the racial minorities for whom the exclusionary patterns of mental health services delivery has become a painful reality.

Conclusion

The thrust for Neighborhood-Based Mental Health will provide great challenges and opportunities to neighborhood leaders, researchers, therapists, allied professionals, and the users. Approval of increased funding for NBMH from federal, state and local governments will not come easily or voluntarily since, to a significant degree, the present allocation of resources reflects the priorities of those who strongly control the allocations. Therefore, the adherents for NBMH will have to articulate their goals based on the increasing evidence that NBMH can achieve the Five As (Accessibility, Availability, Appropriateness, Acceptability, and Accountability) with greater efficiency and effectiveness than the conventional models.

At this juncture, an important caveat should be raised to avoid misleading inferences that CMHCs are purposely being unresponsive to the needs of racial and ethnic groups. The blanket generalization about CMHCs is no more universally true than any other stereotype, for there are exemplary CMHC models that have taken major steps to achieve the Five As. In addition, a number of CMHCs have increased the range and quantity of mental health services, substantially reduced the need for care at state hospitals, and increased minority representation on community governing-advisory boards while providing training so that these members become responsive to the true needs of the consumers. The essence of this chapter is to raise the consciousness, sensitivity, and commitment toward the development of culturally and linguistically relevant mental health services.

The recent momentous passage by Congress (August 1981) of the

Alcohol, Drug Abuse and Mental Health (ADM) Block Grant establishes a broad new departure in federal/state relationships, i.e., it allows states substantial flexibility in the use of federal financial assistance with minimum federal requirements. Within this changed political and legislative environment and the restructuring of the federal/state relationships, creative strategies must be developed in order to: assure the most appropriate, effective, and efficient utilization of ADM care; assure residents access to needed mental health services of acceptable quality at reasonable costs; and to encourage the use of services in the least restrictive setting. In order to ensure more effective results from NBMH, it is crucial that racial minorities actively participate in the development and implementation of ADM services with the appropriate state and local entities.

The problems of inadequate and inappropriate mental health services to racial and ethnic minorities, like any festering sore, will not be cured by neglect. The task of implementing NBMH will be demanding, especially in a period when increased competition between groups for decreasing public resources can trigger intergroup animosities and fragmentation. However, because there is solidarity among racial and ethnic groups in their disagreement about the relevancy of the conventional models, there is much to be gained by federal, state, and local governments as well as CMHCs and citizens groups in taking decisive action for the establishment of a NBMH policy. Such a policy meets the needs not only of racial minorities but of white ethnic population groups as well (Biegel & Sherman, 1979).

For racial and ethnic minorities, the 1980s could mean a period when organizations rooted in ethnicity are given an opportunity to work with government for the actualization of this new paradigm—Neighborhood-Based Mental Health.

19

Natural Support Networks and the Welfare State: Some Ethical Considerations

Harold Lewis

The fellowship that we have come to associate with the Garden of Eden is ideally what most people would wish to see in their own neighborhoods. Unhappily, as Janice Perlman observes, neighborhoods today do not resemble Edens. Often they are inhospitable and lacking in sociability, reflecting a major gap in our democratic strivings. Citing the call to arms of the French Revolution—Liberty, Equality, Fraternity—Ms. Perlman notes that some societies have done well at achieving liberty, but not so well at achieving equality. Other societies have moved much farther toward equality, but have fared rather poorly on liberty. No society has really done very well at developing fraternity. She sees as the essential function of neighborhood organization the building of fraternity, that is, the transformation of individual self-interest into collective mutual concern (Perlman, 1979).

But neighborliness does not necessarily include a concern for the rights of strangers, those who are not indigenous to or those who are recent arrivals in the community. From the perspective of those who may enjoy its kindred spirit, a neighborhood may have some of the attributes of Eden, but from the perspective of the excluded, it can easily be mistaken for a jungle. Whether neighborhoods produce sociability or discordance depends primarily on the quality of the smaller constituent units that make up the local informal support networks and the wider community's disposition toward them (Wellman, 1979b). The

An earlier version of this paper was presented at the Helping Networks and the Welfare State Symposium, Toronto, May 6, 1979, sponsored by the University of Toronto, School of Social Work.

protection of the rights of the stranger, however, depends primarily on the legal provisions incorporated into the formal welfare structure.

It is interesting to surmise what rule was followed in Eden, when it came to sharing the Apple. From what can be deduced, the rule followed was grounded in the belief that one should treat the other as one would want to be treated in his or her place. In Kant's formulation, "I ought never to act except in such a way that I can also will that my maxim should become a universal law," or as Marx would have it, "From each according to his ability, to each according to his needs." Of course, efforts to formulate a rule that would recapture the fairness implicit in Eden have challenged our greatest minds. Currently, the rule we in the United States have evolved for sharing the Apple does not suggest an abiding interest in a fraternal society, rich in that sought-after virtue, the kindred spirit. As best one can determine, our guiding rule for sharing is *from each according to his or her opportunity, to each according to his or her power*. While this rule is disadvantageous to some, it has proven to be very profitable for others. Consider how conveniently it serves the interests of those with power who unflinchingly advocate proposals that would solve problems brought on by inflation by increasing unemployment, and that would seek to stimulate the flagging economy by protecting the profits of the wealthy while reducing the incomes of the poor. It may well be, as the moral philosopher John Rawls suggests, that only when we can conceive of ourselves in an original state of innocence, as might describe Adam and Eve, could we agree on principles for distributive justice that would meet the conditions of fairness implicit in the spirit we call fraternal (Rawls, 1971).

In the real world, where the original state of innocence does not prevail and persons are aware of their attributes and conditions, the rule that operates appears to maximize the opportunities for the most advantaged to help the disadvantaged do what they have learned to do best: that is, to bear the burdens. It seems fairly obvious that if we are to protect and promote justice and enlarge on the fraternal spirit that supports fairness, we will have to change the rule.

This chapter will consider the function of the formal and informal welfare structure and the methods of helping used by the human services professions as they affect rights, promote the fraternal spirit, and influence the rule governing just distribution of benefits—which we call distributive justice—in the welfare system. The analysis will conclude with a rule of conduct that could help achieve the goal of distributive justice as well as a set of principles of practice congenial with this rule which can guide those seeking to design and implement a system of welfare services.

Individualism: Rights

Philanthropy was once described as the wealthy classes' "fire escape," providing the affluent with an exit pass from hell. Supposedly ill-gotten gains were used to finance charitable efforts. In this perception, unjust rules of distribution allowed the haves to withhold from the have-nots their fair share, returning to the poor a minor portion as a means of assuaging their own deserved guilt. Of course, this bitter analogy denigrates the generous impulse we have come to associate with the altruistic intent of the welfare state.

Many rights protecting the less powerful have been incorporated into formal structures financed by public as well as private sources (Kramer, 1979). We have come to depend upon the welfare structure, philanthropic and tax supported, for services as broad as health and social insurance and as narrowly focused as dialysis units. These benefits are perceived as rights for those eligible to use them. Such welfare programs represent considerable progress toward achieving the good life for many. They are the products of much struggle to mitigate the effects of the not-so-golden rule that governs our distributive system. But successes in the political-economic arena can and often do widen the gap between the haves and have-nots, so long as the rules that perpetuate unjust distribution remain unchanged. The same programs that have extended rights have concurrently diminished collective mutual concern.

An analogy may help to clarify this point. Writing in the mid-1930s Bertha Reynolds, one of the "greats" of social work in the United States, observed about psychoanalysis that it had helped the profession to individualize each client and, in the process, to isolate him. The formal welfare structure has similarly focused our attention on the individual, on each person's rights, and in the process diminished the kindred spirit that one hopes will accompany neighborly concerns.

How this lessening comes about is no mystery. One can experience it directly by applying for a public assistance grant in any major city in the United States. You will quickly discover that the eligibility process is concerned with only two of the three categories of ethical imperatives—virtues (honesty, trustworthiness, etc.) and duties. These are to be manifest as you seek to justify your claims, in order to exercise your rights to share in the program's available resources. You are not expected or encouraged to consider imperatives intended to provide for the third category of ethical imperatives—the common good: to concern yourself with the impact of your claims on the claims of other applicants. You may assume, if you think about it at all, that concern for the common good is provided for in the rules under which the program operates. Nor are you likely to challenge this assumption if your own claims seem to receive fair consideration. The belief that if each person pursues his own interests, the interests of all will be advanced, has been deeply ingrained in us through our indoctrination into the virtues of a laissez-faire market economy. This belief may in some situations be true, but few applicants for public assistance would care to prove it false, so long as their interests are being served.

Exceptions to this neglect of the common good do occur, and are noteworthy. When recipients are in control of a service and are responsible for implementing rules of eligibility, the effort may be closer to a mutual-aid situation, as for example in a union-sponsored welfare service or a neighborhood-based cooperative day-care program. In these circumstances, there are psychological and social pressures to consider the common good, particularly as those who allocate resources may be currently or at a future date dependent on the very resources they allocate (Reynolds, 1951).

Fraternalism: Collective Mutual Concern

Concerns for virtue and duties and for individual rights in the formal structures are well founded. Such concerns are a necessary if not a sufficient condition for an ethical and just welfare system. But the diminished pursuit of the common good is problematic. In contrast to the client in his role as public assistance applicant, participants in the informal arena are more often compelled to consider the common good. Informal programs, for example, could not survive if fraternal shared obligations were ignored, and an individualistic perspective took precedence over the collective.

In informal support systems, which may include kith and kin, mutual-help associations, and self-help groups, acting in one's own interest is less likely to result in purely self-serving action, since the intimacy of the relationships such systems require is bound to promote a concern for how one's actions affect the well-being of others as well as oneself. The voluntary nature of membership in such systems promotes commitment and trust in the motives of fellow members, since most are free to vote with their feet should doubts as to intentions develop. In the formal structures, worker authority is often exercised on the basis of claimed expertise. The recipient is expected to trust the superior knowledge of the staff member serving him. Where the recipient is compelled to trust the motives, not just the knowledge, of the worker, the relationship is not one of authority, but is authoritarian (Lewis, 1972). In the informal system, the opposite is true. Trust in the motivation of others promotes shared authority. The knowledge of the collectivity is explored for mutual gain and not perceived as a valid claim for individual authority in the group. When the expert is consulted, the authority of knowledge must first pass the acid test of trustworthiness in motivation, or it is unlikely to influence the work of the collectivity.

Thus, the distrust that often prevails among recipients of services from formal structures is understandable. In the formal structure, resources are chronically in short supply; often even minimal needs cannot be met. As we noted, the eligibility process itself impels one to attend to private ends without too much regard for how this affects the welfare of others. Thus, the programs are not only designed to promote individualistic outlooks, but in their inadequacy press recipients to put self-interest first. In contrast, the informal system promotes a shared experience, which is in itself a potential source for emotional and psychological growth, a natural healing milieu. In the formal system, this milieu is not likely to be present unless a self-help group for recipients is promoted as part of the organization's program.

The informal and formal sectors share many attributes. Each seeks to obtain resources for its constituencies; each permits various arrangements for achieving a balance of support for persons in need. Negotiated allocations of resources are managed by plan, persuasion, and market. Each promotes efforts to monitor the performance of the other. The utilization of helpers, whether voluntary or paid, professional or lay, indigenous or bureaucratic, leads to exchanges and interactions affecting a shared pool of human service practitioners. Both suffer from abuses and misuses and hold the potential for doing much damage as well as good. Our concern, however, is not with these shared attributes, but with their distinctive ethical concerns; that is, the focus on rights in the formal structure, and on the fraternal in the informal. While both will be affected by the general well-being of the society in which they operate, it is illusory in our society to believe that one can readily fulfill the ethical focus of the other or that our society can long survive in a civilized state without both.

The Professional Helper

In the last decade of the nineteenth century in the United States, the term *social worker* gradually replaced that of the *friendly visitor*. This change reflected the newly acquired employee status of helpers, who formerly were largely unpaid volunteers. Workers continued to view their efforts as friendly rather than unfriendly, but also accepted the role of organizational agents, which more accurately described their status. When help was sought from the organization that employed them, the visiting required of these workers served an investigatory purpose and was rarely intended as a social house call. Over time, as social work developed within the bureaucratic structure of the formal welfare system, it incorporated into its practice a sensitivity to its own dependence on organizational resources for its survival, and an awareness of threats to its own as well as a client's well-being, when no contractual assurances of rights and obligations accompanied work and service arrangements. The inevitable preoccupation of social workers with their rights as organization employees coincided with a similar concern of consumers of their agencies' services whose rights often were subordinate to the wishes and intentions of these organizations.

But the employee status of the social worker does not account for the methodological preferences that have come to shape professional social work practice. The organizational context invested each service transaction with constraints common to the action of agents in a bureaucracy. Such constraints were sometimes perceived by workers as strengths to be used creatively in shaping the transaction, and at other times as barriers to sound practice. Approaches to practice sought to incorporate the organizational context into their theoretical frameworks. Nevertheless, the *methods* of practice that often are guided by principles of practice for which theoretical justifications are lacking were far more influenced by their assumptions about attributes of consumers who sought services, the environment in which these consumers lived, and the psychosocial influences that shaped and were in turn shaped by their behaviors, than by their agency context. That these approaches, almost without exception, contrived against the natural tendency for friendships to develop between workers and clients, viewing relationships as professional the more they departed from the fraternal, is thus not attributable primarily to bureaucratic constraints. In fact, most of the preferred approaches were modeled after the practice of individual-, not organizational-, based practitioners, particularly those in the medical and legal profession.

Traditionally, the origins of social work as the dominant professional practice in social welfare organizations in the United States are located in the institutions that evolved from the period of the Poor Laws in the public sector, and from the Charity Organization Society and Settlement Movement in the voluntary sector. The influence of Northern European welfare practices and the dominant Protestant ethic are manifest in our prevalent perceptions of persons who are dependent and the causes of their dependency. The time-is-money mentality favored by the elites in commerce, industry, and finance also contribute to an emphasis on cost-efficiency measures, on what is manufactured and invented rather than on what grows and is discovered. No wonder then that little attention has been given to the associations of the working poor, the ethnic immigrant fraternal associations, the black slavery and post-slavery church and service organizations, the Native American, Spanish and Oriental tribal and communal support systems, and the like, until very recently. Only with the upheaval of the 1960s, with an awakened Black Consciousness, the upsurge of ethnic self-awareness, the effort to organize welfare clients, the rekindling of the women's rights movement dormant since the suffragette period but revived with the massive entrance of women into the world of work, and the significant expansion of welfare programs under the auspices of trade unions, was a "critical mass" reached, forcing a reconsideration of the one-sided nature of the traditional view. Inevitably, conceptions of the client systems and approaches to practice intended to influence them were challenged on many fronts and had to change.

While there is general acceptance of the concept of individual personal dignity in the major belief systems that guide the efforts of communities to provide for those in need, the treatment of paupers and otherwise dependent and handicapped during the period of the Poor Laws through to the end of the nineteenth century hardly reflected this belief, as far as the disadvantaged were concerned. The distinction between the worthy and unworthy poor, the level of support that was provided, and the dim view taken of the moral behavior of clients contributed to the rescue fantasy that permeated the literature of friendly visiting and conspired to deny, in practice, the intrinsic dignity of recipients of aid. The focus of interventions was on their dysfunctional behaviors and attitudes, not their strengths.

In an individualistic-oriented society such as ours, respect for the individual's dignity is often dependent on the economic and political status of the person. The power professionals have accrued because of their specialized knowledge is gained, not only through extensive education, but through the dependent position in which their clients are placed when seeking professional help. Thus clients who have political power and economic resources can and often do use such power to position themselves more favorably in seeking access to professional services and manage to convey the sense of their own worth to would-be helpers who might otherwise trifle with their self-esteem. During the nineteenth century most persons seeking help for welfare-related problems lacked both political and economic power. Those who proffered help had little reason to identify or promote the client's power, which would have given these mendicants a sense of their own worth. Not until the last decade of that century did self-organization among dependent persons into unions and fraternal associations reach a level that constituted significant political and economic power. In these beginnings of fraternal unity, of informal support networks providing their constituents with assistance and self-esteem, are to be found the forerunners of the 1960s. Seeing their need as the by-product of societal as well as personal failure, participants in these groups held expectations of worker skill and attitude that differed from those of the isolated supplicant. While various explanations for these expectations can be offered, it seems more plausible to attribute the current press for professional competence that includes skill in work with informal support systems to the changing power of consumer self-support networks than to a sudden uncovering of new knowledge about such networks or a new concern on the part of the haves for the quality of services to be rendered the have-nots.

The heightened interest in the informal support networks during the past decade has prompted a reexamination of social work helping processes, with new awareness of the potential power in client-systems. Systems, networks, and ecological formulations (Siporin, 1975; Germain and Gitterman, 1978) go much farther than did Mary Richmond when she asked the helper to consider both the individual and the wider self, farther than the second Milford Conference in the early 1930s, which asked the worker to see the client and his situation as the unit of attention. In seeking to incorporate the clients' natural and communal sources of nurturance into the method of helping, these approaches see the wider self and the clients' situations as sources of strength to be tapped: as part of the solution, not only as part of the problem.

The Changing Rule

Inevitably, the entry of new power groupings contending for their special interests and seeking to extend their claims on available resources must force a reevaluation of existing rules, particularly those shaping the pattern of distributive justice in our society. Not immune to changes in the relationship of nations and peoples the world over, yet responding primarily to the shifting pressures at home, welfare systems have moved to the point where their command over some nations' resources suggests to many that they have become welfare states. But a welfare state, no more than a welfare system, is only as just and fair as are the rules by which it makes its allocations. The discussion thus far has suggested a critical function for the informal support networks in shaping the welfare system and professional practice within that system.

Not all who have thought about the issues discussed would agree with these interpretations. While there is evidence in support of the view presented, it is hardly conclusive evidence.

The assertion that the societal context of a welfare system affects the division of labor between the formal and informal sources of support is more certain than the assertion that this context also influences the ethical concerns that distinguish these networks (Litwak & Meyer, 1967). The assertion that service providers may individualize clients and concurrently isolate them is more certain than the assertion that concern for the other necessarily advances the common good. The assertion that professional practice is responsive to bureaucratic influences in formal structures is more certain than the assertion that client power influences professional methods of helping. There is far more support for the view that defines the problems brought by consumers of welfare services as inclusive of situational as well as personal factors, than for the assertion that the situation of the client, including informal support networks, is best conceived as part of the solution, not the problem.

Granted these limitations on what can be asserted with certainty, a direction for rule modification will be proposed. The rule to be sought as an alternative to the existing one (i.e., from each according to his opportunity and to each according to his power) would recognize the need for differential benefits during a period of finite resources and almost limitless need, but would concurrently seek to narrow the gap between the haves and have-nots. It combines two familiar rules into one. The first—from each according to his ability, to each according to his contribution—is intended to satisfy the need for justice in the distributive system. As stated, this rule does not satisfy the condition that assures fairness as well, where fairness compensates for the unequal distribution of endowments persons bring with them at birth, and the great variance in the social condition into which persons are born. To achieve a fair as well as a just society, Donald Howard argues, "The social conscience of today requires that the rear guard of the disadvantaged be brought up as the advance guard of the advantaged proceeds" (Howard, 1969, p. 391). Thus, the second rule should contain an imperative such as that proposed by Rawls—with unequal benefits being justified only when they raise the expectations of the least advantaged (Rawls, 1971).

To summarize, it has been argued that the guiding ethic of a welfare state should promote its major goal-distributive justice. The welfare system through which the Welfare State hopes to achieve this goal consists of a formal structure that stresses those rights essential for a just system and informal support networks that promote a fraternal concern for the common good, essential for a system that is fair as well as just. Professionals in the welfare system have developed methods of work that have helped individualize recipients of service, but concurrently have tended to isolate them. Increased influence of consumers has affected these methods. Finally, a rule has been proposed that could help achieve a goal of the Welfare State—distributive justice. In conclusion, a set of practice principles congenial with this rule is proposed to guide the practice, policies, education, and research of those associated with the operation of the welfare system.

1. In relation to social work practice: The method of helping must seek to enhance the consumers' power through promoting opportunities for linkage to informal support networks, or risk failure in seeking to achieve a sustained change in the consumers' problematic circumstances, concurrently defeating efforts to transform individual self-interest into collective mutual concern.

2. In relation to social welfare policy: The organization of programs and allocation of resources must promote opportunities for consumers of service to develop a collective concern for the common good, or risk perpetuating the isolation and self-oriented behavior that the formal structure now promotes.

3. In relation to social work education: The school milieu in which students are prepared for professional practice must encourage the use of informal support networks in their own education to heighten their appreciation of such cooperative efforts. In both class and field, schools ought to provide opportunities for students to develop skill in helping clients connect appropriately with informal support networks.

4. In relation to knowledge and value clarification: It is necessary to design and study new applications of what we think we know about informal support networks to test the utility of such knowledge, or risk methods of intervention, policies and programs, and educational offerings that are not likely to promote distributive justice, or may even detract from such efforts.

Conclusion

David E. Biegel and
Arthur J. Naparstek

Considerable evidence has been presented in this volume concerning the varied and significant roles that community support systems can play in the mental health system. In this final section we will discuss limitations of community support systems, obstacles to the development of partnerships between mental health professionals and community support system elements, and dangers of a community systems approach in mental health.

Limitations of Community Support Systems

At this point, a few caveats are in order. We must not romanticize community support systems and long for the golden days of yesteryear when family, friends, and community were sufficient to provide for individual needs. To do so would be to err in several ways. In the first place, this is taking a rose-colored and distorted view of the role of such support systems. Mental health institutions developed because of the inability and/or unwillingness of families to provide for the mentally ill in their own homes. In fact, many mentally ill persons were hidden away and mistreated by the community. Community support systems, though capable of performing many useful mental health functions, can also do harm. Families can aggravate the mental health problems of a particular member and can undo the effects of professional treatment upon the patient's return to the family at home. It makes no more sense to ask whether community support systems are effective than to ask, "Is psychotherapy effective?" Rather, we must examine particular support systems serving identified target populations in specific situations.

Second, we live in a complex, technological, urbanized society where both lay and professional services are needed to meet human needs adequately. Failure to recognize this often leads to "either/or" strategies. It is sometimes mistakenly assumed that only the community can offer services to its members or only the professional has the expertise to meet human needs.

Obstacles to Partnerships

An entire part of this book has been devoted to an examination of the relationship of professionals with community support systems. There is general consensus among the volume's contributors that collaborative partnerships/relationships are needed between mental health professionals and lay helping networks. Although some of the difficulties of developing and sustaining partnerships have been discussed, insufficient attention has been paid to this area. We have briefly examined professional behavior, while omitting any mention of responsibilities that community helpers have if partnerships are to be successful. Since we do not wish to leave the reader with the impression that such partnerships are easy to develop and maintain, we will highlight at length some obstacles to partnerships between mental health professionals and "community helpers." In doing so we will make generalizations about each helper group that, while not being universally true, are, we think, fair overall descriptions.

Despite the potentials that exist for linkages, there are significant obstacles to developing partnerships between community and professional helpers. These obstacles reflect both biases and attitudinal and value differences between professional and community helpers. Also, a narrow view of community needs is often held by both professional and community helpers due to their focus or "targeting" on specific population groups or services.

Mental health and human service professionals often think that they have all the answers, expertise, and skill necessary to help people in need and that community residents can provide little assistance since they are not professionally trained. Unfortunately, professionals may, by themselves, be unable to reach many community residents who might never go to a "professional" for help because of reasons of pride or privacy. In addition, professionals may not be fully aware of community values, nor of resources and networks that are already providing support to persons in need. Even more basically, the mental health and human service needs of any community are so tremendous that if community workers stopped helping people, professional systems would become overloaded.

Professionals tend to "aggregate" needs of individuals and to speak about "at-risk" population groups and underserved areas using statistical data, surveys, needs assessment studies, and the like. Community helpers speak about individuals—*that* retired man down the block who needs someone to help him take care of his mentally ill wife; *that* woman with three children needing emotional support. Community helpers are unable to understand why the client is not "eligible" for services—he has problems, doesn't he? Professionals in many ways have less flexibility than community workers. They have caseloads, waiting lists, and rules and regulations to follow.

Community helpers have their biases also. Community helpers are dedicated individuals who help others because they want to and because it brings them pleasure and fulfillment. While their dedication and zeal are a positive asset, they sometimes think that they are the only ones who really care about people, the only ones who really want to help. They feel that professionals are more interested in their rules and regulations than in helping people. Besides, professionals work just nine to five, and *we* community helpers are on call all the time, is a commonly heard statement. Community helpers fail to realize that professionals do care and want to help people as much as informal helpers do, but oftentimes they are constrained by agency or government regulations, which they themselves alone cannot change. Community helpers sometimes fail to see that worker and agency are not one and the same.

Community helpers are often intimidated by professionals and uncomfortable around them. This makes mutual trust harder to achieve. In summary, community helpers and mental health and human service professionals often have difficulty working together. They talk different languages. As we have said, the professional talks of community needs, the community helper talks of the needs of individual residents. Community helpers do not have access to "data" as do professionals, and thus their only way of discussing community-wide needs is on an intuitive or gut-level basis. Professionals find it difficult to respond, and a lack of communication results. Differences in education and training and in class and ethnic background often make community helpers and professionals uncomfortable with each other as well.

Another set of obstacles to partnerships between professionals and community helpers stems from the lack of information that individual helpers often have about the services provided by other helpers, professional and community. Of critical importance is the fact that not only are professional helpers unaware of the important roles played by lay helpers, but lay helpers themselves often do not fully appreciate the scope, magnitude, and helpfulness of the services they provide. This lack of linked helping networks is evident on both an intra- and inter-network level. Examples of this from our research on Baltimore, Maryland, and Milwaukee, Wisconsin, through the Neighborhood and Family Services Project include the Catholic priest in a parish who is unaware of the counseling roles of other Catholic clergy in nearby parishes; or the two administrators of mental health clinics who had never met each other despite the fact that they served the same neighborhood; or the natural helper who is unaware of another helper only several blocks away performing similar roles. On an inter-network level the general lack of awareness by lay and professional helpers of mutual and/or complementary roles prevents any effective linking of services (Naparstek et al., 1979). It is essential then that realistic assessments be made of the obstacles that may inhibit partnerships so strategies can be developed to overcome them. We have presented a capacity-building "process" strategy to enhance neighborhood networks (see chapter 17), but since community support systems are so diverse, multiple strategies for professional/community collaboration must be articulated. This is an important area for further research.

Dangers of a Community Support Systems Approach

There are a number of dangers in emphasizing the role of community support systems in mental health. Interventions by professionals that are not carefully conceived and carried out can cause more harm than good. Professionals who are working, for example, with natural helpers might make the natural helpers aware of their lack of education or training and then these helpers may begin referring the people they have been helping to the professional, instead of continuing to work with them. Or competition either on an intra- or inter-agency level may ensue around working with natural helpers. In a situation of which we have knowledge, a family counseling unit of a large agency began working with natural helpers. After a number of months of successful efforts, another unit of this multiservice agency found out about the intervention and felt that it was just the strategy they were looking for in their program. They went to this same community and contacted these very same natural helpers. The family counseling unit was furious, feeling that this would harm their efforts so carefully built after months of work. As the concept of community support systems gets popular, such fighting may occur between agencies as well. Since natural helpers are usually identified only after slow and careful community work, one agency may do the discovering and then others may come who want to reap the benefits. In the Neighborhood and Family Services Project, various agencies were always trying to utilize community helpers the project "discovered" for their agencies' own purposes. This is not to say, however, that cooperation within and between agencies cannot be achieved; it can and should be an important goal of those working with community support systems.

Community support systems can be harmed by professionals even when such systems are not the target of the intervention. Several years ago, one of the editors helped develop a home care program for the elderly sponsored by a large sectarian social service agency. The objective of the program was to provide light housekeeping and chore services to the elderly homeowners to help them live independently and reduce the necessity for nursing home care. It was a very worthwhile preventive project. Unfortunately, despite intensive planning with other agencies to target services to those most in need and to avoid duplication and overlap of services, the effort bypassed, through ignorance, the informal helpers—friends, neighbors, and other lay helpers who were already performing many of the same roles the agency workers intended to play. The result, we found out much later, was that a number of community helpers stopped their efforts, feeling they were not needed anymore. In actuality, our program soon had a waiting list and if we had known what to do, we could have worked very closely with existing helpers to maximize the number of persons being served.

These issues are raised here because we want readers who are interested in working with community support systems to do so carefully. This book is not designed as a "how-to" text on working with support systems. Those persons interested in doing so and not knowledgeable in this area should do further reading and also consult with others who have the needed expertise.

We must be careful not to base major program or policy efforts on inadequate bases of research about community support systems. For example, though much evidence exists documenting the correlation between social support and positive mental health status, findings have been based on cross-sectional analyses from which causal inferences cannot be made. There are several longitudinal studies underway at present aimed at exploring this question, but results are not in as yet. Therefore, there is a danger that we will use existing knowledge that fits our ideological framework about support systems without careful enough scrutiny.

There is a danger that community support systems will be used as a rationale to cut needed professional services. We strongly concur with the admonition of the Community Support Systems Task Panel of the President's Commission on Mental Health (1978b) that it would be a grave error to proceed in this direction.

A Closing Note

Too often in the past mental health and human service programs have promised more than they can deliver. The same mistake should not be repeated in regard to the benefits of a community support systems approach in mental health. Community support systems will not "revolutionize" mental health nor solve all the problems of service delivery in the mental health system. The important roles that it can play should not be underestimated, however.

We have just scratched the surface in our knowledge about community support systems. Much more work needs to be done in this area. It is important that knowledge-building efforts continue and expand in the future, while at the same time program and policy changes should be implemented based upon existing knowledge about community support systems.

References

Abad, V. A model for delivery of mental health services to Spanish-speaking minorities. *American Journal of Orthopsychiatry*, 1974, *44*, 584–595.

Abrahams, R.B. Mutual help for the widowed. *Social Work*, 1972, *17*, 54–61.

Abrahams, R.B. Mutual helping: Styles of caregiving in a mutual aid program. In G. Caplan & M. Killilea (Eds.), *Support systems and mutual help*. New York: Grune & Stratton, 1976.

Abrams, P. Community care: Some research problems and priorities. In J. Barnes & N. Connelly (Eds.), *Social care research*. London: Bedford Square Press, 1978, pp. 78–100.

Abrams, P. Social change, social networks and neighborhood care. *Social Work Services*, 1979, *22*, 12–23.

Abzug, R.H. The black family during reconstruction. In N.I. Huggins, M. Kelson, & D.M. Fox (Eds.), *Key issues in the Afro-American experience*. New York: Harcourt Brace Jovanovich, 1971.

Acosta, F.X. Barriers between mental health services and Mexican Americans: An examination of a paradox. *Community Psychology*, 1979, *7*, 503–520.

Acosta, F.X., Yamamoto, J., & Evans, L.A. *Effective psychotherapy for low income and minority patients*. New York: Plenum Press, in press.

Action for mental health. Report of the Joint Commission on Mental Illness and Health. New York: Basic Books, 1961.

Adler, H.M., & Hammett, V.O. Crisis, conversion and cult formation: An examination of a common psychosocial sequence. *American Journal of Psychiatry*, 1973, *13*, 861–864.

Agranoff, R. Services integration. In W. Anderson, B. Frieden, & M. Murphy (Eds.), *Managing human services*. Washington, D.C.: International City Management Association, 1977.

Al-Anon. *Living with an alcoholic*. New York: Al-Anon Family Group Headquarters, (rev. 6th ed.), 1975.

Alcoholics Anonymous. New York: Alcoholics Anonymous World Services, Inc., 1955.

Aldrich, H. Centralization versus decentralization in the design of human service delivery systems. In R. Sarri & Y. Hasenfeld (Eds.), *The management of human services*. New York: Columbia University Press, 1978, pp. 51–79.

Alford, R. *Health care politics*. Chicago: University of Chicago Press, 1975.

Alinsky, S.D. The poor and the powerful. *International Journal of Psychiatry*, 1967, *4*(4), 308.

Allport, G. *Pattern and growth in personality*. New York: Holt, Rinehart & Winston, 1961.

Anderson, W.A., & Anderson, N.D. The politics of age exclusion: The adults only movement in Arizona. *The Gerontologist*, 1978, *18*, 6–12.

Andrews, G., Tennant, D., Hewson, V. Life event stress, social support, coping style and risk of psychological impairment. *Journal of Nervous & Mental Disease*, 1978, *166*, 307–316.

Antze, P. The role of ideologies in peer psychotherapy organizations: Some theoretical considerations and three case studies. *Journal of Applied Behavioral Science*, 1976, *12*, 323–344.

Arling, G. The elderly widow and her family, neighbors and friends. *Journal of Marriage & the Family*, 1976, *38*, 757–788.

Arnstein, S. A ladder of citizen participation. *Journal of the American Institute of Planners*, 1969, *35*, 221.

Association Mixta Progresista et al., V. HEW et al. Civ. No. C-72-882-SAE, N.D. California, May 16, 1972.

Aviran, U., & Segal, S.P. Exclusion of the mentally ill. *Archives of General Psychiatry*, 1973, *29*, 136–141.

Back, K.W., & Taylor, R.C. Self-help groups: Tool or symbol? *Journal of Applied Behavioral Science*, 1976, *12*, 295–309.

Bailey, M.B. Al-Anon family groups as an aid to wives of alcoholics. *Social Work*, 1965, *10*, 68–74.

Baker, F. The interface between professional and natural support systems. *Clinical Social Work Journal*, 1977, *5*(2), 139–148.

Bandoli, L.R. Leaderless support groups in child protective services. *Social Work*, 1977, *22*, 150–151.

Bandura, A. *Social learning theory*. Englewood Cliffs, N.J.: Prentice-Hall, 1977.

Bane, M., Lein, L., O'Donnell, L., Steuve, A., & Wells, B. Child-care arrangements of working parents. *Monthly Labor Review*, 1979, *102*(10), 50–56.

Bayley, M. *Community oriented systems of care*. Berkhamsted, England: The Volunteer Centre, 1978.

Bean, M. Alcoholics Anonymous, Part I. *Psychiatric Annals*, 1975, *5*(2), 7–61. (a)

Bean, M. Alcoholics Anonymous, Part II. *Psychiatric Annals*, 1975, *5*(3), 7–57. (b)

Beers, C. *A mind that found itself*. New York: Doubleday, 1948.

Bellah, R.N. Religious evolution. *American Sociological Review*, 1964, *29*(3), 358–374.

Bengtson, V. Ethnicity and aging: Problems and issues in current and social science inquiry. In D.E. Gelfand & A.J. Kutzik (Eds.), *Ethnicity and aging: theory, research, and policy*. New York: Springer Publishing Company, 1979.

Benson, H.B., Rosner, B.A., Marzetta, B.R., & Kleinchuck, H.P. Decreased blood pressure in borderline hypertensive subjects who practiced meditation. *Journal of Chronic Disease*, 1974, *27*, 163–69; *52*, 80–86.

Berger, P., & Neuhaus, R. *To empower people: The role of mediating institutions*. Washington, D.C.: American Enterprise Institute for Public Policy Research, 1977.

Beverley, E.V. Organizations for seniors—what they stand for, what they offer. *Geriatrics*, 1976, *31*(11), 121ff.

Bickel, C. The uniqueness of pastoral counseling. Paper presented at Seventh Annual Clinical-Community Psychology Conference, University of Maryland, Silver Springs, Maryland, 1978.

Biegel, D. The clergy's role in help seeking and receiving in urban ethnic neighborhoods. Paper presented at Seventh Annual Clinical-Community Psychology Conference, University of Maryland, Silver Springs, Maryland, 1978.

Biegel, D. *Neighborhood support systems: People helping themselves*. Washington, D.C.: University of Southern California, Washington Public Affairs Center, 1979.

Biegel, D., & Naparstek, A. The neighborhood and family services project: An empowerment model linking clergy and agency professionals. In A. Jeger & R. Slotnik (Eds.), *Community mental health: A behavioral ecological perspective*. New York: Plenum Press, in press.

Biegel, D., & Naparstek, A. Organizing for mental health: An empowerment model. *Journal of Alternative Human Services*, 1979, *3*(5), 8–14.

Biegel, D., Naparstek, A., & Khan, M. Social support and mental health: An examination of interrelationship. Paper presented at the Annual Convention of the American Psychological Association, Montreal, Canada, 1980.

Biegel, D., & Sherman, W. Neighborhood capacity building and the ethnic aged. In D.E. Gelfand & A.J. Kutzik (Eds.), *Ethnicity and Aging: Theory, Research, and Policy*. New York: Springer Publishing Company, 1979.

Biegel, D., & Spence, B. *Human service policy recommendations to the National Commission on Neighborhoods*. Washington, D.C.: University of Southern California, Washington Public Affairs Center, 1978.

Billingsley, A. *Black families in white America*. Englewood Cliffs, N.J.: Prentice-Hall, 1968.

Blassingame, J.W. *The slave community*. New York: Oxford University Press, 1979.

Bley, N., Dye, D., Goodman, M., & Jensenik, K. Client's Perceptions: A Key Variable in Evaluating Leisure Activities for the Elderly. *Gerontologist*, 1973, *13*, 365–367.

Bloom, B.L. Prevention of mental disorders: Recent advances in theory and practice. *Community Mental Health Journal*, 1979, *15*(3), 179–191.

Boleloucky, Z., & Horvath, M. The SCL-90 rating scale: First experience with the Czech version on healthy male scientific workers. *Activas Nervosa Superior*, 1974, *16*, 115–116.

Bond, G.R., & Lieberman, M.A. The role and function of women's conscious-

ness-raising: Self-help, psychotherapy, or political activation? In C.L.
Heckerman (Ed.), *Women and psychotherapy: Changing emotions in changing times*. New York: Human Sciences Press, 1979.

Bond, H.M. *The education of the Negro in the American social order*. New
York: Prentice-Hall, 1934.

Borkman, T. Experiential knowledge: A new concept for the analysis of self-help
groups. *Social Service Review*, 1976, *50*, 445–456.

Borman, L.D. (Ed.). *Explorations in self help and mutual aid*. Evanston, Ill.:
Northwestern University, Center for Urban Affairs, 1975.

Borman, L.D. Action anthropology and the self-help/mutual aid movement. In
R. Minshaw (Ed.), *Currents in anthropology: Essays in honor of Sol Tax*.
Chicago: Aldine, 1979.

Borman, L.D. *National epilepsy self-help workshop*. Evanston, Ill.: Self-Help
Institute, Center for Urban Affairs, Northwestern University, 1980.

Borman, L.D., Davies, J., & Droge, D. Self-help groups for persons with
epilepsy. In B. Hermann (Ed.), *A multidisciplinary handbook for epilepsy*.
Springfield, Ill.: Charles C Thomas, 1980.

Borman, L.D., & Lieberman, M.A. Conclusion: Contributions, dilemmas, and
implications for mental health policy. In M.A. Lieberman & L.D. Borman
(Eds.), *Self-help groups for coping with crisis*. San Francisco: Jossey-Bass,
1979, pp. 406–430.

Bowles, E. *Self-help groups: Perspectives and directions—an instructional guide
for developing self-help mutual aid groups*. New York: New Careers Training Laboratory, CUNY Graduate Center, 1978.

Boylin, W., Gordon, S.K., & Nehrke, M.F. Reminiscing and ego integrity in
institutionalized elderly males. *The Gerontologist*, 1976, *16*(2), 118–128.

Breslow, L. A quantitative approach to the World Health Organization definition of health: Physical, mental and social well-being. *International Journal
of Epidemiology*, 1972, *1*: 347–355.

Breton, R. Institutional completeness of ethnic communities and the personal
relations of immigrants. *American Journal of Sociology*, 1964, *70*(2), 193–
205.

Brown, V.B. Drug people: Schizoid personalities in search of a treatment. *Psychotherapy: Theory, Research and Practice*, 1971, *8*, 213–215.

Burke, R.J., & Weir, T. Giving and receiving help with work and non-work
related problems. *Journal of Business Administration*, 1975, *6*, 59–78.

Burke, R.J., & Weir, T. Organizational climate and informal helping processes
in work settings. *Journal of Management*, 1978, *4*, 91–105.

Burke, R.J., Weir, T., & Duncan, C. Informal helping processes in work settings. *Academy of Management Journal*, 1976, *19*, 370–377.

Burruel, G. & Chavez, N. Mental health outpatient centers: Relevant or irrelevant to Mexican Americans? In A.B. Tulipan, C.L. Atteneave, & E. King-
ston (Eds.), *Beyond clinic wall*. University, Ala.: University of Alabama
Press, Vol. 5 (Psychiatric Outpatient Centers of America series), 1974.

Bushfield, D.C. A church-sponsored crisis counseling service. In H.J. Clinebell

(Ed.), *Community mental health: The role of church and temple*. Nashville: Abingdon, 1970.

Butler, R. The life review: An interpretation of reminiscence in the aged. *Psychiatry*, 1963, *26*, 65–76.

Butler, R. Looking forward to what? The life review, legacy, and excessive identity. *American Behavioral Scientist*, 1970, *14*, 121–128.

Butler, R., & Lewis, M. *Aging and mental health*. St. Louis: Mosby, 1977.

Campaign for Human Development. *1978 Annual Report*, New York: United States Catholic Conference, 1978.

Cantor, M.H. The informal support system of the "family-less" elderly—who takes over? Paper presented at the 31st Annual Meeting of the Gerontological Society, Dallas, November, 1978.

Cantor, M.H. The informal support system of New York's inner city elderly: Is ethnicity a factor? In D. E. Gelfand & A. J. Kutzik (Eds.), *Ethnicity and aging: Theory, Research, and Policy*. New York: Springer Publishing Company, 1979.

Caplan, G. *The theory and practice of mental health consultation*. New York: Basic Books, 1970.

Caplan, G. *Support systems and community mental health: Lectures on concept development*. New York: Behavioral Publications, 1974.

Caplan, G. Introduction and overview. In G. Caplan & M. Killilea (Eds.), *Support systems and mutual help*. New York: Grune & Stratton, 1976. (a)

Caplan, G. The family as support system. In G. Caplan, & M. Killilea (Eds.), *Support systems and mutual help*. New York: Grune & Stratton, 1976. (b)

Caplan, G., & Killilea, M. *Support systems and mutual help: Multi-disciplinary explorations*. New York: Grune & Stratton, 1976.

Caplan, R.D. Organizational stress and individual strain: A social-psychological study of risk factors in coronary heart disease among administrators, engineers, and scientists. Unpublished doctoral dissertation, The University of Michigan, 1972.

Carson, R.J. *Mental health centers and local clergy: A source book of sample projects*. Washington, D.C.: Community Mental Health Institute, 1976.

Cassel, J. Psychosocial processes and stress: theoretical formulations. *International Journal of Health Services*, 1974, *4*, 471–482.

Cassel, J. The contribution of the social environment to host resistance. *American Journal of Epidemiology*, 1976, *104*, 107–123.

Central Policy Review Staff, DHSS. The wider context. In J. Barnes & N. Connelly (Eds.), *Social care research*. London: Bedford Square Press, 1978, pp. 45–59.

Challis, D. & Davies, B. Community care of the elderly: A new approach. *British Journal of Social Work*, 1980, *10*(1): 1–18.

Chavez, N. Forward. In P.P. Martin (Ed.), *La Frontera perspective: Providing mental health services to Mexican Americans*. Tucson, Ariz.: Pueblo Printers, 1979.

Chellam, G. The disengagement theory: Awareness of death and self-engagement. Unpublished dissertation, Case-Western Reserve University, Cleveland, Ohio, 1964.

Clinebell, H.J., Jr. The local church's contribution to positive mental health. In H.J. Clinebell (Ed.), *Community mental health: The role of church and temple*. Nashville: Abingdon, 1970.

Clinebell, H.J., Jr. *Growth groups*. Nashville: Abingdon, 1977.

Cobb, S. Social support as a moderator of life stress. *Psychosomatic Medicine*, 1976, *38*, 300–314.

Cocozza, J.J., & Steadman, H.J. Community fear of the mentally ill: An obstacle for the community mental health movement. Prepared for presentation at Conference on Community and Policy Research, State University of New York at Albany, 1976.

Cohen, C., & Sokolovsky, J. Social engagement versus isolation: The case of the aged in SRO hotels. *The Gerontologist*, 1980, *20*(1), 36–44.

Collins, A., & Pancoast, D. *Natural helping networks: A strategy for prevention*. Washington, D.C.: National Association of Social Workers, 1976.

Comer, J.P. *Beyond black and white*. New York: Quadrangle/New York Times Books, 1972.

Comer, J.P. The education of inner-city children. *Grants Magazine*, March 1980, *3*(1), 20–27. (a)

Comer, J.P. *School power: Implications of an intervention project*. New York: Free Press, 1980. (b)

Comer, J.P., & Schraft, C.M. Working with black parents. In Richard R. Abidin (Ed.), *Parent education and intervention handbook*. Springfield, Ill.: Charles C Thomas, 1980.

Community Mental Health Centers Act, P.L. 88–164.

Conley, R., Conwell, M., & Arrill, M. An approach to measuring the cost of mental illness. *American Journal of Psychiatry*, 1967, *124*, 63–70.

Costa, P., & Kastenbaum, R. Some aspects of memories and ambitions in centenarians. In D. Charles & W. Looft (Eds.), *Readings in psychological development through life*. New York: Holt, Rinehart & Winston, 1973.

Costello, J. *A summary and integration of evaluation studies conducted in the Baldwin-King school program*. New Haven, Conn.: Yale University Child Study Center, 1973.

Council of Jewish Federations Report. New York, 1977.

Coursey, R., Specter, G., Murrell, S., & Hunt, B. (Eds.). *Program evaluation for mental health: Methods, strategies, and participants*. New York: Grune & Stratton, 1977.

Cowgill, D.O., & Holmes, L.D. (Eds.). *Aging and modernization*. New York: Appleton-Century-Crofts, 1972.

Creer, C., & Wing, J.K. Schizophrenia at home. *National schizophrenia fellowship* (Vol. 78). Surrey, 1974.

Crouch, B. Age and institutional support: Perceptions of older Mexican-Americans. *Journal of Gerontology*, 1972, *27*, 524–529.

Cuellar, J. On the relevance of ethnographic methods: Studying aging in an urban Mexican-American community. In V.L. Bengtson (Ed.), *Gerontological research and community concern: A case study of a multidisciplinary project*. Los Angeles: Andrus Gerontology Center, University of Southern California, 1974.

Cuellar, J. El senior citizens club: The older Mexican-American in the voluntary association. In B. Meyerhoff & A. Simic (Eds.), *Life's career—Aging*. Beverly Hills, Calif.: Sage Publications, 1978.

Cummings, J., & Cummings, E. On the stigma of mental illness. *Community Mental Health Journal*, 1965, *21*(2), 138.

Curry, R., & Young, R.D. Socially indigenous help: The community cares for itself. Paper presented at the meeting of the American Psychological Association, Toronto, September 1978.

Cutler, S. Membership in different types of voluntary associations and psychological well-being. *Gerontologist*, 1976, *16*(4), 335, 339.

Darvill, G. *Bargain or barricade?* Berkhamsted, England: The Volunteer Centre, 1975.

D'Augelli, A.R., Vallance, T.R., Danish, S.J., Young, C.E., & Gerdes, J.L. The community helpers project: A description of a prevention strategy for rural communities. *Journal of Prevention*, in press.

Davis, H.R. Management of innovation and change in mental health services. *Hospital and Community Psychiatry*, 1978, *29*, 649–658.

Davis, M.S. Women's liberation groups as a primary preventive mental health strategy. *Community Mental Health Journal*, 1977, *13*(3), 219–228.

Dean, A., & Lin, N. The stress-buffering role of social support: Problems and prospects for systematic investigation. *Journal of Nervous and Mental Disease*, 1977, *165*, 403–417.

Dean, S.R. The role of self-conducted group therapy in psychorehabilitation: A look at Recovery, Inc. *American Journal of Psychiatry*, 1971, *127*(7), 934–937.

Dentler, R.A., & Erikson, K.T. The functions of deviance in groups. *Social Problems*, 1959, *8*, 98–107.

Derogatis, L. *SCL-90* (revised manual). Baltimore: School of Medicine, Johns Hopkins University, 1976.

Derogatis, L.R., Yevzeroff, H., & Wittelsberger, B. Social class, psychological disorder, and the nature of the psychopathologic indicator. *Journal of Consulting and Clinical Psychology*, 1975, *43*, 183–191.

Devall, B. Gay liberation: An overview. *Journal of Voluntary Action Research*, 1973, *2*(1), 24–35.

Dewar, T. The professionalization of the client. *Social Policy*, 1978, *8*(4), 4–9.

DHEW, Office for Civil Rights, Region IX. DHEW findings on the Title VI compliance status of California welfare agencies, 1973.

Dinitz, S., & Beran, N. Community mental health as a boundary-less and boundary-busting system. *Journal of Health and Social Behavior*, 1971, *12*, 99–108.

Dolgoff, R., & Feldstein, D. *Understanding social welfare*. New York: Harper & Row, 1980.

Dominick, G.P. The clergyman's role in the treatment of the alcoholic. In H.J. Clinebell (Ed.), *Community mental health: The role of church and temple*. Nashville: Abingdon, 1970.

Dory, F.J. *Building self-help groups among older persons: A training curriculum to prepare organizers*. New York: New Careers Training Laboratory, CUNY Graduate Center, 1979.

Doughton, M.J. *People power*. Bethlehem, Penn.: Media American, 1976.

DuBois, W.E.B. *The Philadelphia Negro*. New York: Benjamin Bloom, 1899.

DuBois, W.E.B. *The Atlanta University publications*. New York: Arno Press, 1903.

Dubos, R. *Mirage of health*. New York: Harper & Row, 1959.

Dumont, M.P. Self-help treatment programs. *American Journal of Psychiatry*, 1974, *6*, 631–635.

Dumont, M.P. Self help treatment programs. In G. Caplan & M. Killilea (Eds.), *Support systems and mutual help*. New York: Grune & Stratton, 1976.

Dunlop, B. Expanded home-based care for the impaired elderly: Solution or pipe-dream? *American Journal of Public Health*, 1980 *70*(5), 514–519.

Durkheim, E. *Suicide* (1897). Translated, G. Simpson (Ed.). Glencoe, Ill.: The Free Press, 1951.

Durlak, J.A. Comparative effectiveness of paraprofessional and professional helpers. *Psychological Bulletin*, 1979, *86*, 80–92.

Durman, E.C. The role of self-help in service provision. *Journal of Applied Behavioral Science*, 1976, *12*, 433–443.

Edmunson, E.D., Bedell, J.R., Archer, R.P., & Gordon, R.E. Integrating skill building and peer support in mental health treatment: The early intervention and community network development projects. In A. M. Jeger & R. S. Slotnick (Eds.), *Community mental health: A behavioral-ecological perspective*. New York: Plenum Press, 1981.

Eisenberg, L. The perils of prevention: A cautionary note. *New England Journal of Medicine*, 1977, *297*, 1230–1232.

Eisenberg, L., & Parron, D. Strategies for the prevention of mental disorders. *Healthy people: The surgeon general's report on health promotion and disease prevention, background papers* (DHEW PHS Pub. No. 79-55071A). Washington, D.C.: U.S. Government Printing Office, 1979, pp. 135–55.

Enright, M.F., & Parsons, B.V. Training crisis intervention specialists and peer group counselors as therapeutic agents in the gay community. *Community Mental Health Journal*, 1976, *12*, 383–291.

Equal Opportunities Commission (EOC). The experience of caring for elderly and handicapped dependents. Manchester, England: EOC, March, 1980.

Erikson, E. Identity and the life cycle. *Psychological Issues I*, 1959, Monograph I.

Erikson, E. *Childhood and society*. New York: W.W. Norton, 1963.

Fairweather, G.W., Sanders, D., Cressler, D., & Maynard, H. *Community life for the mentally ill: an alternative to hospitalization*. Chicago: Aldine, 1969.

Fawcett, S.B., Fletcher, R.K., & Mathews, R.M. Applications of behavior analysis in community education. In D. Glenwick & L.A. Jason (Eds.), *Behavioral community psychology: Progress and prospects*. New York: Prager, 1980.

Fawcett, S.B., Fletcher, R.K., Mathews, R.M., Whang, P.L., Seekins, T., & Merola, L.S. Designing behavioral technologies with community self-help organizations. In A.M. Jeger & R.S. Slotnick (Eds.), *Community mental health: A behavioral-ecological perspective*. New York: Plenum Press, in press.

Festinger, L. *A theory of cognitive dissonance*. Stanford, Calif.: Stanford University Press, 1957.

Field Research Corporation. *In pursuit of wellness*. Report to Office of Prevention, Department of Mental Health, State of California, March, 1979.

Finan, B.G. Special report on inequities in mental health service delivery. Human Sciences Research, Inc., March 28, 1975, prepared for NIMH, Center for Minority Group Studies.

Francisco, R. Third World population in California. Sacramento, Office of the Lieutenant Governor, 1977. Unpublished.

Frazier, E.F. *The Negro family in the United States*. Chicago: University of Chicago Press, 1939.

Frazier, E.F. *The Negro church in America*. New York: Schocken Books, 1963.

French, J.R.P., Jr. Person–role fit. In A. McLean (Ed.), *Occupational stress*. Springfield, Ill.: Charles C Thomas, 1974.

Froland, C. Formal and informal care: Discontinuities in a continuum. *Social Service Review*, 1980, 54(4), 572–587.

Froland, C., & Pancoast, D.L. (Eds.). *Networks for helping: Illustrations from research and practice*. Portland, Ore.: Portland State University, 1979.

Froland, C., Pancoast, D.L., Chapman, N.J., & Kimboko, P.J. *Professional partnerships with informal helpers: Emerging forms*. Paper presented at the meeting of the American Psychological Association, New York, September 1979.

Froland, C., Parker, P., & Bayley, M. Relating formal and informal care: Reflections on initiatives in England and America. Paper presented to First World Congress of International Association of Voluntary Action Researchers, Brussels, Belgium, June 22, 1980.

Gabriel, R. *Ethnic factor in the urban policy*. New York: MSS Information Corporation, 1973.

Gallup Opinion Index. *Religion in America*. Princeton, N.J.: American Institute of Public Opinion, 1978.

Gans, H. *The urban villagers*. New York: Free Press, 1961.

Gans, S., & Horton, G. *Integration of human services*. New York: Praeger, 1975.

Garb, J.R., & Stunkard, A.J. Effectiveness of a self-help group in obesity control. *Archives of Internal Medicine*, 1974, *134*, 716–720.

Gartner, A. A powerful new trend. *Self-Help Reporter*, 1980, 4(3), 1–2.

Gartner, A., & Riessman, F. *Self-help in the human services*. San Francisco: Jossey-Bass, 1977.

Gelfand, D., & Fandetti, D. Urban and suburban white ethnics: Attitudes towards care of the aged. *Gerontologist*, 1980, *20*, 588–594.

Gelfand, D.E. & Gelfand, J.R. Senior centers and support networks. In D. Biegel & A. Naparstek (Eds.), *Community support systems and mental health: Research, practice, and policy*. New York: Springer Publishing Company, 1981.

Genovese, E. *Roll Jordan roll: The world the slaves made*. New York: Pantheon, 1974.

Germain, C.B., & Gitterman, A. *The life model of social work practice*. New York: Columbia University Press, 1978.

Gershon, M., & Biller, H., *The other helpers*. Lexington, Mass.: Lexington Books, 1976.

Gilbert, N. Assessing service delivery methods: Some unsettled questions. *Welfare in Review*, 1973, *10*, 25.

Giordano, J. Group identity and mental health. *International Journal of Mental Health*, Summer 1976, 5, 5–15.

Gladstone, F.J. *Voluntary action in a changing world*. London: Bedford Square Press, 1979.

Glaser, E.M., & Marks, J.B. Putting research to work. *Rehabilitation Record*, 1966, 7(6), 6–10.

Glass, D. *Behavior patterns, stress and coronary disease*. New Jersey: L. Erlbaum Associates, 1977.

Glazer, N. The limits of social policy. *Commentary*, 1971, 52(3), 51–58.

Glazer, N.S., & Moynihan, D.P. *The Negroes, Puerto Ricans, Jews, Italians, and Irish of New York City*. Cambridge, Mass.: MIT Press, 1963.

Glick, P. The future marital status and living arrangements of the elderly. *Gerontologist*, 1979, *19*, 301–309.

Glock, C., & Stark, R. *Religion and society in tension*. Chicago: Rand-McNally, 1965.

Goffman, E. *Asylums*. Garden City, N.Y.: Doubleday, 1961.

Goffman, E. *Stigma: Notes on the management of spoiled identity*. New York: Aronson, 1974.

Goldberg, G. Untrained neighborhood workers in a social work program. In A. Pearl & F. Riessman (Eds.), *New careers for the poor*. New York: Free Press, 1965, pp. 125–144.

Goldman, H.H., Sharfstein, S., & Frank, R.G. Equity and parity in psychiatric care. National Institute of Mental Health, 1980, unpublished.

Goldstein, E.G. Knowledge base of clinical social work. *Journal of the National Association of Social Workers*, 1980, 25, 174–175.

Gollub, J., & Waldhorn, S. *Local governance approaches to social welfare problems*. Menlo Park, Calif.: SRI International, 1979.

Gordon, R., Edmunson, E., Bedell, J., & Goldstein, N. Reducing hospitalization of state mental patients: Peer management for support. *Journal of the Florida Medical Association*, 1979, *66*, 927–933.

Gore, S. The effect of social support in moderating the health consequences of unemployment. *Journal of Health and Social Behavior*, 1978, *19*, 157–165.

Gorman, M. The challenge of change. *Mental Hygiene*, 1975, *59*(4), 10–12.

Gottlieb, B.H. Lay influences on the utilization and provision of health services. *Canadian Psychological Review*, 1976, *17*, 126–136.

Gottlieb, B.H. The development and application of a classification scheme of informal helping behaviors. *Canadian Journal of Behavioral Science*, 1978, *10*, 105–115.

Gottlieb, B.H. Opportunities for collaboration with informal support systems. In S. Cooper & W.F. Hodges (Eds.), *The field of mental health consultation*. New York: Human Sciences Press, in press.

Gourash, N. Help-seeking: A review of the literature. *American Journal of Community Psychology*, 1978, *6*, 413–423.

Granovetter, M. The Strength of Weak Ties, *American Journal of Sociology*, 78 (May), 1973, 1360–1380.

Greeley, A. *Why can't they be like us?* New York: E.P. Dutton, 1971.

Greenberg, M. The Jewish component: Jewish family and children's service. Paper presented at the National Symposium: An analysis of the Jewish component of Jewish communal service. Baltimore, Maryland, University of Maryland School of Social Work and American Jewish Committee, February, 1978.

Gross, H. The effect of race and sex on the variation of diagnosis and disposition in a psychiatric emergency room. *Journal of Nervous and Mental Diseases*, 1969, *48*(6), 638–642.

Gussow, Z., & Tracy, G.S. The role of self-help clubs in adaptation to chronic illness and disability. *Social Science and Medicine*, 1976, *10*, 407–414.

Gutman, H.A. *The black family in slavery and freedom, 1750–1925*. New York: Pantheon Books, 1976.

Gutowski, M., & Feild, T. *The graying of suburbia*. Washington, D.C.: The Urban Institute, 1979.

Guttmann, D. Use of informal and formal supports by the ethnic aged. In D.E. Gelfand and A.J. Kutzik (Eds.), *Ethnicity and aging: Theory, research, and policy*. New York: Springer Publishing Company, 1979.

Guttmann, D., Kolm, R., Mostwin, D., Kestenbaum, S., Harrington, D., Mullaney, J., Adams, K., Suziedelis, G. & Varga, L. *Informal and formal support systems and their effect on the lives of the elderly in selected ethnic groups, Final Report*. AoA Grant 90-A-1007. Washington, D.C.: The Catholic University of America, 1979.

Guttmann, D., Kolm, R., Mostwin, D., Kestenbaum, S., Harrington, D., Mullaney, J., Adams, K., Suziedelis, G., & Varga, L. *The impact of needs, knowledge ability and living arrangements on decision making of the elderly, Final Report*. AoA Grant 90-A-522. Washington, D.C.: The Catholic University of America, 1977.

Hadley, R., & McGrath, M. *Going local*. London: Bedford Square Press, 1980.

Hallowitz, E., & Riessman, R. The role of the indigenous non-professional in a community mental health neighborhood service center program. *American Journal of Orthopsychiatry*, 1967, *37*(4), 766–778.

Hamburg, B., & Killilea, M. Relation of social support, stress, illness and use of health services. *U.S. Surgeon General's report: Background papers*. Washington, D.C.: U.S. Government Printing Office, 1979.

Hapgood, D. *The screwing of the average man*. New York: Bantam, 1978.

Hardin, G. The tragedy of the commons. *Science*, 1968, *162*, 1243–1248.

Hardy, A.B. *Agoraphobia: Symptoms, causes, treatment*. Menlo Park, Calif.: Terrap, Inc., 1976.

Harlow, E. Sexual liberation doesn't always mean freedom. *Working Woman*, 1979, *4*, 47–52.

Harms, Ernest. Aftercare of the psychiatric patient: An 1847 view. *American Journal of Psychiatry*, 1968, *125*(5), 694–695.

Hatanaka, H.K., Watanabe, B.Y., & Ono, S. The utilization of mental health services in the Los Angeles area. In W.H. Ishikawa & N.H. Archer (Eds.), *Service delivery in pan Asian communities*. San Diego: Pacific Asian Coalition, 1975.

Hatfield, Agnes B. The family as partner in the treatment of mental illness. *Hospital and Community Psychiatry*, 1979, *30*(5), 338–340.

Haugk, K. Unique contributions of churches and clergy to community mental health. *Community Mental Health Journal*, 1976, *12*(1), 20–28.

Haugk, K. *The Stephen series*. St. Louis: Pastoral Care Team Ministries, 1978.

Havelock, R., Guskin, A., Frohman, M., Havelock, M., Hill, M., & Huber, J. *Planning for innovation through the dissemination and utilization of knowledge*. Ann Arbor: Institute for Social Research, University of Michigan, 1971.

Havelock, R.G., & Havelock, M.C. *Training for change agents*. Ann Arbor: University of Michigan, 1973.

Healthy people: The surgeon general's report on mental promotion and disease prevention (DHEW PHS Pub. No. 79-55071). Washington, D.C.: U.S. Government Printing Office, 1979.

Henderson, S., Byrne, D., Duncan-Jones, P., Adcock, S., Scott, R., & Steele, G.P. Social bonds in the epidemiology of neurosis: A preliminary communication. *British Journal of Psychiatry*, 1978, *132*, 463–466.

Henry, S., & Robinson, D. Understanding Alcoholics Anonymous. *The Lancet*, 1978, *1*, 372–375.

Hester, R. Toward professionalism or voluntarism of pastoral care. *Pastoral Psychology*, 1976, *24*(4), 305–316.

HEW Task Force on the Report to the President from the President's Commission on Mental Health. *Report*. Washington, D.C.: U.S. Government Printing Office, 1979.

Hill, R.B. *The strengths of black families*. New York: Emerson Hall Publishers, 1971.

Hirschowitz, R.G. Groups to help people cope with the task of transition. In R.G. Hirschowitz & B. Levy (Eds.), *The changing mental health scene*. New York: Spectrum Publications, 1976.

Hogan & Hartson. Letter to HEW Secretary Califano, Washington, D.C., November 21, 1978.

Holahan, C.J., Wilcox, B.C., Spearly, J.L., & Campell, M.D. The ecological perspective in community mental health. *Community Mental Health Review*, 1979, *4*, 1, 3–8.

Holmes, T., & Rahe, R. The social adjustment rating scale. *Journal of Psychosomatic Research*, 1967, *11*, 213–218.

Holtmann, A. Alcoholism and the economic value of a man. *Review of Social Economy*, 1965, *23*, 143–153.

Horizon House Institute. *Community careers: An assessment of the life adjustment of former mental hosptial patients*. Philadelphia: Horizon House Institute, 1975.

Howard, D.S. *Social welfare: Values, means and ends*. New York: Random House, 1969.

Huey, K. Conference report: Developing effective links between human service providers and the self-help system. *Hospital and Community Psychiatry*, 1977, *28*, 767–770). (a)

Huey, K. Developing effective links between human service providers and the self help system. *Hospital and Community Psychiatry*, 1977, *28*(10), 767–770. (b)

Hughes, J.M. Adolescent children of alcoholic parents and the relationship of Alateen to these children. *Journal of Consulting and Clinical Psychology*, 1977, *45*(5), 946–947.

Hugman, B. *Act natural*. London: Bedford Square Press, 1977.

Humphreys, L. *Out of the closets: The sociology of homosexual liberation*. Englewood Cliffs, N.J.: Prentice-Hall, 1972.

Hurvitz, N. The origins of the peer self-help psychotherapy group movement. *Journal of Applied Behavioral Science*, 1976, *12*, 283–294.

Hurvitz, N. Peer self-help psychotherapy groups and their implications for psychotherapy. *Psychotherapy: Theory, Research and Practice*, 1970, *7*, 41–49.

Illich, I. *Medical nemesis: The expropriation of health*. London: Calder & Boyars, 1975.

Iscoe, I. Community psychology and the competent community. *American Psychologist*, 1974, *29*, 607–613.

Jackson, A., Berkowitz, H., & Farley, G.K. Race as a variable offsetting the involvement of children. *Journal of the American Academy of Child Psychiatry*, 1974, *13*(1), 20–31.

Jackson, J.J. Sex and social class variation in black aged parent–adult relationships. *Aging and Human Development*, 1971, *2*, 96–107.

Jacobs, J. *The death and life of great American cities*. New York: Random House, 1961.

Jacques, M.E., & Patterson, K.M. The self-help group model: A review. *Rehabilitation Counseling Bulletin*, 1974, *17*, 48–58.

Jacquet, C.H., Jr. (Ed.). *Yearbook of American and Canadian Churches, 1977*. Nashville: Abingdon, 1977.

Jahoda, M. *Current conceptions of positive mental health*. New York: Basic Books, 1958.

Janowitz, M., & Suttles, G. The social ecology of citizenship. In R. Sarri & Y. Hasenfeld (Eds.), *The management of human services*. New York: Columbia University Press, 1978, pp. 80–115.

Jeger, A.M., & Slotnick, R.S. (Eds.). *Community mental health: A behavioral-ecological perspective*. New York: Plenum Press, 1981.

Jessor, R., & Jessor, S. *Problem behavior and psycho-social development: A longitudinal study on youth*. New York: Academic Press, 1977.

Joint Commission for Accreditation of Hospitals (JCAH). *Principles for Accreditation of Community Mental Health Service Programs*. Chicago: JCAH, 1976.

Kadushin, A. *Consultation in social work*. New York: Columbia University Press, 1977.

Kant, I. *Groundwork of the metaphysics of morals*. New York: Harper & Row, 1964, p. 98.

Kaplan, B.H. A note on religious beliefs and coronary heart disease. *Journal of the South Carolina Medical Association*, 1976, *XV*(5), supplement, 60–64.

Kaplan, B., Cassel, J., & Gore, S. Social support and health. *Medical Care*, 1977, *15*, 47–58.

Karno, M. The enigma of ethnicity in a psychiatric clinic. *Archives of General Psychiatry*, 1966, *14*, 516–520.

Karno, M., & Edgerton, R.B. Perception of mental illness in a Mexican-American community. *Archives of General Psychiatry*, 1969, *20*, 233–238.

Kasarda, J., & Janowitz, M. Community attachments in mass society. *American Sociological Review*, 1974, *39*(3), 328–339.

Katz, A.H. *Parents of the handicapped*. Springfield, Ill.: Charles C Thomas, 1961.

Katz, A.H. Application of self-help concepts in current social welfare. *Social Work*, 1965, *10*, 68–74.

Katz, A.H. Self-help organizations and volunteer participation in social welfare. *Social Work*, 1970, *15*(1), 51–60.

Katz, A.H. Self-help groups. *Social Work*, 1972, *17*(6), 120–121.

Katz, A.H. A discussion of self-help groups: Haven in a professional world? Paper presented at the Mediating Structures Project Conference on Professionalization, May 1979.

Katz, A.H., & Bender, E.I. Self-help groups in Western society: History and prospects. *Journal of Applied Behavioral Science*, 1976, *12*, 265–282. (a)

Katz, A.H., & Bender, E.I. *The strength in us*. New York: New Viewpoints, 1976. (b)

Katz, D. Gutek, B., Kahn, R., & Barton, E. *Bureaucratic encounters*. Ann Arbor: University of Michigan Press, 1975.

Keller, S. *The urban neighborhood*. New York: Random House, 1968.

Kelly, J.G. 'Tain't what you do, it's the way that you do it. *American Journal of Community Psychology*, 1979, *7*, 244–258.

Ketterer, R.F., Bader, B.C., & Levy, M.R. Strategies and skills for promoting mental health. In R.H. Price, R.F. Ketterer, B.C. Bader, & J. Monahann (Eds.), *Prevention in mental health*. Beverly Hills: Sage, 1980.

Killilea, M. Mutual help organizations: Interpretations in the literature. In G. Caplan & M. Killilea (Eds.), *Support systems and mutual help*. New York: Grune & Stratton, 1976.

Kiresuk, T., & Sherman, R. Goal attainment scaling: A general method for evaluating comprehensive community mental health programs. *Community Mental Health Journal*, 1968, *4*, 443–453.

Kiritz, S., & Moos, R.H. Physiological effects of social environments. *Psychosomatic Medicine*, 1974, *36*, 96–114.

Kirshbaum, H.R., Harveston, D.S., & Katz, A.H. Independent living for the disabled. *Social Policy*, 1976, *7*(2), 59–60.

Kitano, H. *Japanese American mental illness, changing perspectives in mental illness*. New York: Holt, Rinehart & Winston, 1969.

Klein, D.C. & Goldston, S.E. (Eds.). *Primary prevention: An idea whose time has come* (DHEW PHS Pub. No. (ADM) 77--47). U.S. Government Printing Office, 1977.

Kleinman, M.A., Mantell, J.E., & Alexander, E.S. Collaboration and its discontents: The perils of partnership. *Journal of Applied Behavioral Science*, 1976, *12*, 403–410.

Klerman, G.C., & Borus, J.F. Research and evaluation. In L.B. Macht, L.S. Donald, & S. Sharfstein (Eds.), *Neighborhood psychiatry*. Lexington Mass.: Lexington Books, 1977.

Klerman, G.L. Report to the National Advisory Mental Health Council, December, 1979, unpublished.

Klerman, G.L. Depression and adaptation. In R. Freidman & M. Katz (Eds.), *The psychology of depression*. New York: Winston-Wiley, 1974, pp. 127–156.

Kline, L.Y. Some factors in the psychiatric treatment of Spanish Americans. *American Journal of Psychiatric Research*, 1969, *125*, 1674–1681.

Kohl, G.J. Self-help module on three senses: Vision, hearing, and taste. Long Island Self-Help Clearinghouse, New York Institute of Technology, Old Westbury, N.Y., 1979.

Kohl, G.J., & Marcus, C.R. Suggested play activities to enhance the motor, language, and social skills in infants and preschoolers. Long Island Self-Help Clearinghouse, New York Institute of Technology, Old Westbury, N.Y., 1979.

Kolm, R. Ethnicity in social work and social work education: Some theoretical considerations. In R. Kolm, M. Flynn, D. Mostwin, D. Harrington, E. Ryle, L. Carrigan, & D. Guttmann (Eds.), *Appreciation of ethnic pluralism in education for social work*. Washington, D.C.: The Catholic University of America, 1977.

Kolm, R. Issues of Euro-American elderly in the '80s. Paper presented at the National Center for Urban Ethnic Affairs, Washington, D.C., July, 1980.

Kramer, R.M. Future of the voluntary service organization. In S. Pflanczer & T.J. Kinney (Eds.), *Social policy and services: A process oriented reader*. Albany, N.Y.: Continuing Education Project, School of Social Welfare, State University of New York, 1979.

Kreissman, D., & Joy, V. Family response to the mental illness of a relative: A review of the literature. *Schizophrenia Bulletin*, 1974, *10*, 34–59.

Kulys, R., & Tobin, S.S. Older people and their "responsible others." *Social Work*, 1980, *25*(2), 138–145.

Lalonde, M. A new perspective on the health of Canadians. Ottawa, Canada: Government of Canada, 1974.

Lamb, H.R., & Zusman, J. Primary prevention in perspective. *American Journal of Psychiatry*, 1979, *136*, 12–17.

Larson, J., Norris, E., & Kroll, J. *Consultation and its outcome: Community mental health centers*. Palo Alto, Calif.: American Institutes for Research, 1976.

Lau v. Nichols, 414 U.S. 563, 1974.

Lazarus, R.S. *Psychological stress and the coping process*. New York: McGraw-Hill, 1966.

Leat, D. *Limited liability?* Berkhamsted, England: The Volunteer Centre, 1979.

Lee, D.T. Therapeutic type: Recovery, Inc. In A.H. Katz & E.I. Bender (Eds.), *The strength in us*. New York: New Viewpoints, 1976.

Lee, E. Mental health services for the Asian Americans: Problems and alternatives. In *Civil Rights, Issues of Asian and Pacific Americans. Myths and Realities*. Washington, D.C.: U.S. Government Printing Office, 1980.

Lee, T. Urban neighborhood as a socio-spatial schema. *Human Relations*, 1968, *21*(3), 241–268.

Lehmann, S. Community and psychology and community psychology. *American Psychologist*, 1971, *26*, 554–560.

Leighninger, L. The generalist–specialist debate in social work. *Social Service Review*, 1980, *54*(1), 1–12.

Leighton, D.C., Hurding, J.S., Macklin, D.B., McMillan, A.M., & Leighton, A.H. *The character of danger: The Sterling County study. Psychiatric symptoms in selected communities*. New York: Basic Books, 1963.

Lenrow, P. Dilemmas of professional helping. In Wispe (Ed.), *Sympathy, altruism and helping*. Cambridge, Mass.: Harvard University Press, 1976.

Lerner, M.P. Stress at the workplace: The approach of the Institute for Labor and Mental Health. Unpublished manuscript, Institute for Labor and Mental Health, Oakland, California, 1980.

Levenson, H. *Organizational diagnosis*. Cambridge, Mass.: Harvard University Press, 1972.

Levin, M., Tulkin, S., Intagliata, J., Perry, J., & Whitson, E. The paraprofessional: A brief social history. Department of Psychology, SUNY, Buffalo, March, 1978, unpublished.

Levine, I.M., & Herman, J. The new pluralism. In M. Friedman (Ed.), *Overcoming middle class rage*. Philadelphia: Westminster Press, 1971.

Levitz, L.S., & Stunkard, A.J. A therapeutic coalition for obesity: Behavior modification and patient self-help. *American Journal of Psychiatry*, 1974, *34*, 423–427.

Levy, L.H. Processes and activities in groups. In M.A. Lieberman & L.D. Borman (Eds.), *Self-help groups for coping with crisis*. San Francisco: Jossey-Bass, 1979.

Levy, L.H. Self-help groups: Types and psychological processes. *Journal of Applied Behavioral Science*, 1976, *12*, 310–322.

Levy, P. *The eclipse of community: Queen Village*. Philadelphia: Institute for Study of Civic Values, 1978.

Lewis, H. Morality and politics of practice. *Social Casework*, 1972, *3*(7), 404–417.

Lewis, M., & Butler, R. Life review therapy: Putting memories to work. *Geriatrics*, 1974, *29*, 165–173.

Libertoff, K. Natural helping networks in rural youth and family services. Paper presented at the meeting of the American Psychological Association, New York, September, 1979.

Lieberman, G. Children of the elderly as natural helpers. *American Journal of Community Psychology*, 1978, *6*(5), 489–498.

Lieberman, M.A., & Bond, G.R. The problem of being a woman: A survey of 1,700 women in consciousness-raising groups. *Journal of Applied Behavioral Sciences*, 1976, *12*, 363–379.

Lieberman, M.A., & Bond, G.R. Self-help groups: Problems of measuring outcome. *Small Group Behavior*, 1978, *9*(2), 221–241.

Lieberman, M.A., & Borman, L.D. (Eds.). *Self-help groups for coping with crisis*. San Francisco: Jossey-Bass, 1979.

Lieberman, M.A., & Borman, L.D. Self-help and social research. *Journal of Applied Behavioral Science*, 1976, *12*, 455–463.

Lieberman, M.A., & Mullan, J.T. Does help help? The adaptive consequences of obtaining help from professionals and social networks. *American Journal of Community Psychology*, 1978, *6*, 499–517.

Lightfoot, S. *Worlds apart*. New York: Basic Books, 1978.

Likert, R. *New patterns of management*. New York: McGraw-Hill, 1961.

Likert, R. *The human organization*. New York: McGraw-Hill, 1967.

Lin, N., Simeone, R., Ensel, W., & Kuo, W. Social support, stressful life events and illness: A model and an empirical test. *Journal of Health and Social Behavior*, 1979, *20*, 108–119.

Lipman, E. Pastoral counseling and psychology. Paper presented at Seventh Annual Clinical-Community Psychology Conference, University of Maryland, Silver Springs, Maryland, 1978.

Litwak, E. Voluntary associations and neighborhood cohesion. *American Sociological Review*, 1961, *26*(2), 258–271.

Litwak, E. Agency and family linkages in providing neighborhood services. In D. Thursz & J.L. Vigilante (Eds.), *Reaching people: The structure of neighborhood services*. Beverly Hills: Sage, 1978.

Litwak, E. Support networks and the disabled: The transition from the community to institutional setting. Paper presented at the meeting of the Gerontological Society, Washington, D.C., 1979.

Litwak, E., & Meyer, H.J. A balance theory of coordination between bureaucratic organizations and community primary groups. *Administrative Science Quarterly*, 1967, *11*, 31–58.

Litwak, E., & Szelenyi, I. Primary group structures and their functions: Kin, neighbors, and friends. *American Sociological Review*, 1969, *34*, 465–481.

Lonsdale, S., Flowers, J., & Saunders, B. *Long term psychiatric patients: A study in community care*. London: Personal Social Services Council, 1980.

Lorion, R.P. Patient and therapist variables in the treatment of low income patients. *Psychological Bulletin*, 1973, *79*, 263–270.

Lowenthal, M. Social isolation and mental illness in old age. In B. Neugarten (Ed.), *Middle age and aging*. Chicago: University of Chicago Press, 1968.

Lowenthal, M.F., & Robinson, B. Social networks and isolation. In R.H. Binstock & E. Shanas (Eds.), *Handbook of aging and the social sciences*. New York: Van Nostrand Reinhold, 1976.

Lowenthal, M., Thurner, M., & Chiriboga, D. *Four stages of life*. San Francisco: Jossey-Bass, 1975.

Lowinger, P.L., & Dobie, S. Attitudes and emotions of the psychiatrist in the initial interview. *American Journal of Psychotherapy*, 1966, *20*, 17–32.

Madison, P. Have grouped, will travel. *Psychotherapy: Theory, Research and Practice*, 1972, *9*, 324–327.

Maguire, L. Factors in successful treatment outcome in community mental health. Dissertation for the University of Michigan in Social Work and Psychology. Ann Arbor: University Microfilms, International, 1979.

Mann, P. *An approach to urban sociology*. London: Routledge & Kegan Paul, 1965.

Mann, P. The neighborhood. In R. Gutman & D. Popenoe (Eds.), *Neighborhood, city and metropolis*. New York: Random House, 1970.

Marcus, C.R. You and your medications *or* how to become a better informed drug consumer. Long Island Self-Help Clearinghouse, New York Institute of Technology, Old Westbury, N.Y., 1979.

Margolis, P.M., & Favazza, A.R. Mental health and illness. In *Encyclopedia of Social Work*. Washington, D.C.: National Association of Social Workers, 1977.

Marshall, V. Awareness of finitude and developmental theory in gerontology: Some speculations. Paper presented at the University of California, Berkeley Conference on Death and Dying, 1973.

McCall, R.J. MMPI factors that differentiate remediably from irremediably obese women. *Journal of Community Psychology*, 1973, *1*, 34–36.

McCall, R.J. Group therapy with obese women of varying MMPI profiles. *Journal of Clinical Psychology*, 1974, *30*, 466–470.

McCall, R.J., Siderits, M.A., & Fadden, T.F. Differential effectiveness of informal group procedures in weight control. *Journal of Clinical Psychology*, 1977, *2*, 351–355.

McClung, F.B., & Stunden, A.A. *Mental health consultation to programs for children: A review of the data collected from selected U.S. sites* (U.S. Public Health Service Publication No. 2066). Washington, D.C.: National Clearinghouse for Mental Health Information, 1970.

McCready, W. Social utilities in a pluralistic society. In P. Cafferty & L. Chastang (Eds.), *The diverse society: Implications for social policy*. Washington, D.C.: National Association of Social Workers, 1976.

Meier, A., & Rudwick, E. *From plantation to ghetto*. New York: Hill & Wang, 1976.

Mendel, W. The education of the consultant. In W. Mendel & P. Solomon (Eds.), *The psychiatric consultant*. New York: Grune & Stratton, 1968.

Meyer, Adolph. *The problem of the state in the care of the insane* (Vol. IV). In E. Winters (Ed.), *The collected papers of Adolph Meyer*. Baltimore: Johns Hopkins Press, 1952.

Miller, L.K., & Miller, O. Reinforcing self-help group activities of welfare recipients. *Journal of Applied Behavior Analysis*, 1970, *3*, 57–64.

Miller, P.M. Behavior modification and Alcoholics Anonymous: An unlikely combination. *Behavior Therapy*, 1978, *9*, 300–301.

Mindel, C. Multigenerational family households: Recent trends and implications for the future. *Gerontologist*, 1979, *19*, 456–464.

Mitchell, O.C. (Ed.). *Social networks in urban situations*. New York: Oxford University Press, 1969.

Moline, R.A. The therapeutic community and milieu therapy: A review and current assessment. *Community Mental Health Review*, 1977, *2*(5), 1–13.

Moos, R.H. Major features of a social ecological perspective. In R.S. Slotnick, A.M. Jeger, & E.J. Trickett (Eds.), *Social ecology in community psychology*. Special issue APA Division of Community Psychology Newsletter, Summer, 1980.

Morales, A. The need for non-traditional mental health programs in the barrio. In M.J. Casas & S.E. Keefe (Eds.), *Family and mental health in the Mexican American community, Los Angeles*. Los Angeles: Spanish-speaking Mental Health Research Center, Monograph #7, 1978.

Moroney, R.M. *Family and the state: Considerations for social policy*. London: Longman, 1976.

Mowrer, O.H., & Vattano, A.J. Integrity groups: A context for growth in honesty, responsibility, and involvement. *Journal of Applied Behavioral Science*, 1976, *12*, 419–431.

Murase, K. Delivery of social services to Asian Americans. In *Encyclopedia of Social Work*. Washington, D.C.: National Association of Social Workers, 1977.

Myerhoff, B., & Tufte, V. Life history as integration: An essay on an experiential model. *The Gerontologist*, 1975, *15*(6), 137–140.

Myers, J., & Bean, L. *A decade later: A follow up to social class and mental health*. New York: John Wiley and Sons, 1968.

Naparstek, A. *Policy options for neighborhood empowerment*. Dayton, Ohio: Academy for Contemporary Problems, 1976.

Naparstek, A., & Biegel, D. Partnership building in mental health and human services: A community support systems approach. In Subcommittee on Health and the Environment, Committee on Interstate and Foreign Commerce, House of Representatives, *Community support for mental patients*. Washington, D.C.: U.S. Government Printing Office, 1979.

Naparstek, A., & Biegel, D. Community support systems: An alternative approach to mental health service delivery. In U. Rueveni, R. Speck, & J. Speck (Eds.), *Interventions: Healing human systems*. New York: Human Sciences Press, in press.

Naparstek, A., Biegel, D., Sherman, W., Andreozzi, J., & Coffey, J. *The community mental health empowerment model: Assumptions underlying the model/review of the literature*. Washington, D.C.: University of Southern California, Washington Public Affairs Center, 1978.

Naparstek, A., Biegel, D., Sherman, W., Andreozzi, J. & Coffey, J. Neighborhood and family services project. First year annual report. University of Southern California, Washington Public Affairs Center, 1977, unpublished.

Naparstek, A., Biegel, D., & Spence, B. Community analysis data report, volume I, first level analysis. *Catalogue of selected documents in psychology*. Manuscript #1964, November, 1979.

National Center for Health Statistics (NCHS). *Home care for persons 55 years and over*. Vital and Health Statistics Series 10-No. 73, DHEW Pub. No. (HSM) 72-1062, 1972.

National Commission on Neighborhoods. *People building neighborhoods*. Washington, D.C.: U.S. Government Printing Office, 1979.

National Conference on Catholic Charities. *Annual survey, 1979*. Washington, D.C.: NCCC, 1980.

National Conference on Social Welfare. *The future of social services in the United States*. Washington, D.C.: NCSW, 1977.

National Council on the Aging. *Senior centers: A report of senior group programs in America*. Washington, D.C.: NCOA, 1975.

National Institute of Mental Health, Division of Biometry and Epidemiology, Chart Book, 1975 data, unpublished.

Neugarten, B.L., & Hagestad, G.O. Age and the life course. In R. Binstock & E. Shanas (Eds.), *Handbook of aging and the social sciences*. Princeton, N.J.: Van Nostrand Reinhold, 1976.

Norman, J. Consciousness-raising: Self-help in the women's movement. In A.H. Katz & E.I. Bender (Eds.), *The strength in us*. New York: New Viewpoints, 1976.

Norton, D., Morales, J., & Andrews, E. The neighborhood self-help project. Occasional Paper No. 9, School of Social Service Administration, University of Chicago, Chicago, Ill., 1980.

Novak, M. *The rise of the unmeltable ethnics*. New York: Macmillan, 1973.

Nuckolls, K., Cassel, J., & Kaplan, B. Psycho-social assets, life crisis and the prognosis of pregnancy. *American Journal of Epidemiology*, 1972, 95, 431–441.

Nuttal, E.V., Nuttal, R.L., Polit, D., & Clark, K. Assessing adolescent mental health needs: The views of consumers, providers and others. *Adolescence,* 1977, *12,* 277–285.

O'Donnell, E., & Sullivan, E. Service delivery and social action through the neighborhood center: A review of research. In H. Demone and D. Harshberger (Eds.), *Human service organizations,* New York: Behavioral Publications, 1974, pp. 133–158.

Ohio Public Interest Campaign. Training of displaced workers and human service trainers. Unpublished manuscript, Ohio Public Interest Campaign, Cleveland, Ohio, 1978.

Older Americans Act of 1978. Washington, DC: Administration on Aging, 1978.

Overall, B., & Aaronson, N. Expectation of psychotherapy in patients of lower socioeconomic class. *American Journal of Orthopsychiatry,* 1963, *33,* 421.

Owan, T. Improving productivity in the public sector by use of bilingual–bicultural staff. *Social Work Research and Abstracts,* 1978, *14,* 10–18.

Owan, T. Asian Americans: A case of benighted neglect. National Conference on Social Welfare, San Francisco, 1975. Unpublished.

Pargament, K.I., Steele, R., Mitchell, R., & Schlien, B. Psychology and religion: Building a partnership to meet human needs. Paper presented at the American Psychological Association, New York, September, 1979.

Pargament, K.I., Tyler, F., & Steele, R. The church/synagogue and the psychosocial competence of the member: An initial inquiry into a neglected dimension. *American Journal of Community Psychology,* 1979, *7,* 649–664.

Parker, R.A. *The state of care.* Richard Titmuss Memorial Lecture, University of Jerusalem, April, 1980.

Parsons, T. *The structure of social action.* New York: McGraw-Hill, 1937.

Pelletier, K.R. *Mind as healer, mind as slayer: A holistic approach to preventing stress disorders.* New York: Delacorte Press, 1977.

Perlman, J. Grassroots participation from neighborhood to nation. In S. Langton (Ed.), *Citizen participation.* Lexington, Mass.: Lexington Books, 1978, pp. 65–80.

Perlman, J.E. Grassroots empowerment and government response. *Social Policy,* Sept./Oct. 1979, 16–21.

Peterson, Ronald. What are the needs of chronic mental patients? In J.A. Talbott (Ed.), *The chronic mental patient: Problems, solutions, and recommendations for a public policy.* Washington, D.C.: American Psychiatric Association, 1978, p. 44.

Pilisuk, M., & Froland, C. Kinship, social networks, social support and health. *Social Science and Medicine,* 1978, *12*(B), 273–280.

Pinneau, S.R., Jr. Effects of social support on psychological and physiological strains. Unpublished doctoral dissertation, The University of Michigan, 1975.

Piven, F.F., & Cloward, R.A. Social advocacy type: The national welfare rights organization. In A.H. Katz & E.I. Bender (Eds.), *The strength in us.* New York: New Viewpoints, 1976.

Pokorney, A.D., & Overall, J.E. Relationship of psychopathology to age, sex, ethnicity, education, and marital status in state hospital patients. *Journal of Psychiatric Research*, 1970, 7, 143–152.

Powell, T.J. The use of self-help groups as supportive reference communities. *American Journal of Orthopsychiatry*, 1973, 45(2), 756–764.

President's Commission on Mental Health. *Report to the President from the President's Commission on Mental Health* (Vol. I). Washington, D.C.: U.S. Government Printing Office, 1978. (a)

President's Commission on Mental Health. *Task Panel Reports* (Vol. II–IV). Washington, D.C.: U.S. Government Printing Office, 1978. (b)

Proceedings first annual conference on prevention, the Alcohol, Drug Abuse and Mental Health Administration (DHEW ADM). Washington, D.C.: U.S. Government Printing Office, 1980.

Ramirez, D.G. *A review of the literature on the underutilization of mental health services by Mexican Americans: Implications for future research and service delivery*. San Antonio, Texas: Intercultural Research Association, 1980.

Rapoport, L. Consultation: An overview. In R. Morris (Eds.), *Consultation in social work practice*. New York: National Association of Social Workers, 1963.

Rapoport, L. Consultation. In R. Morris (Ed.), *Encyclopedia of social work*. New York: National Association of Social Workers, 1971.

Rappaport, J. *Community psychology: Values, research, and action*. New York: Holt, Rinehart, & Winston, 1977.

Rawls, J. *A theory of justice*. Cambridge Mass.: Harvard University Press, 1971.

Rein, M. Decentralization and citizen participation in social services. *Public Administration Review*, 1972, 32, 687–700.

Renne, K. Measurement of social health in a general population survey. *Social Science Research*, 1974, 3, 25–44.

Reynolds, B. *Social work and social living*. New York: Citadel Press, 1951.

Riessman, F. Self-help and the professional. Keynote Address, Conference on the Self-help Movement and Human Service Professionals: New Ways of Working Together, Long Island Self-Help Clearinghouse, New York Institute of Technology, Old Westbury, N.Y., January 18, 1979.

Riessman, F. The "helper" therapy principle. *Social Work*, 1965, 10, 27–32.

Riessman, F. How does self help work? *Social Policy*, 1970, 7(2), 41–46.

Rittel, H., & Webber, M. Dilemmas in a general theory of planning. *Policy Sciences*, 1973, 4, 155–169.

Robinson, J.P., Shauer, P.R., Rusk, J.G., & Head, K.D. *Measures of political attitudes*. Ann Arbor, Mich.: Institute for Social Research, 1973.

Robinson, T. *In worlds apart*. London: Bedford Square Press, 1978.

Roeppel, C., Director, Office of Prevention, California State Department of Mental Health, personal communication, 1980.

Rogawski, A. Teaching consultation techniques in a community agency. In W. Mendel & P. Solomon (Eds.), *The psychiatric consultation*. New York: Grune & Stratton, 1968.

Rogers, E.M., & Shoemaker, F.L. *Communication of innovations*. New York: Free Press, 1971.

Rosenberg, M. *Society and adolescent self-image*. Princeton, N.J.: Princeton University Press, 1965.

Rosenmayr, L. The family—a source of hope for the elderly? In E. Shanas & M.B. Sussman (Eds.), *Family bureaucracy and the elderly*. Durham, N.C.: Duke University Press, 1977.

Rosenthal, D., & Frank, J. Fate of psychiatric clinic outpatients assigned to psychotherapy. *Journal of Nervous and Mental Diseases, 127*, 1958, 330–343.

Rosow, I. *Socialization to old age*. Berkeley and Los Angeles: University of California Press, 1974.

Rosten, L. (Ed.). *Religions of America: Ferment and faith in an age of crisis*. New York: Simon & Schuster, 1975.

Russell, G., & Salterwhite, B. It's your turn in the sun. *Time,* October 16, 1978, pp. 48–61.

Ryan, W. *Blaming the victim*. New York: Random House, 1971.

Sanchez, A.J. An analysis of the barrio as a socio-cultural environment and its informal needs-meeting resources. Doctoral dissertation, University of California, Berkeley, 1977.

Sarason, S.B. *The psychological sense of community: Prospects for a community psychology*. San Francisco: Jossey-Bass, 1974.

Sarason, S.B. *The creation of settings and the future societies*. San Francisco: Jossey-Bass, 1972.

Sarason, S.B., Carroll, C.F., Maton, K., Cohen, S., & Lorentz, E. *Human services and resource networks*. San Francisco: Jossey-Bass, 1977.

Sarason, S.B., & Lorentz, E. *The challenge of the resource exchange network*. San Francisco: Jossey-Bass, 1979.

Sargent, J.D., Green, E.E., & Walter, E.D. Preliminary report on use of autogenic feedback in the treatment of migraine and tension headaches. *Psychosomatic Medicine*, 1973, *35*, 129–135.

Scherer, J. *Contemporary community*. London: Tavistock Publications, 1972.

Schofield, W. *Psychotherapy: The purchase of friendship*. Englewood Cliffs, N.J.: Prentice-Hall, 1964.

Schumacher, E. *Small is beautiful: Economics as if people mattered*. New York: Harper & Row, 1973.

Schure, M., Leif, A., Slotnick, R.S., & Jeger, A.M. *People helping people: A directory of Long Island self-help organizations*. Old Westbury, N.Y.: New York Institute of Technology Press, 1980.

Schwartz, J.C. From a community mental health center: Shared reflections. *Journal of Religion and Health,* 1978, *17*(1), 31–38.

Segal, J. Research in the service of mental health: A summary of the report of the NIMH Research Force Staff and Coordinating Committee with H. Yahraes, 1974, unpublished.

Self, N.D. The pastor as linking person. *The Center Letter, 10*(1), Naperville, Ill.: Center for Parish Development, January, 1980.

Sennett, R. *The uses of disorder: Personal identity and city life.* New York: Vintage Books, 1970.

Shanas, E. The family as a social system in old age. *The Gerontologist,* 1978, *18*(4), 169–174.

Shapiro, D., Tursky, B., & Gershon, E. Effects of feedback and reinforcement on the control of human systolic blood pressure. *Science,* 1969, *163,* 588–90.

Sharfstein, S.S. Neighborhood psychiatry: A new community approach. *Community Mental Health,* 1974, *10,* 77–82.

Sharfstein, S.S. Will community mental health service survive in the 1980s? *American Journal of Psychiatry,* 1978, *135:*11, 1363–1365.

Shatan, C.F. The grief of soldiers: Vietnam combat veterans self-help movement. *American Journal of Orthopsychiatry,* 1973, *43*(4), 648–649.

Shaw, M.E., & Wright, J.M. *Scales for the measurement of attitudes.* New York: McGraw-Hill, 1967.

Sheehy, G. *Predictable crises of adult life.* New York: E.P. Dutton, 1974.

Sheldon, A. On consulting to new, changing, or innovative organizations. *Community Mental Health Journal,* 1971, 7(1), 62–71.

Sherman, W., & Haskell, C. *Partnerships for effective action: Capacity building for neighborhood revitalization.* Washington, D.C.: University of Southern California, Washington Public Affairs Center, 1980.

Silverman, P.R. The widow as a caregiver in a program of preventive intervention with other widows. *Mental Hygiene,* 1970, *54,* 540–547.

Silverman, P.R. Widowhood and preventive intervention. *The Family Coordinator,* 1972, *20,* 95–102.

Silverman, P.R. Mutual help. In R.G. Hirschowitz & B. Levy (Eds.), *The changing mental health scene.* New York: Spectrum Publications, 1976.

Silverman, P.R. *Mutual help groups: A guide for mental health workers* (DHEW Pub. No. 78-646). Washington, D.C.: U.S. Government Printing Office, 1978.

Silverman, P.R. The mental health consultant as linking agent. In D. Biegel & A. Naparstek (Eds.), *Community support systems and mental health: Research, practice and policy.* New York: Springer Publishing Company, 1982.

Silverman, P.R., & Murrow, H.G. Mutual help during critical role transitions. *Journal of Applied Behavioral Science,* 1976, *12,* 410–418.

Siporin, M. *Introduction to social work practice.* New York: Macmillan, 1975.

Slater, P. *The pursuit of loneliness: American culture at the breaking point.* Boston: Beacon Press, 1970.

Smith, L. Operation bootstrap. In A.H. Katz & E.I. Bender (Eds.), *The strength in us.* New York: New Viewpoints, 1976.

Smith, M.B. Competence and socialization. In M. Clausen (Ed.), *Socialization and society.* Boston: Little, Brown, 1968.

Snyder, P.Z. Neighborhood gatekeepers in the process of urban adaptation: Cross-ethnic commonalities. *Urban Anthropology,* 1976, *5,* 35–51.

Sosin, M. Social welfare and organizational society. *Social Service Review*, 1979, *53*(3), 392–405.

Sotomayer, M. Alternative models of service delivery for the Hispanic elderly. Paper presented to the National Hispanic Conference on Aging and Mental Health, Miami, Florida, 1980.

Spiegel, D. The psychiatrist as a consultant to self-help groups. *Hospital and Community Psychiatry*, 1977, *28*(10), 771–772.

Spiegel, D. Going public and self-help. In G. Caplan & M. Killilea (Eds.), *Support systems and mutual help*. New York: Grune & Stratton, 1976.

Spiegel, D., & Keith-Spiegel, P. (Eds.). *Outsiders USA: Original essays on 24 outgroups in American society*. San Francisco: Rinehart Press, 1973.

Stack, C.B. *All our kin*. New York: Harper & Row, 1974.

Steckler, A., & Herzog, W. How to keep your mandated citizen board out of your hair and off your back. *American Journal of Public Health*, 1979, *69*(8), 809–812.

Steinman, R., & Traunstein, D.M. Redefining deviance: The self-help challenge to the human services. *Journal of Applied Behavioral Science*, 1976, *12*, 347–361.

Strupp, H. *Psychotherapy: Clinical research and theoretical issues*. New York: Aronson, 1973.

Stuart, G. The context of community. Paper presented at the 6th Annual Summer Program on Mental Health Education, Madison, Wisconsin, 1979.

Stuart, R.B. Self-help group approach to self-management. In R.B. Stuart (Ed.), *Behavioral self-management*. New York: Brunner/Mazel, 1977.

Stunkard, A.J. The success of TOPS, a self-help group. *Postgraduate Medicine*, 1972, *51*, 143–147.

Stunkard, A., Levine, H., & Fox, S. The management of obesity, patient self-help and medical treatment. *Archives of Internal Medicine*, 1970, *125*, 1067–1072.

Sue, S. Community mental health services to minority groups: Some optimism, some pessimism. *American Psychologist*, 1977, *32*, 616–624.

Sue, S., Allen, D., McKinney, H., & Hall, J. Delivery of community mental health services to black and white clients. *Journal of Consulting & Clinical Psychology*, 1974, *42*, 794–801.

Sue, S. & McKinney, H. Asian-American in community health care system. *American Journal of Orthopsychiatry*, 1975, *45*(1), 111–118.

Sue, S., Wagner, N., Ja, D., Margullis, C., & Lew, L. Conceptions of mental illness among Asian and Caucasian-American students. *Psychological Reports*, 1976, *38*(3), 703–708.

Sussman, M.B. Relationships of adult children with their parents in the United States. In E. Shanas & G. Streib (Eds.), *Social structure and the family: Generational relations*. Englewood Cliffs, N.J.: Prentice-Hall, 1965.

Sussman, M.B. A reconstituted young-old family: Social and economic supports in family formation. Paper presented at the 31st Annual Meeting of the Gerontological Society, Dallas, November, 1978.

Swenson, C. Social networks, mutual aid, and the life model of practice. In C. Germain (Ed.), *Social work practice: People and environments*. New York: Columbia University Press, 1979.

Tableman, B. Prevention activities at the state level. In R.H. Price, R.K. Ketterer, B.C. Bader, & J. Monahan (Eds.), *Prevention in mental health*. Beverly Hills: Sage, 1980.

Taietz, P. Two conceptual models of the senior center. *Journal of Gerontology*, 1976, *31*(2), 219–222.

Takahashi, T. A social club spontaneously formed by ex-patients who had suffered from anthropophobia [Taijin Kyofu (SHO)]. *International Journal of Social Psychiatry*, 1975, *21*(2), 137–140.

Tax, S. Self-help groups: Thoughts on public policy. *Journal of Applied Behavioral Science*, 1976, *12*, 448–454.

Title VI, Civil Rights Act of 1964, 42 U.S.C. S 2000 et seq. (45C.7.R. S 80 et seq.)

Today in Psychiatry. Mendota: a pact for mental health, 1979, *5*(1).

Torrey, E.G. *The mind game: Witchdoctors and psychiatrists*. New York: Benton Books, 1973.

Toseland, R., & Rasch, J. Factors contributing to older persons' satisfaction with their communities. *The Gerontologist*, 1978 *18*(4), 395–402.

Tracy, G.S., & Gussow, Z. Self-help groups: A grassroots response to a need for services. *Journal of Applied Behavioral Science*, 1976, *12*, 381–396.

Trela, J.E. Social class and association membership: An analysis of age-graded and non-age-graded voluntary participation. *Journal of Gerontology*, 1976, *31*(2), 198–203.

Trela, J.E., & Sokolovsky, J.H. Culture, ethnicity and policy for the aged. In D.E. Gelfand & A.J. Kutzik (Eds.), *Ethnicity and aging: Theory, research, and policy*. New York: Springer Publishing Company, 1979.

True, R.H. Mental health services in a Chinese American community. In W.H. Ishikawa & N.H. Archer (Eds.), *Service delivery in pan Asian communities*. San Diego: Pacific Asian Coalition, 1975.

Turner, J., & TenHoor, W. The NIMH community support program: A pilot approach to a needed social reform. *Schizophrenia Bulletin*, 1978, *4*(3), 319–348.

Tyler, R.W. Social policy and self-help groups. *Journal of Applied Behavioral Science*, 1976, *12*, 444–448.

Vallance, T.R., & Crawford, M. Identifying training needs and translating them into research requirements. In R. Glaser (Ed.), *Training, research and education*. Pittsburgh: University of Pittsburgh Press, 1962.

Vallance, T.R., & Sabre, R. (Eds.). *Mental health services in transition: A policy sourcebook*. New York: Human Sciences Press, 1981.

Vattano, A.J. Power to the people: Self-help groups. *Social Work*, 1972, *17*, 7–15.

Veroff, J., Douvan, E., & Kulka, R. *Americans view their mental health*. Ann Arbor: Survey Research Center, University of Michigan, 1976.

Wagonfield, S., & Wolowitz, H.M. Obesity and the self-help group: A look at TOPS. *American Journal of Psychiatry*, 1968, *2*, 145–148.

Waldman, E., Grossman, A., Hayghe, H., & Johnson, B. Working mothers in the 1970's: A look at the statistics. *Monthly Labor Review*, 1979, *102*(10), 50–56.

Wang, L.S., & Louie, W. The Chinatown aftercare program: A report on a selected group of Chinese patients and their state hospital experience. San Francisco, Department of Public Health, 1979 (unpublished).

Warren, D.I. Neighborhoods in urban areas. *Encyclopedia of Social Work* (Vol. 1). New York: National Association of Social Workers, 1971.

Warren, D.I. *Helping network study data report*. Ann Arbor: Program in Community Effectiveness, University of Michigan, 1976.

Warren, D.I. Neighborhoods in urban areas. In J. Turner (Ed.), *The encyclopedia of social work*. New York: National Association of Social Workers, 1977.

Warren, D.I. Using social networks: A key social bond of urbanites. In D.E. Biegel & A. J. Naparstek (Eds.), *Community support systems and mental health: Research, practice, and policy*. New York: Springer Publishing Company, 1982.

Warren, R.L. *Social research consultation: An experiment in health and welfare planning*. New York: Russell Sage Foundation, 1963.

Webber, M. The urban place and the non-place urban realm. In M. Webber (Ed.), *Explorations in urban structure*. Philadelphia: University of Pennsylvania, 1964.

Weber, M. Science as vocation (1919). In H.H. Gerth and C.W. Mills (Trans. & Eds.), *From Max Weber*. New York: Oxford University Press, 1946.

Wechsler, H. The self-help organization in the mental health field: Recovery, Inc. A case study. In G. Caplan & M. Killilea (Eds.), *Support systems and mutual help*. New York: Grune & Stratton, 1976.

Wechsler, H. The ex-patient organization: A survey. *Journal of Social Issues*, 1960, *16*, 47-53. (a)

Wechsler, H. The self-help organization in the mental health field: Recovery, Inc., a case study. *Journal of Nervous and Mental Disease*, 1960, *131*(30), 297–314. (b)

Weiss, C. *Evaluation research: Methods of assessing program effectiveness*. Englewood Cliffs, N.J.: Prentice-Hall, 1972.

Weiss, R. The provision of social relationships. In Z. Rubin (Ed.), *Doing unto others*. Englewood Cliffs, N.J.: Prentice-Hall, 1974.

Weiss, R.J., & Bergen, B.J. Social support and the reduction of psychiatric disability. *Psychiatry: Journal for the Study of Interpersonal Processes*, 1968, *31*, 107–115.

Weiss, R.S. The fund of sociability. *Transaction*, 1969, *6*, 26–43.

Weiss, R.S. The contributions of an organization of single parents to the well-being of its members. In G. Caplan & M. Killilea (Eds.), *Support systems and mutual help*. New York: Grune & Stratton, 1976.

Welch, M.S. Networking on the job. *Ms*, March, 1980, pp. 85–88.

Wellman, B. The community question: The intimate ties of East Yorkers. *American Journal of Sociology*, 1979, *84*, 1201–1231. (a)

Wellman, B. *What is network analysis?* Research Paper No. 1, Structural Analysis Programme. Toronto: Department of Sociology, University of Toronto, September, 1979. (b)

Wellman, B., & Crump, B., *Networks, neighborhoods and communities*. Research paper no. 77. Toronto: Centre for Urban and Community Studies, University of Toronto, 1978.

Wells, J.A. Differences in sources of social support in conditioning the effect of perceived stress on health. Paper presented at the meeting of the Southern Sociological Association, Atlanta, Georgia, 1977.

Wholey, J.S. *Evaluation: Promise and performance*. Washington, D.C. Urban Institute, 1979.

Windle, C., & Wu, I. The impact of data-based technical assistance to CMHCs underserving ethnic minorities. Draft manuscript, NIMH, 1979.

Wing, J.K., & Olsen, Rolf. *Community care for the mentally disabled*. Oxford: Oxford University Press, 1979.

Winters, W.G., & Schraft, C. *Developing parent-school collaboration: A guide for school personnel*. Hartford, Conn.: Connecticut State Department of Education, Bureau of Pupil Personnel, 1977.

Wittenberg, R.M. Personality adjustment through social action. *American Journal of Orthopsychiatry*, 1948, *14*(2), 219.

Wolfenden Report. *The future of voluntary organizations*. London: Croom Helm, 1978.

Wollert, R.W., Knight, B., & Levy, L.H. Make Today Count: A collaborative model for professionals and self-help groups. *Professional Psychology*, 1980, *11*, 130–138.

Wong, H.Z. Letter to Tom Owan, 1979.

Wong, H.Z. Community mental health services and manpower and training concerns of Asian Americans. Paper presented to the President's Commission on Mental Health, 1977.

Woodson, C.G. *The education of the Negro prior to 1861*. New York: Arno Press, 1968.

Woodson, C.G. *The history of the Negro church*. Washington, D.C.: The Associated Publishers, 1921.

Yalom, I.D. *The theory and practice of group psychotherapy*. New York: Basic Books, 1975.

Yalom, I.D., Bloch, S., Bond, G., Zimmerman, E. & Qualls, B. Alcoholics in interactional group therapy. *Archives of General Psychiatry*, 1978, *35*, 419–425.

Yamamoto, J. Therapy for Asian Americans. *Journal of the National Medical Association*, 1978, *70*, 267–270.

Yamamoto, J., James, Q.C., & Palley, N. Cultural problems in psychiatric therapy. *Archives of General Psychiatry*, 1968, *19*, 45–49.

Index

Index